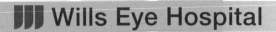

Wills Eye Hospital

COLOR ATLAS & SYNOPSIS OF
Clinical Ophthalmology

Glaucoma

THIRD EDITION

EDITOR
Douglas J. Rhee, MD
Professor and Chairman
Department of Ophthalmology and Visual Sciences
Case Western Reserve University School of Medicine
Director
University Hospitals Eye Institute
University Hospitals of Cleveland
Cleveland, Ohio

SERIES EDITOR
Christopher J. Rapuano, MD
Director and Attending Surgeon, Cornea Service
Co-Director, Refractive Surgery Department
Wills Eye Hospital
Professor of Ophthalmology
Sidney Kimmel Medical College at Thomas Jefferson University
Philadelphia, Pennsylvania

Wills Eye Hospital

COLOR ATLAS & SYNOPSIS OF
Clinical Ophthalmology

Glaucoma

THIRD EDITION

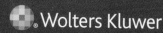

Philadelphia • Baltimore • New York • London
Buenos Aires • Hong Kong • Sydney • Tokyo

Acquisitions Editor: Chris Teja
Editorial Coordinator: Lauren Pecarich
Marketing Manager: Rachel Mante Leung
Production Project Manager: Marian Bellus
Design Coordinator: Stephen Druding
Manufacturing Coordinator: Beth Welsh
Prepress Vendor: S4Carlisle Publishing Services

Third edition

9 8 7 6 5 4 3 2 1

Printed in China

Library of Congress Cataloging-in-Publication Data

Names: Rhee, Douglas J., editor. | Wills Eye Hospital (Philadelphia, Pa.)
Title: Glaucoma / editors, Douglas J. Rhee, MD, Professor and Chairman,
  Department of Ophthalmology and Visual Sciences, Case Western Reserve
  University School of Medicine, Director, University Hospitals Eye
  Institute, University Hospitals of Cleveland, Cleveland, Ohio.
Description: Third edition. | Philadelphia: Wolters Kluwer Health, 2018. |
  Series: Color atlas & synopsis of clinical ophthalmology-Wills Eye
  Hospital | Includes bibliographical references and index.
Identifiers: LCCN 2018007721 | ISBN 9781496363480
Subjects: LCSH: Glaucoma—Atlases.
Classification: LCC RE871 .R48 2018 | DDC 617.7/41—dc23 LC record available at https://lccn.loc.gov/2018007721

LWW.com

To my lovely wife, Tina, I dedicate my contributions to you and am so grateful for your patience and support.
To my daughters, Ashley and Alyssa, I dedicate this book with my hopes for your future happiness and success.
To my father and mother, Dennis and Serena Rhee, in appreciation for your endless love, sacrifice, support, and dedication, I thank you.
To Susan Rhee, for your understanding and kindness. Broadly dedicated to all of my families - Rhee, Chang, Kim, Chomakos, and Joseph.

Contributors

Augusto Azuara-Blanco, PhD, FRCS(Ed), FRCOphth
Professor of Ophthalmology
Centre for Public Health
Queen's University Belfast
Honorary Consultant Ophthalmologist
Department of Ophthalmology
Belfast Health and Social Care Trust
Belfast, United Kingdom

Oscar V. Beaujon-Balbi, MD
Specialist in Ophthalmology
Department of Ophthalmology
Clinica Luis Razetti
Caracas, Venezuela
Oscar Beaujon-Rubin, MD, PhD
Specialist in Ophthalmology
Department of Ophthalmology
Clinica Luis Razetti
Caracas, Venezuela

Nicole Benitah, MD
Private Practice
California

Jacob W. Brubaker, MD
Sacramento Eye Consultants
Sacramento, California

Ronald Buggage, MD
Chief Scientific Officer
Novagali Pharma
Evry, France

Gabriel Chong, MD
Glaucoma Specialist
Raleigh Ophthalmology
Raleigh, North Carolina

Mary Jude Cox, MD
Eye Physicians
Voorhees, New Jersey

Syril Dorairaj, MD, FACS
Associate Professor of Ophthalmology
Consultant Glaucoma, Anterior Segment Surgery
Department of Ophthalmology
Mayo Clinic
Jacksonville, Florida

Francisco Fantes, MD
Associate Professor of Ophthalmology
Bascom Palmer Eye Institute
University of Miami School of Medicine
Miami, Florida

Scott Fudemberg, MD, FACS
Assistant Professor
Department of Glaucoma
Wills Eye Hospital, Sidney Kimmel
    Medical College
Philadelphia, Pennsylvania

JoAnn A. Giaconi, MD
Health Sciences Associate Professor
Department of Ophthalmology
David Geffen School of Medicine, UCLA
Chief of Ophthalmology
Surgery
Veterans Administration
Los Angeles, California

Michael C. Giovingo, MD
Director of Glaucoma Service
Department of Ophthalmology
Cook County Health and Hospital System
Chicago, Illinois

Josh Gross, MD
Department of Ophthalmology
Eugene and Marilyn Glick Eye Institute
Indiana University School of Medicine
Indianapolis, Indiana

Alon Harris, PhD
Professor of Ophthalmology
Letzter Endowed Chair in Ophthalmology
Director of Clinical Research
Professor of Cellular and Integrative Physiology
Department of Ophthalmology
Eugene and Marilyn Glick Eye Institute
Indiana University School of Medicine
Indianapolis, Indiana

Ribhi Hazin, MD
Graduate Student
Harvard School of Public Health
Boston, Massachusetts

Katie Hutchins, MD
Department of Ophthalmology
Eugene and Marilyn Glick Eye Institute
Indiana University School of Medicine
Indianapolis, Indiana

Malik Y. Kahook, MD
Professor of Ophthalmology
Chief, Glaucoma Service & Co-Director,
    Glaucoma Fellowship
Department of Ophthalmology
University of Colorado School
    of Medicine
Aurora, Colorado

L. Jay Katz, MD
Professor
Department of Ophthalmology
Thomas Jefferson University
Director
Glaucoma Service
Wills Eye Hospital
Philadelphia, Pennsylvania

Fabio Lavinsky, MD, MBA
Research Fellow
Department of Ophthalmology
New York University
New York, New York

Daniel Lee, MD
Assistant Professor
Glaucoma Service
Wills Eye Hospital
Philadelphia, Pennsylvania

Ashley G. Lesley, MD
Glaucoma Specialist
Jervey Eye Group
Greenville, South Carolina

**Christopher Kai-Shun Leung, MBChB
(CUHK), MD (CUHK), BMedSc, MSc (Lond),
FCOphth (HK), FHKAM**
Professor
Department of Ophthalmology
    & Visual Sciences
The Chinese University of Hong Kong
Honorary Consultant
Hong Kong Eye Hospital
Kowloon, Hong Kong

Richard A. Lewis, MD
Sacramento Eye Consultants
Sacramento, California

Jeffrey M. Liebmann, MD
Shirlee and Bernard Brown
    Professor of Ophthalmology
Vice-Chair, Department of Ophthalmology
Director, Glaucoma Division
Department of Ophthalmology
Edward S. Harkness Eye Institute
Columbia University College of
    Physicians & Surgeons
Columbia University Medical Center
New York, New York

Michele C. Lim, MD
Professor of Ophthalmology
Department of Ophthalmology & Vision Science
University of California, Davis
Vice Chair and Medical Director
Department of Ophthalmology & Vision Science
UC Davis Medical Center
Sacramento, California

Shan C. Lin, MD
Professor
Director, Glaucoma Service
Department of Ophthalmology
University of California San Francisco
San Francisco, CA

Zinaria Y. W. Liu, MD
Department of Ophthalmology
Elmhurst Hospital Center
Queens, New York

Kimberly V. Miller, MD
Clinical Assistant Professor of Surgery
    (Ophthalmology)
Division of Ophthalmology
The Warren Alpert Medical School of
    Brown University Academic Institution
Director of Glaucoma, Ophthalmology
    Residency Program Director
Division of Ophthalmology
Rhode Island Hospital
Providence, Rhode Island

Marlene R. Moster, MD
Professor
Department of Ophthalmology
Thomas Jefferson University School of Medicine
Attending Surgeon
Department of Glaucoma
Wills Eye Hospital
Philadelphia, Pennsylvania

Jonathan S. Myers, MD
Co-Director
Glaucoma Service
Wills Eye Hospital
Philadelphia, Pennsylvania

Jamie E. Nicholl†
Ophthalmic Photographer
Wills Eye Hospital
Thomas Jefferson Medical College
Philadelphia, Pennsylvania

Claudia L. Pabon, MD
Specialist in Ophthalmology
Department of Ophthalmology
Clinica Luis Razetti
Chief
Department of Ophthalmology
Hospital Francisco A. Risquez
Caracas, Venezuela

Konrad S. Palacios, MD, PhD, FEBO
Chairman of the Glaucoma Service
Department of Ophthalmology
Hospital Universitario de Torrevieja
Torrevieja, Spain

Paul F. Palmberg, MD, PhD
Professor
Department of Ophthalmology
Bascom Palmer Eye Institute
University of Miami School of Medicine
Miami, Florida

George N. Papaliodis, MD
Associated Professor
Department of Ophthalmology
Harvard Medical School
Director of the Ocular Immunology and
    Uveitis Service
Department of Ophthalmology
Massachusetts Eye and Ear Infirmary
Boston, Massachusetts

Sung Chul (Sean) Park, MD
Associate Professor
Department of Ophthalmology
Donald and Barbara Zucker School of Medicine
    at Hofstra/Northwell
Hempstead, New York

Director, Glaucoma Research; Co-Director,
    Glaucoma Fellowship Program
Department of Ophthalmology
Manhattan Eye, Ear and Throat Hospital
    (a division of Lenox Hill Hospital)
New York, New York

Louis R. Pasquale, MD
Professor of Ophthalmology
Department of Ophthalmology
Harvard Medical School
Director, Glaucoma Service
Department of Ophthalmology
Mass Eye and Ear Infirmary
Boston, Massachusetts

Thomas D. Patrianakos, MD
Chair
Department of Ophthalmology
Cook County Health and Hospitals System
Chicago, Illinois

Nathan M. Radcliffe, MD
Glaucoma Specialist and Cataract Surgeon
New York Eye Surgery Center
New York Eye & Ear Infirmary
New York, New York

Douglas J. Rhee, MD
Professor and Chairman
Department of Ophthalmology and
    Visual Sciences
Case Western Reserve University School of Medicine
Director
University Hospitals Eye Institute
University Hospitals of Cleveland
Cleveland, Ohio

Robert Ritch, MD, FACS
Professor of Ophthalmology
Shelley & Steven Einhorn Distinguished Chair
Surgeon Director Emeritus and Chief, Glaucoma
    Services
Department of Ophthalmology
New York Eye & Ear Infirmary of Mount Sinai
New York, New York

José I. B. Sanchis, MD, PhD, FEBO
Chairman
Department of Ophthalmology
Hospital Universitario de Torrevieja
Torrevieja, Spain

† Deceased.

Joel S. Schuman, MD
Professor
Department of Ophthalmology,
   Electrical and Computer Engineering,
   Neuroscience and Physiology and
   Neural Science
New York University
Chairman
Department of Ophthalmology
NYU Langone Health
New York, New York

Geoffrey P. Schwartz, MD
Instructor
Glaucoma Service
Wills Eye Hospital
Jefferson Medical College
Thomas Jefferson University
Philadelphia, Pennsylvania

Louis W. Schwartz, MD
Emeritus Clinical Professor
Department of Ophthalmology
Sidney Kimmel Medical College at
   Thomas Jefferson University
Emeritus Attending Surgeon
Department of Ophthalmology
Wills Eye Hospital
Philadelphia, Pennsylvania

Nathaniel C. Sears, MD
Assistant Professor of Ophthalmology
Department of Ophthalmology
University of Iowa
Iowa City, Iowa

Rajesh K. Shetty, MD
Glaucoma and Cataract Specialist
Florida Eye Specialists
Jacksonville, Florida

Brent Siesky, PhD
Research Associate
Assistant Director of the Glaucoma Research
   and Diagnostic Center
Department of Ophthalmology
Eugene and Marilyn Glick Eye Institute
Indiana University School of Medicine
Indianapolis, Indiana

Arthur J. Sit, SM, MD
Associate Professor
Vice Chair, Clinical Practice
Glaucoma Fellowship Director
Department of Ophthalmology
Mayo Clinic
Rochester, Minnesota

Marisse M. Solano, MD
Research Associate
Department of Ophthalmology/Glaucoma
University of California San Francisco
San Francisco, California

George L. Spaeth, MD
Director, Glaucoma Research Center
Esposito Research Professor
Wills Eye Hospital
Jefferson Medical Center
Philadelphia, Pennsylvania

Angela V. Turalba, MD, MMS
Assistant Professor Part-time
Department of Ophthalmology
Harvard Medical School
Chief
Department of Ophthalmology and Visual
   Services
Atrius Health
Boston, Massachusetts

Tara A. Uhler, MD
Program Director
Department of Ophthalmology
Thomas Jefferson University/Wills Eye Hospital
Associate Professor
Department of Ophthalmology
Thomas Jefferson University
Philadelphia, Pennsylvania

Laura A. Vickers, MD
Glaucoma Fellow
Department of Ophthalmology
UCLA Jules Stein Eye Institute
Los Angeles, California

Steven D. Vold, MD
Medical Director
Vold Vision, PLLU
Fayetteville, Arkansas

Konrad W. S. Wenyon, MD, PhD
Chairman of the Ophthalmological
    Department (Retire)
Department of Ophthalmology
Hospital Cesar Rodriguez
Puerto La Cruz, Venezuela

Gadi Wollstein, MD
Professor
Department of Ophthalmology
New York University School of Medicine
New York, New York

About the Series

The beauty of the atlas/synopsis concept is the powerful combination of illustrative photographs and a summary approach to the text. Ophthalmology is a very visual discipline that lends itself wonderfully to clinical photographs. Whereas the seven ophthalmic subspecialties in this series—Cornea, Retina, Glaucoma, Oculoplastics, Neuro-ophthalmology, Uveitis, and Pediatrics—employ varying levels of visual recognition, a relatively standard format for the text is used for all volumes.

The goal of the series is to provide an up-to-date clinical overview of the major areas of ophthalmology for students, residents, and practitioners in all the health care professions. The abundance of large, excellent-quality photographs (both in print and online) and concise, outline-form text will help achieve that objective.

Christopher J. Rapuano
Series Editor

Preface

Color Atlas & Synopsis of Clinical Ophthalmology—Wills Eye Hospital—Glaucoma attempts to cover as many of the glaucoma syndromes as possible. No condition appears identical in all cases. Therefore, many different representative images are presented for the more common conditions in an attempt to reflect the diversity of presentations.

In this third edition, we have added new material to encompass the evolving techniques and technologies of the surgical management of glaucoma, updated text to reflect new treatment paradigms, and updated images throughout this edition. I hope you will find this atlas to be a useful reference and an aid to your clinical endeavors.

Douglas J. Rhee
Editor

Acknowledgments

I would like to thank the many authors and contributors who participated in this endeavor. I believe that the diversity of representations is one of the strengths of this book.

Contents

SECTION II: CLINICAL SYNDROMES

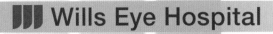

Wills Eye Hospital

COLOR ATLAS & SYNOPSIS OF
Clinical Ophthalmology

Glaucoma

THIRD EDITION

Section I ■ Glaucoma Diagnosis

Introduction to Glaucoma Diagnosis

Douglas J. Rhee ■

The term *glaucoma* is from the Greek *glaukos,* which means "watery blue." It was first mentioned in the Hippocratic Aphorisms around 400 BC. However, it was considered a disease of the crystalline lens for several hundred years following. "The scientific history of glaucoma began the day on which cataracts were put in their correct place" (Albert Terson, 1867–1935). The correct anatomic location of cataracts is credited to Pierre Brisseau (1631–1717) in 1707. Elevation of intraocular pressure (IOP) as a sign of glaucoma was first mentioned in Breviary (1622) by Richard Banister (1570–1626). Discovery of the ophthalmoscope, by Hermann von Helmholtz (1821–1894) in 1851, and its subsequent use by Edward Jaeger (1818–1884) led to the belief that the optic nerve was also involved. Cupping of the optic nerve as a sign of glaucoma was confirmed by anatomist Heinrich Muller in the late 1850s. Von Graefe is credited with having first described contraction of the visual field and paracentral defects in glaucoma in 1856.

In recent history, glaucoma had been defined by having an IOP above 21 mm Hg (i.e., more than two standard deviations above the mean IOP from a population-based survey of IOP, 16 ± 2 mm Hg). Later research indicated that the majority of people with IOPs above 21 mm Hg do not develop glaucomatous visual field loss (e.g., Ocular Hypertension Treatment Study). In addition, up to 40% of patients with documented glaucomatous visual field loss never achieve IOPs higher than 21 mm Hg (e.g., Baltimore Eye Survey). Our modern concept of primary open-angle glaucoma (POAG) is a description of the constellation of signs frequently seen in "glaucoma" that incorporate IOP as well as characteristic optic nerve and visual field changes. The hallmark of the diagnosis of glaucoma is progressive change in the optic nerve or visual field, or both, over time. Many glaucoma specialists believe that the syndrome of POAG probably encompasses many diseases with a final common pathway. Our most recent genetic investigations indicate that POAG is polygenic, in which minor alterations of numerous genes contribute to create the syndrome. All genetic mutations that are inherited in a Mendelian pattern account for less than approximately 10% of all POAGs. Our definition of glaucoma will no doubt continue to evolve as our understanding of the disease increases.

A modern definition for glaucoma is as follows: a pathologic condition in which there is a progressive loss of ganglion cell axons causing visual field damage that is related to IOP. Currently, we look to evaluate the following components when making the diagnosis of glaucoma: history, presence or absence of risk factors, IOP, optic nerve examination, and visual field testing.

This section covers the various methods for obtaining the information used for both diagnosing glaucoma and following the adequacy of treatment.

BIBLIOGRAPHY

Allingham RR, Liu Y, Rhee DJ. The genetics of primary open-angle glaucoma: a review. *Exp Eye Res.* 2009;88:837–844.

Blodi FC. Development of our concept of glaucoma. In: *Basic and Clinical Science Course,* Section 10. San Francisco, CA: American Academy of Ophthalmology; 1996.

Kass MA, Heuer DK, Higginbotham EJ, et al. The Ocular Hypertension Treatment Study: a randomized trial determines that topical ocular hypotensive medication delays or prevents the onset of primary open-angle glaucoma. *Arch Ophthalmol.* 2002;120:701–713.

Kronfeld PC. Glaucoma. In: Albert DM, Edwards DD, eds. *History of Ophthalmology.* Cambridge, MA: Blackwell Science; 1996:203–223.

Mikelberg FS, Drance SM. Glaucomatous visual field defects. In: Ritch R, Shields MB, Krupin T, eds. *The Glaucomas.* St. Louis, MO: Mosby-Year Book; 1996:523–537.

Sommer A, Tielsch JM, Katz J, et al. Relationship between intraocular pressure and primary open angle glaucoma among white and black Americans: the Baltimore eye survey. *Arch Ophthalmol.* 1991;109:1090–1095.

Basics of Aqueous Flow and the Optic Nerve

Arthur J. Sit and Douglas J. Rhee ■

AQUEOUS FLOW

Importance of Intraocular Pressure

Having a basic understanding of the physiology of the eye is helpful to understanding the pathophysiology, diagnosis, and management of glaucoma. Many clinicians and scientists now believe that several factors are involved in the pathogenesis of glaucoma, such as apoptosis, altered blood flow to the optic nerve, and possible autoimmune reactions. However, intraocular pressure (IOP) remains one of the most important risk factors for the disease syndromes. In addition, lowering of the IOP is the only rigorously proven treatment for glaucoma. Although we have some understanding of the physiology of IOP, we do not yet fully understand how the eye regulates IOP at the cellular and molecular levels. However, fundamental research continues to further our understanding of the molecular mechanisms. Someday, we may have the answer to what many patients have asked—what exactly causes glaucoma? As we identify the normal molecular processes, we can elucidate the pathophysiologic mechanisms to directly intervene and disrupt the dysregulation—otherwise known as "disease-modifying" therapy.

Brief Summary of Aqueous Physiology and Intraocular Pressure

Aqueous is formed in the ciliary processes (pars plicata region of the retina) (Fig. 2-1A–D). The epithelial cells of the inner nonpigmented layer are felt to be the site of aqueous production (Fig. 2-2A and B). Aqueous is produced by a combination of active secretion, ultrafiltration, and diffusion. Many of the IOP-lowering agents work by decreasing aqueous secretion in the ciliary body.

Aqueous then flows through the pupil and into the anterior chamber, nourishing the lens, cornea, and iris (Fig. 2-3). Aqueous drains through the anterior chamber angle, which contains the trabecular meshwork (TM) and ciliary body face (Fig. 2-4A and B).

Between 60% and 90% of aqueous outflow is through the TM—the so-called conventional pathway—with the remaining 10% to 40% through the ciliary body face—the so-called uveoscleral or alternative pathway. The TM is thought to be the region where regulation of aqueous humor outflow takes place. Within the TM, especially under conditions of elevated

IOP, the juxtacanalicular area appears to have the highest resistance to outflow (Fig. 2-5).

IOP is physiologically determined by the rate of aqueous production in the ciliary body, resistance to outflow through the conventional outflow tract (TM and Schlemm canal [SC]), resistance to outflow through the unconventional outflow tract (uveoscleral outflow), and episcleral venous pressure. In the Goldmann equation [IOP $= (F/C) + P_v$], P_v is the episcleral venous pressure, F is the rate of aqueous formation, and C is the facility of outflow, which roughly corresponds to the inverse of the total resistance to outflow. As one can imagine, elevations of episcleral venous pressure can result in an elevated IOP (Fig. 2-6).

With open-angle glaucomas, the pathophysiology is increased aqueous drainage resistance through the TM. With primary open-angle glaucoma (POAG), there is an alteration of juxtacanalicular extracellular matrix homeostasis, TM and SC endothelial cell cytoskeleton causing cellular stiffness, and TM cellularity. With POAG, the aqueous humor has an elevated level of transforming growth factor beta-2. Certain proteins or their functions—such as myocilin, gremlin, secreted frizzled-related protein (sFRP) (aka frizzled protein), cochlin, secreted protein acidic and rich in cysteine (SPARC) (aka osteonectin), and serum amyloid A—have been shown to be important to the IOP elevation in POAG. Selectin E may be a unique marker for POAG. With pseudoexfoliation glaucoma, the pseudoexfoliative material accumulates in the juxtacanalicular extracellular matrix increasing outflow resistance; there is also an elevation of transforming growth factor beta-1 in the aqueous humor of patients with pseudoexfoliation glaucoma. With pigment dispersion glaucoma, the ingested debris from the pigmented iris epithelial cells causes TM endothelial cell death, and the denuded TM beams fuse to increase the outflow resistance. With steroid-induced glaucoma, there is an alteration of extracellular matrix within the juxtacanalicular region, but distinct in electron microscopic features and components than POAG, as well as alterations to TM and SC cell cytoskeleton that causes an elevation of outflow resistance.

Measurement of Aqueous Humor Dynamics

As discussed earlier, the basis of IOP can be described by the Goldmann equation. Because most research suggests that the amount of uveoscleral outflow is relatively insensitive to changes in pressure,[1] the Goldmann equation can be modified as: IOP $= (F - U)/C + P_v$, where P_v represents the episcleral venous pressure, F is the rate of aqueous formation, U is the rate of aqueous outflow through the pressure-insensitive uveoscleral pathway, and C is the outflow facility. Each of these parameters can be measured except U, which must be calculated from IOP and the remaining variables.

Outflow facility is measured clinically using tonography. The concept of tonography involves placing a weighted tonometer on the surface of the eye, causing an elevation in IOP, and measuring the rate at which IOP returns to its baseline value over a fixed time interval (usually 2 or 4 minutes).[2] Different devices can be used for tonography measurements, including weighted pneumatonometers or electronic Schiotz tonometers. These devices share the characteristic of being able to record IOP continuously over the measurement interval, either on a paper chart or electronically (Fig. 2-7). Regardless of the device, all share the same limitations including the assumption that aqueous humor production rate, episcleral venous pressure, and outflow facility are constant during the measurement interval.[3] In normal individuals, outflow facility is typically between 0.23 and 0.33 µL/min/mm Hg.[4]

Aqueous humor production rate is measured using fluorophotometry.[5,6] With this technique, a fluorescein depot is established in the cornea using eye drops. Over time, the fluorescein is removed from the cornea because it diffuses into the anterior chamber and is carried away by aqueous humor flow. The rate of fluorescein removal can be estimated using a fluorophotometer to measure the change over time of fluorescence in the cornea and anterior chamber (Fig. 2-8). This information can then be used to calculate the rate of aqueous humor flow, assuming that diffusion into the posterior segment is minimal (around 10% or less). Using this technique, the mean aqueous humor production rate is typically found to range from 2.2 to 3.1 μL per minute.[7]

Episcleral venous pressure is currently the most difficult parameter to measure in aqueous humor dynamics. Noninvasive measurement involves identifying an episcleral vein, placing a clear pressurized membrane on the vein, increasing the pressure within the chamber, and observing the response. The amount of pressure required to produce a response, such as compression, can be used to estimate the episcleral venous pressure (Fig. 2-9). The earliest stages of compression correspond with the correct episcleral venous pressure, but the use of a subjective end point can lead to uncertainty in the measurement. Normal values reported for mean episcleral venous pressure have ranged from 7 to 14 mm Hg.[8-11]

REFERENCES

1. Alm A, Nilsson SF. Uveoscleral outflow—a review. *Exp Eye Res.* 2009;88(4):760–768.
2. Grant WM. Tonographic method for measuring the facility and rate of aqueous flow in human eyes. *Arch Ophthal.* 1950;44(2):204–214.
3. Brubaker RF. Goldmann's equation and clinical measures of aqueous dynamics. *Exp Eye Res.* 2004;78(3):633–637.
4. Becker B. Tonography in the diagnosis of simple (open angle) glaucoma. *Trans Am Acad Ophthalmol Otolaryngol.* 1961;65:156–162.
5. Jones RF, Maurice DM. New methods of measuring the rate of aqueous flow in man with fluorescein. *Exp Eye Res.* 1966;5(3):208–220.
6. McLaren JW, Brubaker RF. A two-dimensional scanning ocular fluorophotometer. *Invest Ophthalmol Vis Sci.* 1985;26(2):144–152.
7. McLaren JW. Measurement of aqueous humor flow. *Exp Eye Res.* 2009;88(4):641–647.
8. Phelps CD, Armaly MF. Measurement of episcleral venous pressure. *Am J Ophthalmol.* 1978;85(1):35–42.
9. Toris CB, Yablonski ME, Wang YL, Camras CB. Aqueous humor dynamics in the aging human eye. *Am J Ophthalmol.* 1999;127(4):407–412.
10. Zeimer RC, Gieser DK, Wilensky JT, Noth JM, Mori MM, Odunukwe EE. A practical venomanometer. Measurement of episcleral venous pressure and assessment of the normal range. *Arch Ophthalmol.* 1983;101(9):1447–1449.
11. Sit AJ, McLaren JW. Measurement of episcleral venous pressure. *Exp Eye Res.* 2011;93:291–298.

BIBLIOGRAPHY

Bill A. The drainage of aqueous humor. *Invest Ophthalmol Vis Sci.* 1975;14:1–3.

Bill A, Phillips CI. Uveoscleral drainage of aqueous humour in human eyes. *Exp Eye Res.* 1971;12:275–281.

Grant WM. Further studies on facility of flow through the trabecular meshwork. *Arch Ophthalmol.* 1958;60: 523–533.

Maepea O, Bill A. Pressures in the juxtacanalicular tissue and Schlemm's canal in monkeys. *Exp Eye Res.* 1992;54:879–883.

Maepea O, Bill A. The pressures in the episcleral veins, Schlemm's canal and trabecular meshwork in monkeys: Effects of changes in intraocular pressure. *Exp Eye Res.* 1989;49:645–663.

Moses RA, Grodzki WJ, Etheridge EL, Wilson CD. Schlemm's canal: The effect of intraocular pressure. *Invest Ophthalmol Vis Sci.* 1981;20:61–68.

Pederson JE, Gaasterland DE, MacLellan HM. Uveoscleral aqueous outflow in the rhesus monkey: importance of uveal reabsorption. *Invest Ophthalmol Vis Sci.* 1977;16:1008–1017.

Seiler T, Wollensak J. The resistance of the trabecular meshwork to aqueous humor outflow. *Graefes Arch Clin Exp Ophthalmol.* 1985;223:88–91.

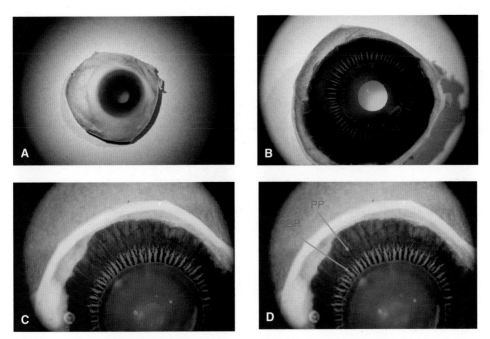

FIGURE 2-1. **Gross dissection of a cadaver eye. A.** Anterior segment from a cadaver eye, frontal view. **B.** Same anterior segment turned over, looking from behind the lens. The lens is still supported by the zonular fibers extending from the ciliary body processes. **C.** Higher magnification view of the ciliary body process. This region is called the pars plicata. The pars plana is peripheral to the pars plicata. **D.** Same image as panel **C**, where CBP = ciliary body processes and PP = pars plana.

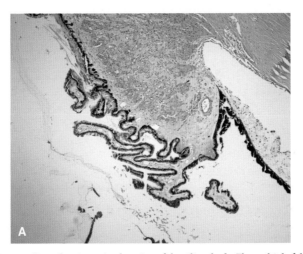

FIGURE 2-2. **A.** Hematoxylin and eosin–stained section of the ciliary body. The multiple folds help increase the overall surface area.

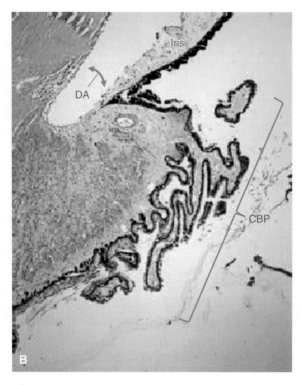

FIGURE 2-2. (*continued*) **B.** Same image as panel **A**, where CBP = ciliary body processes and DA = drainage angle.

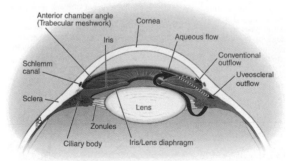

FIGURE 2-3. Route of aqueous flow. Schematic diagram showing the route of aqueous from the ciliary body to the outflow tract. (From Rhee DJ, Budenz DL. Acute angle-closure glaucoma. In: *The Clinics Atlas of Office Procedures*. Philadelphia, PA: Saunders; 2000:267–279.)

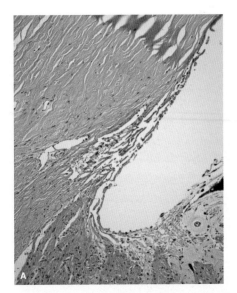 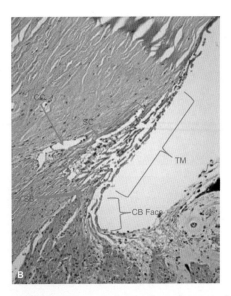

FIGURE 2-4. **A.** Hematoxylin and eosin–stained section of the anterior chamber angle showing the outflow tracts of the eye. The conventional outflow pathway consists of seven layers of TM beams (corneoscleral and uveal TM), the juxtacanalicular region, Schlemm canal, collecting channels, and episcleral veins. The uveoscleral pathway consists of the uveal face, with flow eventually moving into the choroidal space. This pathway is not well understood. There is evidence to show that the aqueous drains out of the vortex veins and through the scleral wall. **B.** Same image as panel **A**, where CC = collecting channel, SC = Schlemm canal, SS = scleral spur, TM = trabecular meshwork, and CB face = ciliary body face.

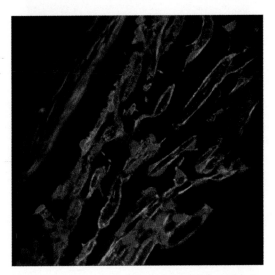

FIGURE 2-5. **Confocal microscopy of the juxtacanalicular region of the trabecular meshwork (TM).** Green (fluorescein labeled) indicates staining for a nonspecific secreted matricellular protein. Red (Texas red labeled) indicates staining for smooth muscle actin (within the TM endothelial cells), whereas the blue DAPI (a fluorescent stain for nuclei) stains for nuclear material. These smaller, bubble-shaped nuclei correspond to the cells of the inner wall of Schlemm canal, whereas the elongated nuclei correspond to the TM endothelial cells. One can see that the uveal and corneoscleral TM consists of endothelial cell–lined beams, whereas the juxtacanalicular region is an amorphous area of extracellular matrix and TM endothelial cells.

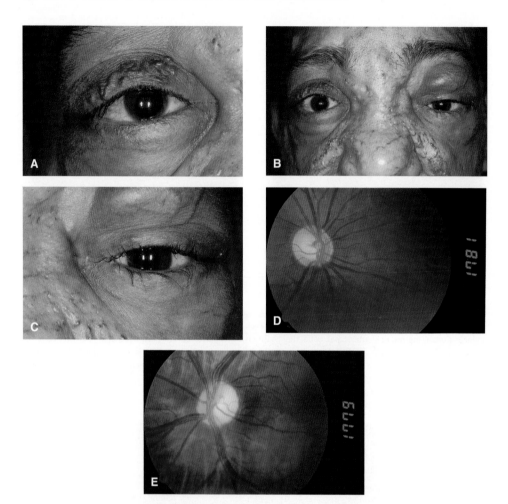

FIGURE 2-6. Extreme example of neglected bilateral carotid cavernous sinus fistula. A–C. The chronic elevation of venous pressure has resulted in dilation of all the downstream venous channels with lid involvement. The patient had elevated intraocular pressure with moderate generalized cupping in the right optic nerve (**D**) and inferior notch in the left optic nerve (**E**).

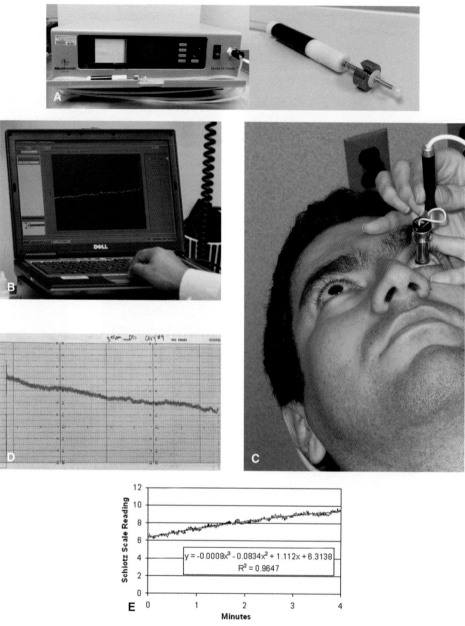

$$y = -0.0009x^3 - 0.0834x^2 + 1.112x + 6.3138$$
$$R^2 = 0.9647$$

FIGURE 2-7. Measurement of facility using tonography. A. Pneumatonometer with weight for pneumatonography (Model 30 Classic, Medtronic Solan, Jacksonville, FL). **B.** Digital Schiotz tonometer recording to computer (Mayo Clinic, Rochester, MN). **C.** Performing Schiotz tonography on a subject. **D.** Paper chart recording of intraocular pressure (IOP) over a 4-minute interval. The slow decay in pressure is recorded as an increase in the Schiotz scale. A curve is manually drawn through the data to determine the rate of IOP decay. **E.** Recording of IOP and curve fitting of data from a 4-minute tonography measurement, using a digital Schiotz tonometer. The scale is reversed compared with the paper chart.

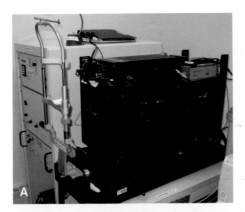
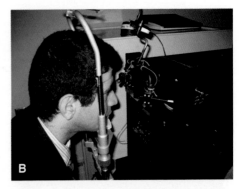

FIGURE 2-8. Measurement of aqueous humor production rate. A. Scanning two-dimensional anterior segment fluorophotometer (Mayo Clinic, Rochester, MN). **B.** Performing fluorophotometry on a subject to measure fluorescein concentration in the cornea and anterior chamber.

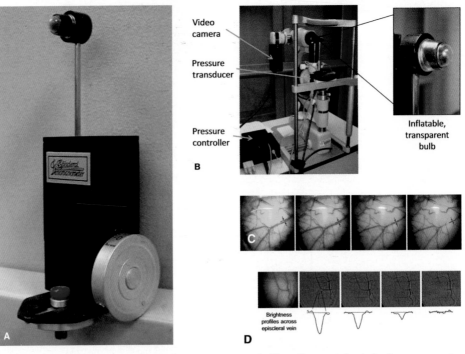

FIGURE 2-9. Measurement of episcleral venous pressure. A. Manually operated episcleral venomanometer (Eyetech Ltd, Morton Grove, IL). **B.** Automated episcleral venomanometry system (Mayo Clinic, Rochester, MN). **C.** Sequence of images showing compression of an episcleral vein (between *arrows*) during the process of venomanometry. The amount of pressure required to create an appropriate compression is used to estimate episcleral venous pressure. This can be performed subjectively with direct visualization. **D.** Objectively using software to determine the amount of compression from baseline (Mayo Clinic, Rochester, MN).

OPTIC NERVE

The optic nerve consists of all the axons from the ganglion cell layer of the retina. The optic nerve is the site of damage in glaucoma (**Figs. 2-10** and **2-11**). Functionally, optic nerve damage causes visual field changes. Without treatment, an elevated IOP can result in progressive loss of the visual field, eventually leading to blindness. The various patterns of optic nerve change and means of measuring the functional status of the optic nerve are described in more detail in subsequent chapters.

BIBLIOGRAPHY

Sit AJ, McLaren JW. Measurement of episcleral venous pressure. *Exp Eye Res.* 2011;93:291–298.

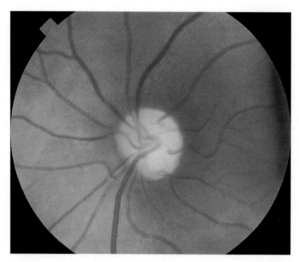

FIGURE 2-10. Photograph of the optic nerve showing an inferior notch from a patient with glaucoma. Note the relative absence of pallor. (Courtesy of L. Jay Katz, MD, Wills Eye Hospital, Philadelphia, PA.)

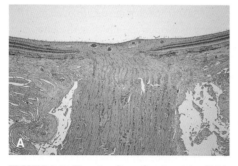 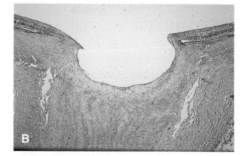

FIGURE 2-11. Hematoxylin and eosin–stained histopathologic section of optic nerves. A. Normal optic nerve. **B.** Optic nerve from advanced glaucoma (bean pot cup). (Courtesy of Ralph J. Eagle, MD, Wills Eye Hospital, Philadelphia, PA.)

Tonometry

Rajesh K. Shetty ∎

INTRODUCTION

Tonometry is the measurement of the intraocular pressure (IOP; the pressure within the eye). Most of the instruments used in tonometry rely on deforming an area of the cornea with a small amount of force that is used to calculate the IOP. Tonometers can be divided into types that applanate, or flatten, the cornea and those that indent it. The accuracy of either type of tonometer assumes that all eyes have a similar ocular rigidity, corneal thickness, and ocular blood flow.

GOLDMANN APPLANATION TONOMETER

Applanation tonometry is based on the Imbert–Fick law that the IOP is equal to the amount of force needed to flatten a spherical surface divided by the applanated area. Goldmann applanation, the gold standard and the most commonly used form of tonometry, was introduced in 1954. This device can be used only in patients seated at a slit lamp. The cornea is viewed through a prismatic doubling device in the center of a cone-shaped head that is obliquely illuminated with a cobalt blue light (Fig. 3-1). Although the patient's head is held steady, the applanation head is gently placed against a fluorescein-stained, anesthetized cornea (Fig. 3-2). The examiner sees a split image of the tear film meniscus around the tonometer head. These fluorescein rings just overlap when the pressure at the head equals the IOP. The graduated dial on the side measures the force in grams, which is converted into millimeters of mercury by multiplying by 10.

With a circular applanation surface 3.06 mm in diameter, the surface tension of the tear film counteracts the force needed to overcome the rigidity of the cornea, allowing the amount of force applied to equal the IOP. The tip flattens the cornea less than 0.2 mm, displaces 0.5 μL of aqueous, increases the IOP by 3%, and provides a reliable measurement of ±0.5 mm Hg. In corneas with high astigmatism (greater than 3 diopters), the flattest corneal meridian should be placed at 45 degrees to the axis of the cone. This can be done simply by placing the red line on the tonometer tip at the same axis of the minus (or flattest) cylinder of the eye.

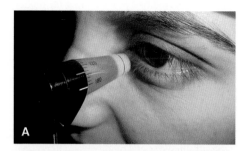

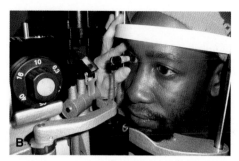

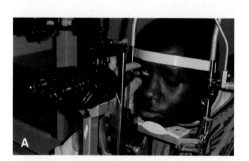

FIGURE 3-1. Goldmann tonometer. Example of a Goldmann tonometer mounted on a Haag-Streit slit lamp. **A.** The *red lines* seen on the cone can be aligned to the axis of negative cylinder in patients with high astigmatism. **B, C.** Cobalt blue illumination of the tonometer tip allows for visualization of the fluorescein-containing tear film.

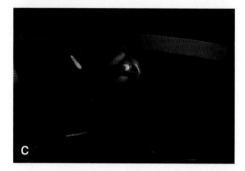

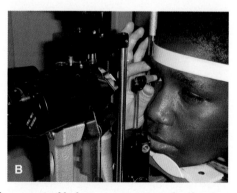

FIGURE 3-2. Applanation technique. A. An individual demonstrating blepharospasm on attempted applanation. **B.** Successful contact between the tonometer tip and the cornea, with the examiner demonstrating the proper technique of placing supporting traction only on the orbital rims, not on the globe itself.

SCHIÖTZ TONOMETER

Introduced in 1905, the Schiötz tonometer is the classic indentation tonometer and requires the patient to be supine (Fig. 3-3). As opposed to applanation tonometry, the amount of indentation of the cornea by the Schiötz tonometer is proportionate to the IOP. This deformation, however, creates an unpredictable and relatively large intraocular volume displacement. The 16.5-g Schiötz tonometer has a base weight of 5.5 g that is attached to the plunger. This weight may be increased to 7.5, 10, or 15 g for higher ocular pressures. The calibrated footplate of the tonometer is placed gently on the anesthetized cornea, and the free vertical movement of the attached plunger determines the scale reading. To estimate IOP, conversion tables based on empirical data from both human cadaver eyes and in vivo studies are available. The tables assume a standard ocular rigidity such that in eyes with altered scleral rigidity (e.g., after retinal detachment surgery), the Schiötz measurement may not be accurate.

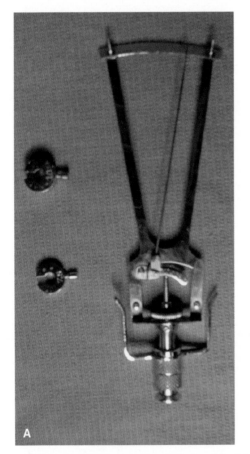
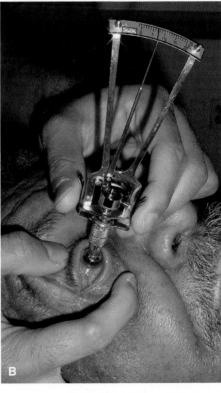

FIGURE 3-3. **Schiötz tonometer. A.** Image of the Schiötz tonometer with the 7.5- and 10-g weights shown. **B.** Schiötz indentation tonometry can be used only on patients in a supine position.

PERKINS TONOMETER

This handheld Goldmann-type applanation tonometer is especially useful in infants and children (Fig. 3-4). The light source is battery powered, and the instrument can be used in either a vertical or a supine position. The force of corneal applanation varies by rotating a calibrated dial with the same conical measuring device as the Goldmann tonometer.

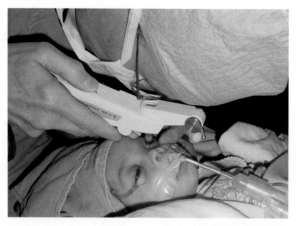

FIGURE 3-4. **Perkins tonometer.** Perkins tonometry is commonly used in the examination of infants under anesthesia.

TONO-PEN

The handheld Tono-Pen© (Mentor Ophthalmics, Santa Barbara, CA) can measure IOP in either a seated or a supine patient (Fig. 3-5). This technique is especially useful in patients with scarred or edematous corneas, those unable to be examined at a slit lamp, or in pediatric patients. With a Mackay–Marg-type tonometer such as the Tono-Pen, the effects of corneal rigidity are transferred to a surrounding sleeve so that the central plate measures only the IOP. A microprocessor in the Tono-Pen that is connected to a strain-gauge transducer measures the force of the 1.02-mm–diameter central plate as it applanates the corneal surface. Measurements of 4 to 10 readings will give a final readout with a variability between the lowest and the highest acceptable readings of less than 5%, 10%, 20%, or greater than 20%.

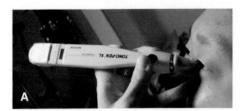
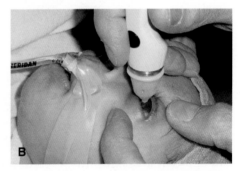

FIGURE 3-5. **Tono-Pen©. A.** The Tono-Pen XL is a handheld device that does not require a slit lamp. **B.** Proper placement of the Tono-Pen is 90 degrees perpendicular to the surface of the cornea. The small diameter of the Tono-Pen makes it also useful in children.

PNEUMOTONOMETER

This handheld device can also be used without a slit lamp, with the patient seated or supine, and on eyes with irregular corneal surfaces (Fig. 3-6). Like the Tono-Pen, this Mackay–Marg-type tonometer has its sensing surface in the center, with an adjacent surrounding rim that transfers the force needed to overcome corneal rigidity. The central sensing area is a silastic diaphragm that caps an air-filled plunger. When this flexible diaphragm is applied to the cornea, gas escape from the plunger is impeded, allowing the air pressure to rise until it balances the IOP. An electronic transducer measures the air pressure in the chamber.

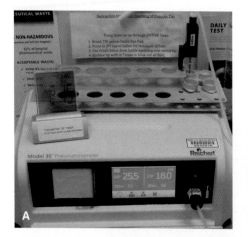

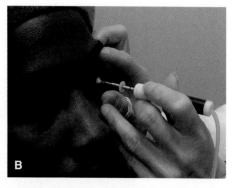

FIGURE 3-6. **Pneumotonometer. A.** The pneumotonometer readout includes a paper tracing with the average intraocular pressure in mm Hg, which demonstrates the relationship to the patient's pulse. **B.** The tip must be held perpendicular to the cornea, with the fingers not exerting force on the globe.

DYNAMIC CONTOUR TONOMETRY

Dynamic contour tonometer (DCT) or Pascal tonometer has a concave pressure-sensing tip (10.5 mm radius of curvature) that is slightly flatter than that of the average human cornea (Fig. 3-7). Because the contour of the 7-mm transducer head matches that of the cornea, there is minimal distortion of the cornea. The 1.7-mm piezoresistive pressure sensor at the center of the concavity measures the IOP at the cornea 100 times per second with less than 1 g of appositional force.

Published studies suggest that DCT may be less dependent than applanation tonometry on central corneal thickness, corneal curvature, astigmatism, anterior chamber depth, and axial length. IOP measured by DCT correlates with Goldmann applanation tonometry; however, DCT may have significantly higher readings. Variability between observers and with the same observer over time may be less with this device than with applanation tonometry. It is possible to measure both the diastolic and the systolic IOPs and determine the difference between the two, that is, the ocular pulse amplitude. Ocular pulse amplitude is an indirect measure of choroidal perfusion and may have a role in the pathophysiology of glaucoma.

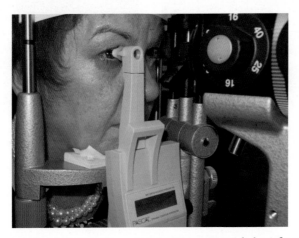

FIGURE 3-7. Dynamic contour tonometer. Dynamic contour tonometry may be less influenced by the structural characteristics of the eye.

ICARE TONOMETER

This portable rebound tonometer is a novel device for the noninvasive measurement of IOP (Fig. 3-8). Within a rod-shaped probe, a magnetized wire with a blunt plastic tip transiently touches the corneal surface and bounces back. A solenoid within the device measures the speed of the probe's rebound. The higher the IOP, the faster the rebound is. Six measurements are taken, and the average IOP value is calculated. IOP measurements correlate well with Goldmann applanation tonometry in normal individuals and are also not independent of corneal properties. The main advantage of the Icare tonometer is that there is no need for topical anesthesia. A version that allows patients to self-monitor may allow for repeatable, reliable diurnal IOP curves at home.

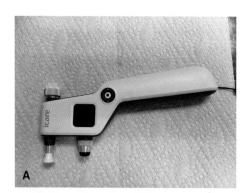
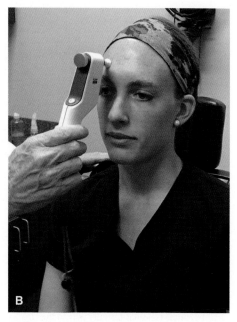

FIGURE 3-8. **Icare tonometer. A.** Icare tonometer relies on rebound tonometry measurements that can be taken without the use of topical anesthesia. **B.** The probe should be horizontal to the ground for the best accuracy.

Gonioscopy

Oscar V. Beaujon-Balbi and Oscar Beaujon-Rubin ■

INTRODUCTION

Gonioscopy is an examination of great importance for the evaluation, diagnosis, and treatment of the patient with glaucoma. Its main purpose is visualization of the configuration of the anterior chamber angle. Under normal circumstances, the structures of the anterior angle cannot be seen directly through the cornea because of the optical phenomenon known as total internal reflection. Briefly, this phenomenon refers to optical physics, whereby light that is reflected from the anterior chamber angle is bent internally within the cornea at the cornea–air interface. The gonioscopy lens (or goniolens) eliminates this effect by placing the lens–air interface at a different angle, making it possible to observe the light reflected from the structures of the angle.

Gonioscopy can be direct or indirect, depending on the lens employed, with a magnification of 15 to 20 times normal.

DIRECT GONIOSCOPY

● Direct gonioscopy refers to a "direct" view of the angle. A lens is used to overcome the internal reflectance of light in the cornea to allow visualization of the angle. Thus, one would examine the nasal angle by looking in the same direction; this is in contradistinction to looking at a mirror to examine the angle opposite to the mirror.

● The Koeppe lens is an example of a direct gonioscopy instrument (Fig. 4-1). It requires a magnification device (microscope) and a separate light source.

● The patient needs to be in a supine position.

● Direct gonioscopy lenses are often used in the operating room for angle surgery, such as goniotomy or *ab interno* trabeculotomy. At the present, we are using the Volk Trascend Vold Gonio Surgical Lens. This goniolens has a grasping ring that allows the surgeon to move the eye without tilting the patients head or microscope offering a clear view of the angle structures. Its has a floating lens with a image magnification of 1.2x and contact diameter of 9 mm (Fig. 4-2).

Advantages

● Direct gonioscopy is useful in patients with nystagmus and irregular corneas.

● Direct gonioscopy is useful for examination in children at the office under topical anesthesia. If necessary, they can be sedated, and the Koeppe lens allows examination of both the angle and the posterior pole.

- Direct gonioscopy allows a wide and panoramic evaluation of the angle that enables comparison between the different sectors and between both eyes if two lenses are placed simultaneously.

- Direct gonioscopy allows retroillumination, which is of great importance in differentiating congenital and acquired abnormalities of the angle (Fig. 4-3).

Disadvantages

- Direct gonioscopy requires that the patient be in the supine position.

- It is technically more difficult to perform.

- It requires a separate light source and magnification device (microscopy) with less optic quality than the examination made at the slit lamp (Fig. 4-4).

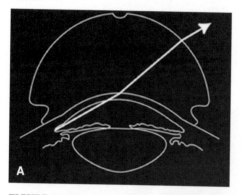
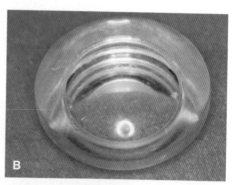

FIGURE 4-1. **Direct gonioscopy instruments. A.** Direct gonioscopy. **B.** Koeppe lens.

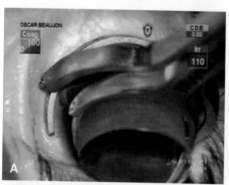
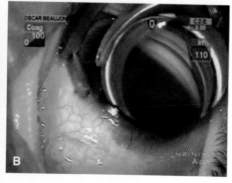
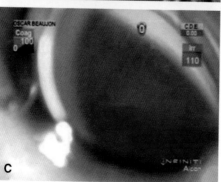

FIGURE 4-2. **Transcend Volk Gonio (TVG) goniolens.** Its grasping outer ring allows the surgeon to move the eye with minimal movement of the patient's head or microscope tilting. **A.** Placement of grasping platform of 15 mm diameter at limbus. **B.** Movement of the goniolens with handle. **C.** Visualization of the angle structures.

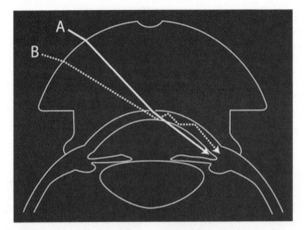

FIGURE 4-3. **Retroillumination.** Retroillumination with the Koeppe lens. **A.** Light reflection from angle structures **B.** Internal corneal scattering of light.

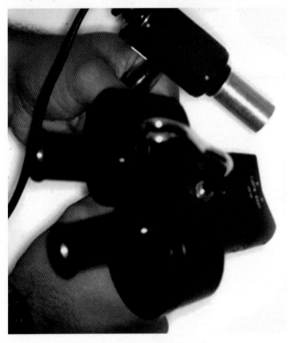

FIGURE 4-4. **Barkan's device.** Barkan's optical and illumination device.

INDIRECT GONIOSCOPY

• The angle is visualized with a lens that has one or more mirrors, allowing the evaluation of the structures opposite to the mirror employed. For evaluating the nasal quadrant, the mirror is placed temporally, but the superior and inferior orientation of the image is maintained. The examination is performed using the slit lamp.

• Since the introduction of Goldmann's indirect concept with the one-mirror goniolens, multiple lenses have been developed (Table 4-1).

■ Lenses are available with two mirrors that enable examination of all quadrants with rotation of 90 degrees of the lens. Other lenses, with four mirrors, allow evaluation of the entire angle without rotation.

■ The Goldmann and similar lenses have a contact surface with a curvature radius and diameter higher than the cornea, requiring the use of a viscous coupling substance. Zeiss and similar lenses do not require any coupling substance, because the radius of curvature is similar to that of the anterior cornea. These lenses also have a smaller contact surface diameter, and the tear film fills the cornea–lens space (Fig. 4-5).

• Proper selection of the type of goniolens is crucial to perform an effective gonioscopy. To aid this selection, some aspects should be considered. Without using a goniolens, the anterior chamber depth can first be estimated using the van Herick–Shaffer method. If a wide-open angle is suspected, any lens could be employed because there is no element that would prevent visualization of the angle (Fig. 4-6).

• If a shallow angle is suspected, it is preferable to use a one- or two-mirror Goldmann or a Zeiss lens. The mirrors of these goniolenses are higher and closer to the center, enabling visualization of the structures that would be otherwise occluded by the anterior displacement of the lens–iris diaphragm.

■ To better explain this concept, see Figure 4-7. Imagine an observer standing at point A who wants to see a house that is situated behind a hill. The hill in this example resembles the iris convexity. To solve the problem, the observer could go to a higher point, B, that enables him to see the house, or move closer to the center (top of the hill), point A', or even better, go to point B', which allows complete observation of the house and surrounding elements.

TABLE 4-1. Characteristics of Goniolenses

Lens	Corneal Diameter (mm)	Radius (mm)	Peripheral Curve (mm)	Distance to Center (mm)	Mirror Height (mm)
Goldmann, three mirrors	12	7.4	3	7	12
Goldmann, one mirror	12	7.4	1.5	3	17
Zeiss, three mirrors	11	7.7	3.5	7	20
Zeiss, four mirrors	9	7.85	—	5	12
Allen Thorpe	10	8.15	—	5	7
Sussman OS4M	9	—	—	—	15

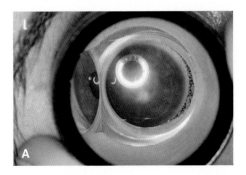

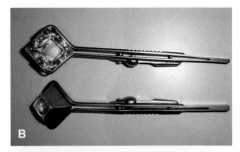

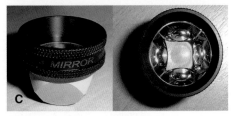

FIGURE 4-5. **Types of goniolenses. A.** Indirect gonioscopy using a Goldmann one-mirror lens. **B.** Zeiss four-mirror type of indirect goniolens, which uses a handle. **C.** Sussman four-mirror type of indirect goniolens, which is handheld.

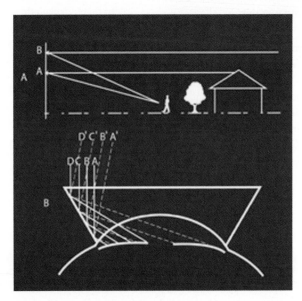

FIGURE 4-6. **Diagram of an open-angle configuration.** This figure shows that with an open angle, you can view any object in a reflective mirror, regardless of the height or distance from the center, because you do not have any interference.

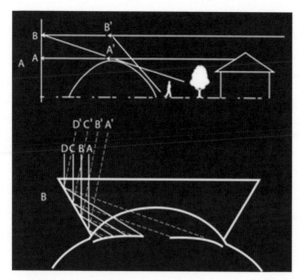

FIGURE 4-7. Observer and obstacle. This figure shows that when there is an obstruction in this example, the hill in part **A**, resembling the convex iris of a narrow angle with gonioscopy. In this case is better to be higher as B that allows to see the tree but not the person or closer as A´or closer and higher as B´. In part **B**, letters A, B, C and D shows the structures saw with the mirrow.; with gonioscopy, the convex iris of a narrow angle, it is better to be higher and closer to the center. This is analogous to using a goniolens whose mirrors are higher and closer to the center.

ESTIMATING THE ANTERIOR CHAMBER DEPTH

● Before evaluating the anterior chamber angle configuration, the van Herick–Shaffer technique is used to estimate the anterior angle depth. The procedure is performed while evaluating the patient with the slit lamp. With the thinnest slit beam possible, the cornea is illuminated perpendicularly near the temporal limbus (creating an optical section) and viewed at 50 to 60 degrees from the slit incidence. To estimate the anterior chamber depth, the ratio between the cornea–iris distance and the corneal thickness is observed.

  ▪ If the separation of the cornea–iris is more than 50% of the corneal thickness, the anterior chamber is most likely deep with a wide-angle configuration (Fig. 4-8A and B). On the other hand, if it is less than 50%, a narrow angle is suspected (Fig. 4-8C and D).

● The angle can be graded as follows:

  ▪ Grade 0 (closed)—when the iris is contacting the corneal endothelium

  ▪ Grade I—when the space between the iris and the cornea is less than 25% of corneal thickness

  ▪ Grade II—when the space is 25%

  ▪ Grade III—when it is 25% to 50%

  ▪ Grade IV—when it is higher than 50%

● This technique does not substitute gonioscopy, but it can be of great help in estimating the amplitude of the anterior chamber, especially in patients with opacities or cloudy corneas.

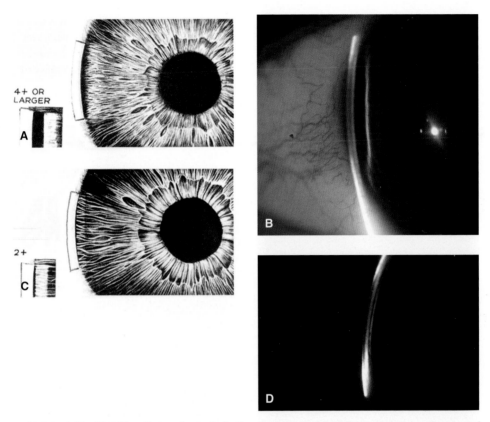

FIGURE 4-8. Van Herick's technique for angle depth estimation. A. Schematic showing proper placement of the slit beam; magnified view shows that the depth of the anterior chamber (AC) (black) is greater than 50% of the corneal slit beam (white), estimating a wide angle. **B.** Demonstration of the preceding placement in a live patient. In this example, the AC depth is approximately 90% of the corneal slit beam. **C.** Schematic showing proper placement of the slit beam; magnified view shows that the AC depth (black) is less than 50% of the corneal slit beam (white), estimating a narrow angle. **D.** Demonstration of the preceding placement in a live patient. In this example, the AC depth is approximately 10% to 15% of the corneal slit beam.

ANTERIOR SEGMENT IMAGING

● The use of imaging devices, such as ultrasound biomicroscopy (UBM) and optical coherence tomography (OCT), has been of great help to evaluate the angle configuration. Both technologies allow the observer to measure the angle amplitude and offer details and relation of structures. The UBM is crucial in iris plateau diagnosis and cases of corneal edema or opacities, for example, before keratoplasty (Fig. 4-9). Even in the presence of high quality and magnification of the images, gonioscopy is still needed. These technologies should be used as complementary tests (Fig. 4-10).

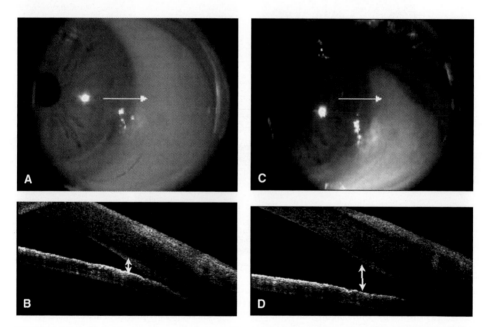

FIGURE 4-9. **Optical coherence tomography on a 60-year-old woman with an occludable angle configuration.** **A.** *Arrow* shows the area studied and magnified in B. **B.** Note apposition of the iris to the trabecular meshwork. **C.** *Arrow* shows the same area studied after laser. **D.** Note the widening of the angle between the iris and the peripheral cornea.

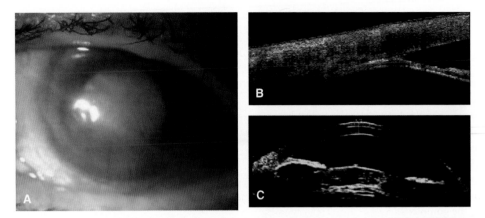

FIGURE 4-10. **A 65-year-old woman with bullous keratopathy secondary to angle-closure glaucoma. A.** Corneal fibrosis with vascularization obscures the view. In this case, gonioscopy is not suitable. **B.** Nasal angle closed by optical coherence tomography. **C.** Same angle closed as demonstrated by ultrasonic biomicroscopy.

TECHNIQUE

• A drop of anesthetic is administered to both eyes, and the examination is performed at the slit lamp. Depending on the lens employed, a viscous coupling substance may be required. The goniolens must be placed gently on the eye, while trying to avoid distortion of the intraocular elements (**Figs. 4-11** and **4-12**). To obtain a good view of the angle, the incidence of the light beam must be perpendicular to the mirror of the goniolens.

• Some adjustments on the slit lamp have to be made as the evaluation is performed:

■ To evaluate the superior and inferior angles, the patient is asked to look at the light source.

■ To evaluate the nasal and temporal angles, the illumination source is inclined forward and the goniolens is shifted slightly downward, and the patient is asked to look to the side being evaluated.

• These simple technical details are vital to enable evaluation of narrow angles and to identify the different elements of the angle, especially Schwalbe line.

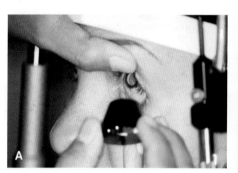

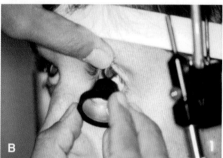

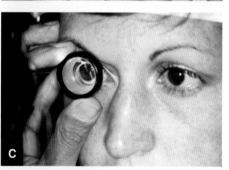

FIGURE 4-11. **Goldmann goniolens. A–C.** Placing of a Goldmann one-mirror–type goniolens.

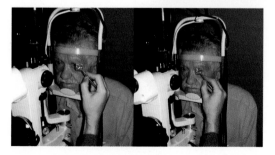

FIGURE 4-12. **Zeiss goniolens.** Placing of a Zeiss-type goniolens.

ELEMENTS OF THE ANGLE ANATOMY

- In Figure 4-13, the different elements to be identified during gonioscopy are illustrated. The angle extends from the last iris fold to Schwalbe line. The angle structures can be divided into two groups:

  - A fixed portion that includes Schwalbe line, the trabecular meshwork, and the scleral spur

  - A mobile portion that includes the anterior–superior face of the ciliary body and the iris insertion, with its last fold

- The examiner must make a general inspection to identify some important aspects:

  - Iris plane—this can be planar on wide angles and very convex on narrow angles.

  - Last iris fold and its distance from Schwalbe line—these two elements are used to estimate the amplitude of the angle. The superior angle portion is generally narrower than the other portions.

  - Iris root—this represents the insertion on the ciliary body. It is the thinnest portion, and the most easily displaced with elevation of the posterior chamber pressure.

In myopic eyes, the iris is larger and thinner, with numerous crypts, and is usually inserted more posterior on the ciliary body. On the other hand, in hyperopic eyes, the iris tends to be thicker and its insertion is more anterior than in emmetropic eyes, resulting in a narrower angle configuration.

- Iris nodules, cysts, nevi, or foreign bodies (Fig. 4-14).

- Most of the time, it is easy to identify one element, making it possible to discern the others. For example, Figure 4-15 shows the Schlemm canal filled with blood. This is a frequent observation in patients with low intraocular pressure or those with increased pressure in the episcleral veins. *An elevation in episcleral venous pressure can occur* when the examiner presses the lens too strongly onto the sclera during gonioscopy.

- Pathologically, it can occur in cases of secondary glaucoma, such as those caused by increased episcleral venous pressure, Sturge-Weber syndrome, carotid cavernous fistula, or in some cases of iridocyclitis in which the venous pressure of congestive eyes could be elevated, causing a passage of the blood from the venous system to Schlemm canal.

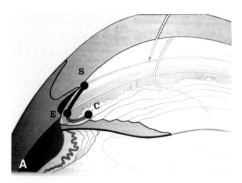

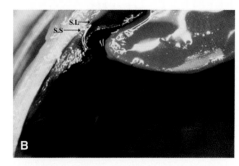

FIGURE 4-13. **Angle structure elements. A.** Schwalbe line (S), scleral spur (E), and ciliary body (C). **B.** Angle structure elements in a human cadaver eye. S.L., Schwalbe line; S.S., scleral spur.

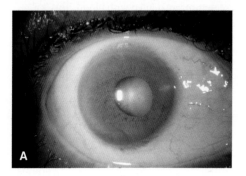

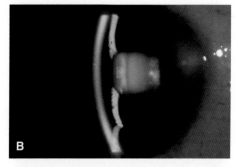

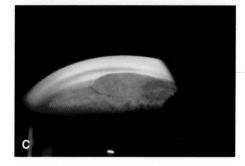

FIGURE 4-14. **Iris cyst. A.** Slit-lamp photograph showing an iris mass inferiorly. **B.** Slit beam showing the same. **C.** Gonioscopic view of the inferior angle showing the cystic mass. The cystic nature of this mass was confirmed by ultrasound biomicroscopy (not shown).

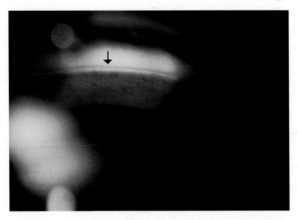

FIGURE 4-15. **Schlemm canal.** Schlemm canal filled with blood (*arrow*).

IDENTIFICATION OF ANGLE STRUCTURES

- Schwalbe line represents the end of the Descemet membrane and marks the anterior limit of the angle. In some patients, Schwalbe line can be thickened with protrusion to the anterior chamber, which has been termed posterior embryotoxon (Fig. 4-16).

- Pigment frequently deposits around Schwalbe line because it marks the transition between the corneal and scleral curvatures. This change of curvature produces a step that facilitates deposition of pigment and other materials. If Schwalbe line is not visible, it can easily be localized by aiming a thin slit beam on the angle. This beam gives reflexes on both the anterior and the posterior surfaces of the cornea. The inner reflection line corresponds to the posterior surface of the cornea and is contiguous with the angle structures and iris surface. The outer line, corresponding to the anterior cornea, ends just where Schwalbe line is located, at the point where both light beams are joined (Figs. 4-13A and 4-17). This maneuver is very important for evaluating a narrow angle and differentiating it from a closed angle (Fig. 4-18).

- In Figure 4-19, the following elements can be observed:

  ▪ Trabecular meshwork that extends from the scleral spur to Schwalbe line

  ▪ Schlemm canal, situated just anterior to the scleral spur. The scleral spur has a grayish appearance in young patients and becomes more pigmented with age. In the figure, a pigment band is evident, corresponding to the pigmented trabecular meshwork.

  ▪ Scleral spur, a whiter line just inferior to the trabecular meshwork. This serves as the insertion to the longitudinal portion of the ciliary muscle.

  ▪ Last iris fold and anterior insertion of the ciliary body. The position where it is inserted determines in major part the amplitude of the chamber angle. The visible portion of the ciliary body extends from its insertion to the scleral spur and is covered anteriorly by trabecular meshwork, termed *uveal meshwork.*

- Sometimes, this tissue is formed of wide and multiple bands that insert on the scleral spur, but they may also extend over the trabecular meshwork. The last ones are called *iris processes* (Fig. 4-20). Iris processes can overpass the trabecular meshwork, coating the angle, and insert onto Schwalbe line, representing a minor manifestation of abnormal embryologic development (Fig. 4-21).

- It is important to avoid confusing iris processes with peripheral anterior synechiae, which are products of adherence of the peripheral iris to any of the angle structures, most often Schwalbe line or the peripheral cornea. Peripheral anterior synechiae are observed as tents passing over the angle (Fig. 4-22B).

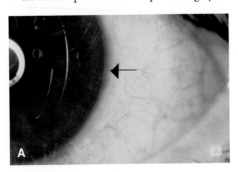
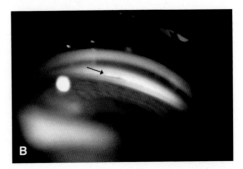

FIGURE 4-16. **Schwalbe line. A.** Posterior embryotoxon (*arrow*). **B.** Schwalbe line in gonioscopy (*arrow*).

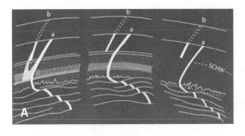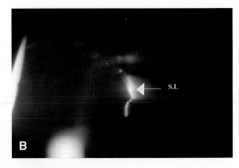

FIGURE 4-17. **Schwalbe line. A.** Schwalbe line localization using the edges of the corneal slit beam. The different beam reflexes are shown; "b" corresponds to anterior cornea and "a" to posterior cornea. **B.** Gonioscopic view demonstrating that Schwalbe line is located where the anterior and posterior light reflexes of the corneal slit beam converge. S.L., Schwalbe line (*arrow*). (**A**, Reproduced with permission from Beaujon-Rubin O, ed. *Glaucoma Primario: Diagnostico & Tratamiento*. Caracas, Venezuela: Venezuelan Society of Ophthalmology; 1983.)

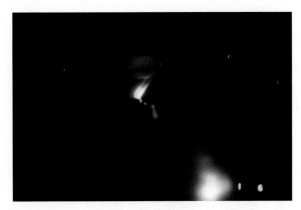

FIGURE 4-18. **Schwalbe line.** Schwalbe line localization using the corneal slit beams in a narrow angle.

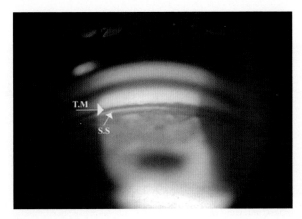

FIGURE 4-19. **Gonioscopy.** Open angle. S.S., scleral spur; T.M., trabecular meshwork.

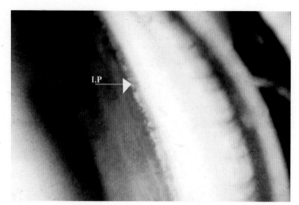

FIGURE 4-20. Iris processes. Gonioscopic view of the anterior chamber angle demonstrating iris processes (I.P.; *arrow*).

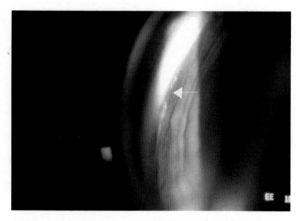

FIGURE 4-21. Iris processes. Iris processes inserting onto Schwalbe line (*arrow*).

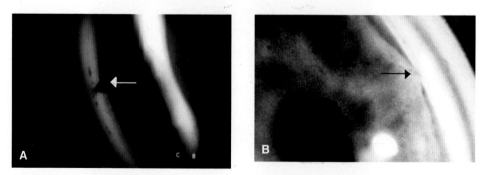

FIGURE 4-22. Peripheral anterior synechiae. A and **B.** Examples of peripheral anterior synechiae (*arrows*).

CLASSIFICATION OF THE ANGLE

● Among the objectives of gonioscopy is to determine the amplitude of the angle and the type of glaucoma, that is open-angle or closed-angle. Each type has a different epidemiology, physiopathology, treatment, and prevention.

● Shaffer's classification (Fig. 4-23) estimates the angle amplitude between the last iris fold and the trabecular meshwork–Schwalbe line as follows:

- Grade IV—45 degrees
- Grade III—30 degrees
- Grade II—20 degrees; angle closure is possible.
- Grade I—10 degrees; angle closure is likely.
- Slit—angle is less than 10 degrees; angle closure is more likely.
- Closed—iris is stuck to the meshwork (Fig. 4-24).

● Spaeth's classification adds detail regarding peripheral iris and the effects of indentation on the configuration of the angle (Fig. 4-25).

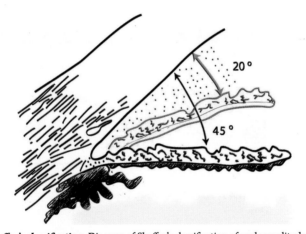

FIGURE 4-23. **Shaffer's classification.** Diagram of Shaffer's classification of angle amplitude.

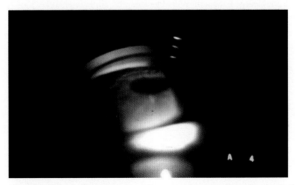

FIGURE 4-24. **Narrow angle.** Aspect of the narrow angle on gonioscopy. Note the marked convexity of the iris, sometimes referred to as iris bowing. The angle structures are difficult to visualize.

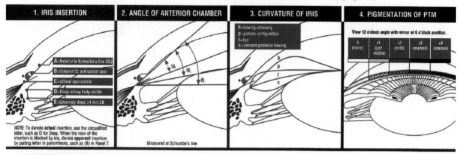

GONIOSCOPIC EVALUATION *(Spaeth Grading System)*

| 1. IRIS INSERTION | 2. ANGLE OF ANTERIOR CHAMBER | 3. CURVATURE OF IRIS | 4. PIGMENTATION OF PTM |

A=Anterior to Schwalbe's line (SL)
B=Between SL and scleral spur
C=Scleral spur visible
D=Deep: ciliary body visible
E=Extremely deep: >1 mm CB

NOTE: To denote actual insertion, use the unqualified letter, such as D for Deep. When the view of the insertion is blocked by iris, denote apparent insertion by putting letter in parentheses, such as (B) in Panel 7.

Measured at Schwalbe's line

b=bowing anteriorly
p=plateau configuration
f=flat
c=concave posterior bowing

View 12 o'clock angle with mirror at 6 o'clock position.

| 0 (none) | +1 (just visible) | +2 (mild) | +3 (marked) | +4 (intense) |

COSOPT is indicated for the reduction of elevated intraocular pressure (IOP) in patients with open-angle glaucoma or ocular hypertension who are insufficiently responsive to beta blockers (failed to achieve target IOP determined after multiple measurements over time). The IOP-lowering effect of COSOPT b.i.d. was slightly less than that seen with the concomitant administration of 0.5% timolol b.i.d. and 2.0% dorzolamide t.i.d.

COSOPT is contraindicated in patients with (1) bronchial asthma; (2) a history of bronchial asthma; (3) severe chronic obstructive pulmonary disease (see WARNINGS); (4) sinus bradycardia; (5) second- or third-degree atrioventricular block; (6) overt cardiac failure (see WARNINGS); (7) cardiogenic shock; or (8) hypersensitivity to any component of this product.

A

GONIOSCOPIC EVALUATION *(Spaeth Grading System)*
Examples

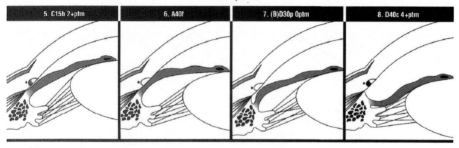

| 5. C15b 2+ptm | 6. A40f | 7. (B)D30p 0ptm | 8. D40c 4+ptm |

www.cosopt.com

Before prescribing COSOPT, please read the accompanying full Prescribing Information.

Provided as a service by Merck & Co., Inc.

MERCK © 2001 Merck & Co., Inc. All rights reserved.   20104466(1)-04/01-COS   Printed in USA

B

FIGURE 4-25. **Spaeth's classification. A** and **B.** Spaeth's classification, which provides additional information and detail. (Courtesy of Dr. George L. Spaeth, Wills Eye Hospital, Philadelphia, PA.)

PIGMENT DEPOSITION AND GONIOSCOPY

● The amount of pigment deposition in the angle varies widely among individuals. Sometimes the pattern can serve as a diagnostic tool to determine the underlying mechanism. Some examples are described next.

Pigmentary Glaucoma

● In this condition, a highly dense band of brown pigment is deposited on the trabecular meshwork in a homogeneous manner (Fig. 4-26A). This pigment is observed on the posterior lens capsule and on the corneal endothelium (Krukenberg spindle) (Fig. 4-26B).

Lens Pseudoexfoliation

● This entity occurs when material of amorphous substance is deposited on and anterior to Schwalbe line in an undulating pattern known as Sampaolesi sign (Fig. 4-27).

● The material also deposits on the lens zonule and can be observed during gonioscopy (Fig. 4-28).

Uveitis

● In cases of uveitis, irregular areas of pigment deposits can be observed, giving an appearance of a "dirty" angle (Fig. 4-29).

Angle-Closure Glaucoma

● In cases of angle-closure glaucoma, a patchy area of pigment may be observed on any angle structure, an indication that the iris was stuck at that place but a permanent adherence did not develop. The presence of a patchy pigment and a narrow angle can be an indication of a previous episode of acute angle-closure glaucoma (Fig. 4-30).

● Vascularization is usually absent on the angle. Sometimes, small branches of the ciliary body's arterial circle can be observed. These branches are usually covered by the uveal meshwork and form a circumferential serpiginous pattern or can be observed radially toward the iris sphincter.

● In neovascular glaucoma, abnormal vessels cross over the ciliary body and arborize the trabecular meshwork. Contraction of myofibrils of the fibroblasts that accompany the abnormal vessels causes peripheral anterior synechiae and angle closure (Fig. 4-31).

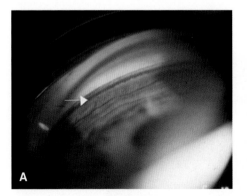
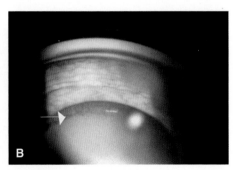

FIGURE 4-26. **Pigmentary glaucoma. A.** Pigmentary deposition on the trabecular meshwork (*arrow*) in an eye with pigment dispersion syndrome. **B.** Pigmentary deposition on the posterior lens capsule (Zentmeyer line, *arrow*) in an eye with pigment dispersion syndrome.

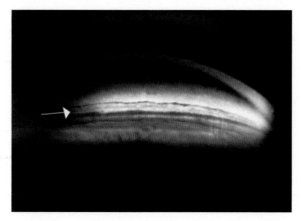

FIGURE 4-27. **Lens pseudoexfoliation.** Sampaolesi sign (*arrow*).

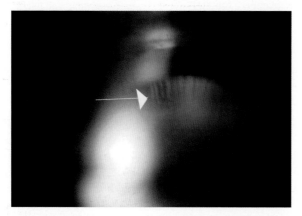

FIGURE 4-28. **Lens pseudoexfoliation.** Deposit of pseudoexfoliation material on the lens zonule (*arrow*).

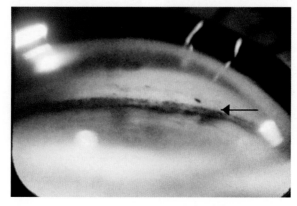

FIGURE 4-29. **Uveitis.** Irregular pigment deposits on the angle in a patient with uveitis (*arrow*).

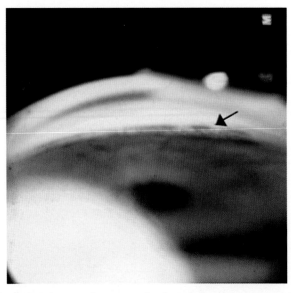

FIGURE 4-30. **Angle-closure glaucoma.** Pigment patches formed after angle-closure crisis (*arrow*).

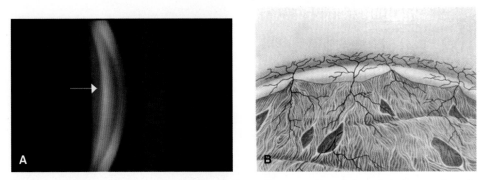

FIGURE 4-31. **Neovascular glaucoma. A.** Fibrovascular membrane over the angle (*arrow*). At this stage, the angle is open but occluded. There is marked corneal edema, giving a hazy view. **B.** Diagram of a fibrovascular membrane growing over the angle and causing peripheral anterior synechiae from contraction in neovascular glaucoma.

IRIDOCORNEOENDOTHELIAL SYNDROME (ICE SYNDROME)

● Iridocorneoendothlial syndrome is a group of three entities that have in common changes on the iris, corneal endothelium, and progressive closure of the anterior chamber angle. Typically unilateral, it affects young adults and is more frequent in females. Glaucoma is often associated. Essential iris atrophy is

characterized by holes and multiple atrophic tears of the iris. Chandler syndrome has less iris involvement but more corneal edema with corectopia and peripheral synechiae (**Figs. 4-32A** and **B.**). The intraocular pressure can get high values, and glaucoma develops as the disease progresses with retinal nerve fiber layer and ganglion cell complex involvement in OCT and visual field defects (**Figs. 4-32** to **4-34**).

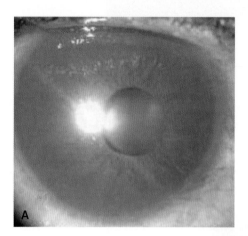

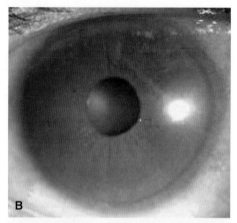

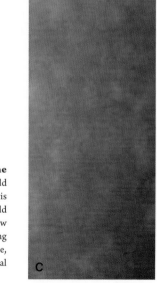

FIGURE 4-32. Chandler syndrome with unilateral glaucoma. A. Note a mild corectopia with some areas of peripheral iris atrophy in the affected right eye with mild central corneal edema. **B.** The normal fellow eye. **C.** Specular microscopic image showing corneal endothelial changes with loss of size, shape, and density in affected eye. **D.** Normal endothelium.

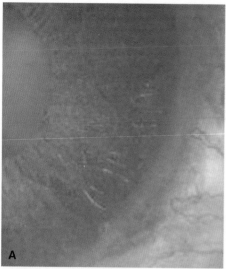

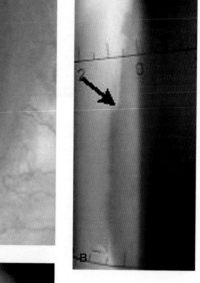

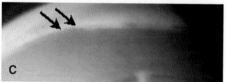

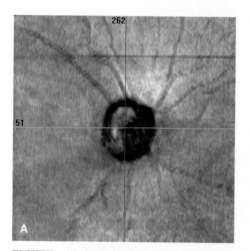

FIGURE 4-33. **Chandler syndrome. A.** Higher magnification of iris atrophy in patient with Chandler syndrome **B** and **C.** Peripheral anterior synechia related to the area of iris atrophy (*black arrows*).

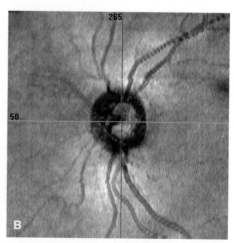

FIGURE 4-34. **Optical coherence tomography (OCT) imaging of patient with Chandlers syndrome in Figures IV and VI. A.** Right optic nerve showing thinning of the retinal nerve fiber layer (RNFL). **B.** Left optic nerve with normal RNFL.

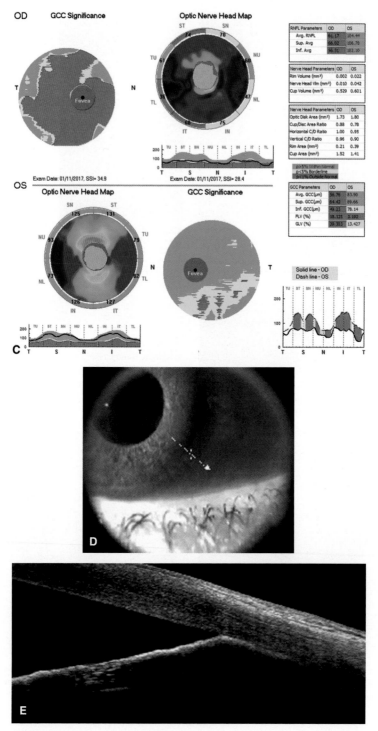

FIGURE 4.34. (*continued*) **C.** Retinal nerve layer defect inferior on right eye. **D** and **E.** Peripheral anterior synechia as seen on anterior segment OCT.

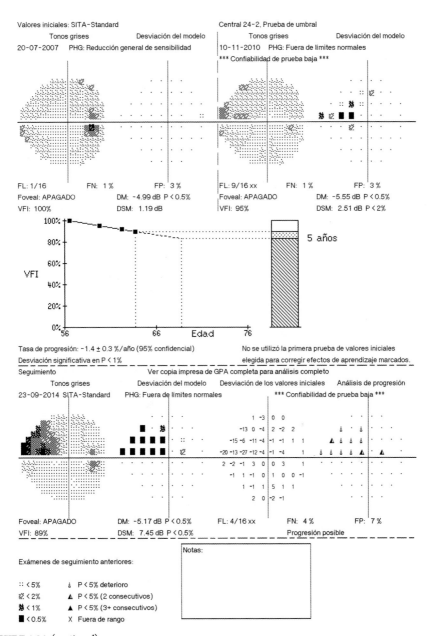

FIGURE 4.34. (*continued*)

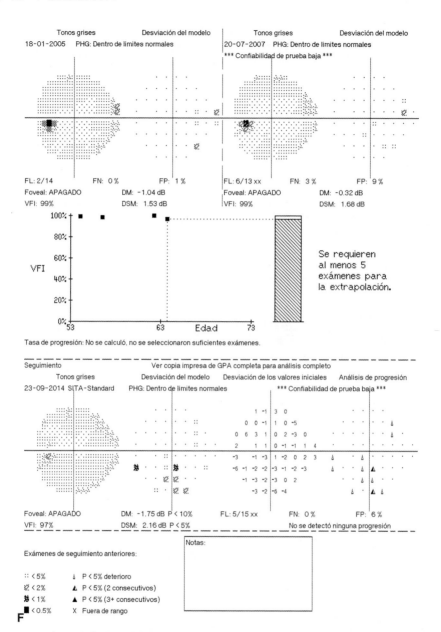

FIGURE 4.34. (*continued*) **F.** Visual field in Chandler syndrome. Note a visual field defect superior nasally area in concordance with the defect in the neuroretinal rim of the optic nerve and OCT RNFL and ganglion cell complex by OCT.

ERROR FACTORS ON GONIOSCOPY

● When performing gonioscopy, the examiner must be aware that some maneuvers alter the precision of the procedure. The gonioscopy lens can deepen the amplitude of the angle if too much pressure is applied to the sclera by forcing a fluid movement toward the angle (Fig. 4-35).

● This indentation gonioscopy is invaluable in evaluating angle-closure glaucoma, especially in differentiating iris apposition from real synechiae. For this maneuver, the Zeiss-type gonioscopy lens is recommended.

■ The procedure, which is called dynamic gonioscopy, employs the mechanical effect on aqueous humor that follows the corneal indentation, enabling the examiner to alter the relative position of the iris in a dynamic way. This maneuver helps to distinguish narrow from closed angles and to determine the risk of closure. An excess of pressure produces folds on Descemet membrane, making evaluation of the angle difficult (Fig. 4-36).

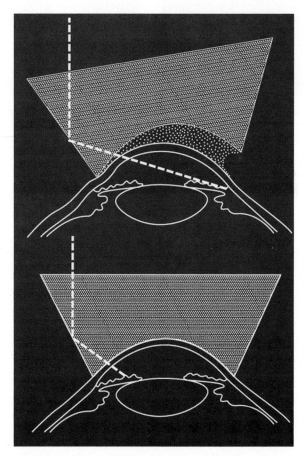

FIGURE 4-35. **Error factors in gonioscopy.** Placing obliquely directed pressure on the sclera.

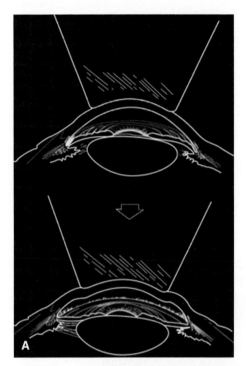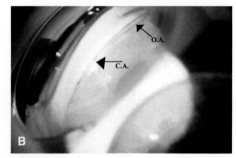

FIGURE 4-36. Dynamic gonioscopy. A. Schematic demonstrating dynamic, compression, or indentation gonioscopy. **B.** Dynamic gonioscopy demonstrating peripheral anterior synechia formation (C.A., closed angle) and chronic angle-closure glaucoma in a patient with narrow angles. Part of the angle is still open (O.A., open angle).

USE OF GONIOSCOPY IN TRAUMA

Contusion Trauma

● When the cornea is hit, a wave of fluid abruptly forms. This wave moves toward the angle because the iris–lens diaphragm acts as a valve, preventing the fluid from going in a posterior direction. This fluid movement can harm the structures of the angle, creating acute lesions that are related to trauma intensity (Fig. 4-37).

● Separation of the iris insertion from the scleral spur, termed *iridodialysis*, causes one of these lesions (Fig. 4-38).

Angle Recession

● Angle recession occurs when the ciliary body is separated, leaving the external wall covered by the longitudinal portion of the ciliary muscle (Fig. 4-39).

Cyclodialysis

● Cyclodialysis is a completed dehiscence of the ciliary body from the sclera, opening a communication pathway to the suprachoroidal space (Fig. 4-40).

● These gonioscopic patterns can be found in the same patient and are frequently accompanied by hyphema.

Iridodialysis

● Iridodialysis occurs when there is separation of the iris insertion from the scleral spur.

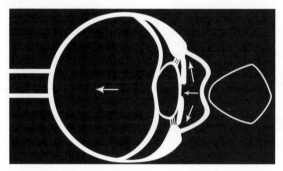

FIGURE 4-37. **Contusion trauma.** Diagram of blunt trauma to the eye. *Arrows* show contusion waves on aquous and vitreous with possible damage to angle, lens, retina and optic nerve.

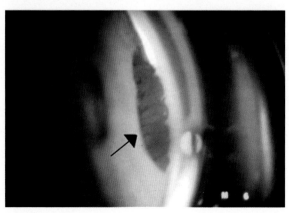

FIGURE 4-38. **Iridodialysis.** The iris root (*arrow*) has fallen, exposing the underlying ciliary body processes.

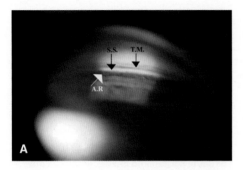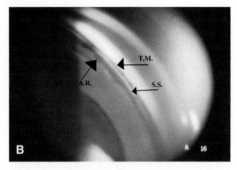

FIGURE 4-39. **Angle recession after trauma. A.** Extensive angle recession after trauma. In this example, the normal angle insertion is not visible, which could fool an examiner into thinking that the angle is normal. **B.** Angle recession after trauma. In this example, there is a smaller degree of angle recession, and the border between the recessed angle and the normal angle is seen. A.R., angle recession; S.S., scleral spur; T.M., trabecular meshwork.

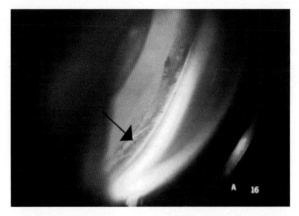

FIGURE 4-40. **Cyclodialysis.** The ciliary body is completely detached, exposing the underlying sclera (*arrow*).

TRAUMATIC INTRAOCULAR FOREIGN BODIES

• In some cases of ocular trauma, a small foreign body can enter the anterior chamber through the sclera or cornea that can be self-sealed. Very gentle gonioscopy could be useful in evaluating the angle structures (Fig. 4-41).

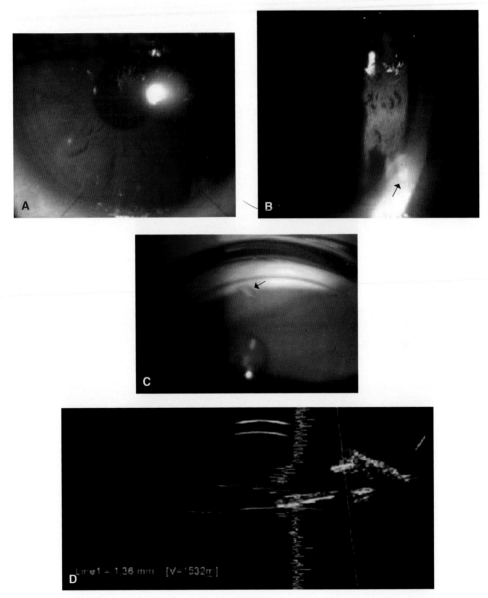

FIGURE 4-41. Intraocular foreign body in a 7-year-old boy. His mother noted that a white dot appeared on his left eye. He had a previous conjunctivitis 2 months before. **A** and **B.** A foreign body present in anterior chamber (*black arrow*) without flare or inflammation. **C.** Gonioscopy showing the foreign body encrusted in the peripheral angle.

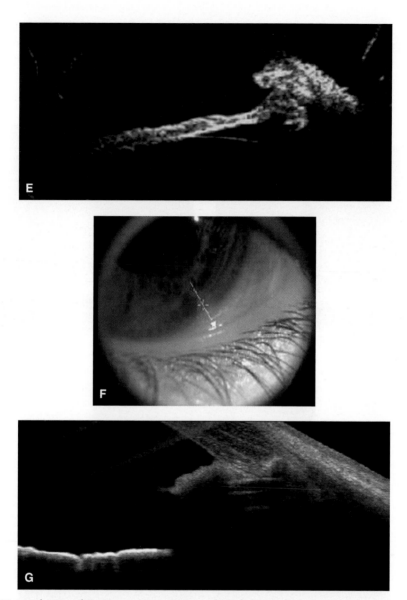

FIGURE 4-41. (*continued*) **D.** Ultrasound biomicroscopy (UBM) showing the hyperechoic image of the foreign body. **E.** UBM of the adjacent peripheral anterior synechiae. **F** and **G.** Optical coherence tomography images of same foreign body.

POSTOPERATIVE EVALUATION

Gonioscopy can be very helpful in evaluating the postoperative status following trabeculectomy and cataract surgery, especially when a complication has occurred or the bleb has failed to form. In some cases, the internal ostium can be occluded by iris or vitreous. At long term, gonioscopy is important in evaluating angle structures (Fig. 4-42).

To perform some of the newer surgical techniques, such as microinvasive glaucoma surgery, the surgeon has to be an expert at evaluating the angle and handling of the surgical goniolens in the operating room. Accurate identification of the angle structures, such as the scleral spur and the trabecular meshwork, is needed (Fig. 4-43).

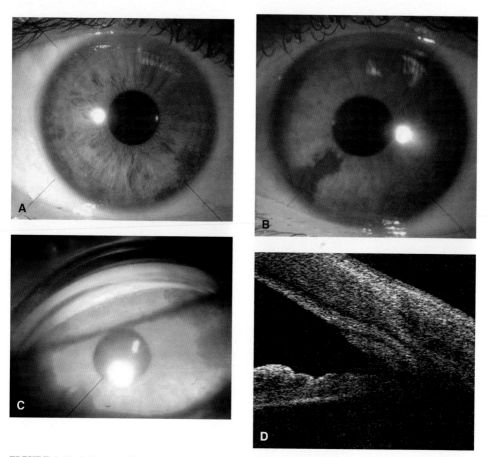

FIGURE 4-42. **A 32-year-old woman with a diagnosis of congenital glaucoma successfully treated with a goniotomy in her left eye at 3 months of life. A.** Normal right eye. **B.** Affected left eye that has mild myopia of −1.50 diopter. **C.** Open-angle visualization of the inferior temporal quadrant that had been surgically treated. **D.** Angle configuration by optical coherence tomography showing the previous incision.

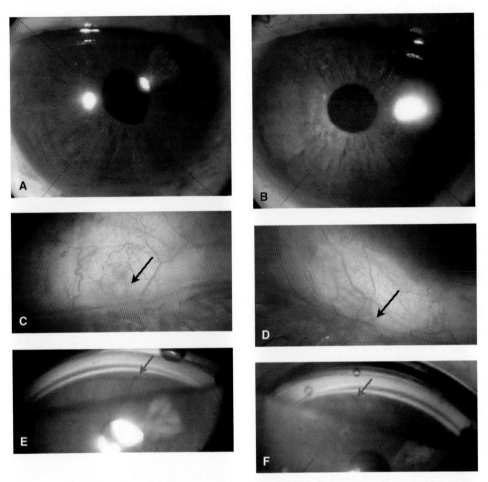

FIGURE 4-43. A 60-year-old man with moderate glaucoma and cataract that was treated with phacoemulsi-fication cataract extraction, intraocular lens implantation, and Xen (Allergan) glaucoma device placement superonasally. A. Slight displacement of pupil toward the entry site of the device in the right eye. B. Central round pupil in left eye. C and D. Subconjunctival visualization of the device (*black arrows*). E. Slight iris incarceration when the device was implanted (*green arrow*). F. Visualization of the device in anterior chamber (*green arrow*).

CHAPTER

5

Anterior Segment Imaging

Sung Chul (Sean) Park, Syril Dorairaj, Jeffrey M. Liebmann, and Robert Ritch ■

INTRODUCTION

Anterior segment ultrasound biomicroscopy ultrasound biomicroscopy (UBM) uses high-frequency transducers (35 to 75 MHz) to provide in vivo imaging of the anterior segment with an axial resolution of 30 to 70 μm and penetration depth of 2 to 7 mm. The structures surrounding the posterior chamber, hidden from clinical observation, can be imaged and their anatomic relationships assessed.

UBM has been used to investigate both the normal structure and disease mechanisms and pathophysiology in many areas of ophthalmology, including glaucoma, cornea, lens, congenital abnormalities, effects and complications of surgical procedures, anterior segment trauma, cysts and tumors, and uveitis. Studies using UBM were initially primarily qualitative, but quantitative studies have become increasingly common.[1] Three-dimensional analysis of UBM images is still in its infancy.

Anterior segment optical coherence tomography (AS-OCT) uses infrared light instead of ultrasound and transmits signals of shorter wavelength (820 to 1,310 nm), which produce images of higher resolution (axial resolution of 5 to 15 μm) than UBM.[2] It enables non-contact imaging because the refractive index between air and tissue is much less than the acoustic impedance between them. Dynamic relationships between the iris, angle wall, and lens can be assessed through real-time limbus-to-limbus cross-sectional images because of its faster scan speed, reducing eye movement artifacts. AS-OCT also provides software for automatic measurement of various cornea and anterior chamber parameters (**Fig. 5-1**). However, the ciliary body is rarely visualized owing to the pigmented posterior layer of the iris, which blocks light penetration. AS-OCT has been used similarly to UBM, but, because of its characteristics, has been more useful in quantitative analysis of the anterior chamber and in corneal disease or surgery, such as keratoplasty.

These imaging devices do not replace conventional slit-lamp biomicroscopy or gonioscopy, but supplement and augment clinical practice and provide invaluable research tools. Characteristics of UBM and AS-OCT are compared in **Table 5-1**.

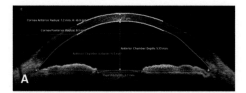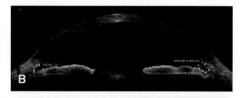

FIGURE 5-1. **Measurement of cornea and anterior chamber parameters using anterior segment optical coherence tomography (AS-OCT).** Corneal thickness, corneal radius of curvature, anterior chamber depth and volume, pupil diameter, and distance between scleral spurs (**A**), as well as anterior chamber angle parameters, such as AOD500 (angle-opening distance at 500 μm from the scleral spur), TISA500 (trabecular–iris space area at 500 μm from the scleral spur), and TIA500 (trabecular–iris angle at 500 μm from the scleral spur) (**B**), can be measured using AS-OCT.

TABLE 5-1. Characteristics of UBM and AS-OCT

	UBM	AS-OCT
Signal source	Ultrasound	Infrared light
Resolution (μm)	~30–70	~5–15
Tissue penetration	Up to 7 mm, ciliary body visualized	Ciliary body rarely visualized
Image width (mm)	4–7	15–16
Tissue contact	Yes (needs fluid coupling medium)	No
Image acquisition time	Slower	Faster
Quantitative analysis	Manual	Automatic

AS-OCT, anterior segment optical coherence tomography; UBM, ultrasound biomicroscopy.

ANGLE-CLOSURE GLAUCOMA

Because of its ability to image the ciliary body, posterior chamber, iris–lens relationships, and angle structures simultaneously, UBM is ideally suited to the study of angle closure. Significant correlations have been found between angle measurements by AS-OCT, UBM, and gonioscopy.[3,4] When assessing a narrow angle for occludability, gonioscopy in a completely darkened room, using the smallest square of light for a slit beam to avoid stimulating the pupillary light reflex, is of utmost importance. The effect of ambient light on the angle configuration is well illustrated by performing UBM under illuminated and darkened conditions (Fig. 5-2).

Because most of the important anterior chamber angle parameters for quantitative measurement are based on the identification of the scleral spur, reliable documentation of the angle dimensions using UBM or AS-OCT is therefore dependent on its precise and repeatable localization. In a UBM or AS-OCT image, the scleral spur can be seen as the innermost point of the line separating the ciliary body and the sclera at its point of contact with the anterior chamber. Although it cannot be visualized with UBM or AS-OCT, the trabecular meshwork is located directly anterior to this structure and posterior to Schwalbe line (Fig. 5-3).

Cornea and angle structures are less distorted during AS-OCT because of its noncontact nature, avoiding artifacts induced by inadvertent pressure on the cornea during gonioscopy or on limbal tissues with the eye cup during UBM. Differentiation of appositional and synechial angle closure in eyes with iridotrabecular contact by indention AS-OCT adds to its clinical utility in the evaluation of patients with angle closure.[5] Anterior chamber depth and volume measured using AS-OCT may be useful parameters for detecting individuals at risk of developing primary angle closure.

Angle closure can be classified by the site of the anatomic structure or force causing iris apposition to the trabecular meshwork. These are defined as blocks originating at the level of the iris (pupillary block), ciliary body (plateau iris), lens (phacomorphic glaucoma), and forces posterior to the lens (malignant glaucoma).

Relative Pupillary Block

Relative pupillary block is responsible for over 90% of the angle closure in Caucasian populations. In pupillary block, resistance to aqueous flow from the posterior to the anterior chamber through the pupil and the resulting increased aqueous pressure in the posterior chamber forces the iris anteriorly (Fig. 5-4A), causing anterior iris bowing and angle narrowing. An anteriorly convex configuration of the entire iris can be imaged using AS-OCT (Fig. 5-5).

Pupillary block may be absolute, if the iris is completely bound to the lens by posterior synechiae, but most often is a functional block, termed *relative pupillary block*. Relative pupillary block usually causes no symptoms. However, if it is sufficient to cause appositional closure of a portion of the angle without elevating intraocular pressure (IOP), peripheral anterior synechiae may gradually form and lead to chronic angle closure (Fig. 5-6). If the pupillary block becomes absolute, the pressure in the posterior chamber increases and pushes the peripheral iris farther forward to cover the trabecular meshwork and close the angle with an ensuing rise of IOP (acute angle closure) (Fig. 5-7).

Laser iridotomy eliminates the pressure differential between the anterior and posterior chambers and relieves the iris convexity. This results in several changes in anterior segment anatomy. The iris assumes a flat or planar configuration (Fig. 5-4B), and the iridocorneal angle widens. The region of iridolenticular contact actually increases, as aqueous flows through the iridotomy rather than the pupillary space.

Plateau Iris

In plateau iris, the ciliary processes are either large or anteriorly situated, or both, so that the ciliary sulcus is obliterated and the ciliary body supports the iris against the trabecular meshwork. The anterior chamber is usually of medium depth and the iris surface only slightly convex. Argon laser peripheral iridoplasty contracts and compresses the peripheral iris, pulling it away from the trabecular meshwork (Fig. 5-8).[6] Although large or anteriorly situated ciliary processes are rarely visualized by AS-OCT, it can be used to confirm a clinical suspicion of plateau iris configuration (Fig. 5-9).[7]

Phacomorphic Glaucoma

Lens enlargement may cause shallowing of the anterior chamber and precipitate acute angle closure by forcing the iris and ciliary body anteriorly. Miotic therapy increases the lens axial length and causes it to move anteriorly, which further shallows the anterior chamber, and may paradoxically worsen the situation (Fig. 5-10). AS-OCT is useful in this condition, because anterior chamber depth, iris configuration, and angle structures can be evaluated at a glance.

Malignant Glaucoma

Malignant (ciliary block) glaucoma is a multifactorial disease in which the following components may play varying roles: (1) previous acute or chronic angle closure, (2) shallow anterior chamber, (3) forward lens movement, (4) pupillary block by the lens or vitreous, (5) zonular laxity, (6) anterior rotation or swelling of the ciliary body, or both, (7) thickening of the anterior hyaloid membrane, (8) vitreous expansion, and (9) posterior aqueous displacement into or behind the vitreous.

UBM reveals a shallow supraciliary detachment, not evident on routine B-scan or clinical examination. This effusion appears to be the cause of the anterior rotation of the ciliary body. Aqueous humor is secreted posterior to the lens (posterior aqueous displacement), increasing vitreous pressure, pushing the lens–iris diaphragm forward, and causing angle closure and shallowing of the anterior chamber (Fig. 5-11). Although changes in the shape or position of the ciliary body cannot be accurately assessed, an anteriorly displaced iris–lens diaphragm and shallow anterior chamber are well demonstrated using AS-OCT (Fig. 5-12).

Pseudophakic Pupillary Block

Anterior chamber inflammation after cataract extraction can lead to posterior synechiae between the iris and a posterior chamber intraocular lens, producing absolute pupillary block and angle closure. Anterior chamber lenses can also underlie pupillary block (Fig. 5-13).

Pseudophakic Malignant Glaucoma

Malignant glaucoma may occur after cataract surgery with posterior chamber intraocular lens implantation. Forward displacement of the vitreous into apposition with the iris and ciliary body, possibly associated with thickening of the anterior hyaloid, has been proposed as the mechanism to account for the posterior diversion of aqueous flow. UBM reveals marked anterior displacement of the intraocular lens (Fig. 5-14). Nd:YAG laser anterior hyaloidotomy may be curative.

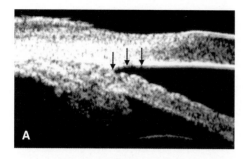
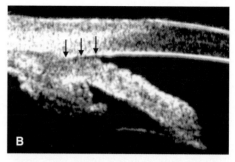

FIGURE 5-2. Effect of ambient light on angle configuration. A. Under light conditions, the angle is open. Aqueous has access to the trabecular meshwork (*arrows*). **B.** In the dark, the angle is capable of occlusion (*arrows*).

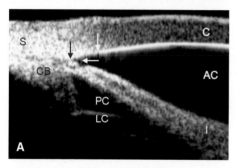
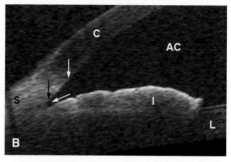

FIGURE 5-3. Anatomy of normal eye. Ultrasound biomicroscopy (**A**) and anterior segment optical coherence tomography (**B**) of normal eye showing anterior chamber (AC), cornea (C), ciliary body (CB), iris (I), lens capsule (LC), posterior chamber (PC), sclera (S), scleral spur (*black arrow*), Schwalbe line (*vertical white arrow*), and angle recess (*horizontal or oblique white arrows*).

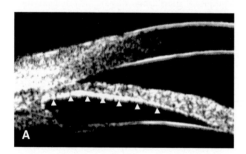
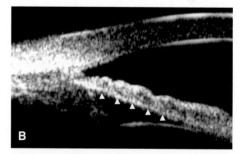

FIGURE 5-4. Iris configuration before and after laser iridotomy (ultrasound biomicroscopy). Convex iris configuration (*arrowheads*) before (**A**) and planar configuration after (**B**) laser iridotomy in an eye with relative pupillary block.

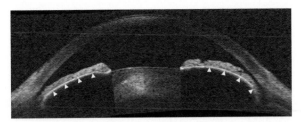

FIGURE 5-5. Iris configuration with relative pupillary block (anterior segment optical coherence tomography). Convex configuration of entire iris (*arrowheads*) is visualized in one frame.

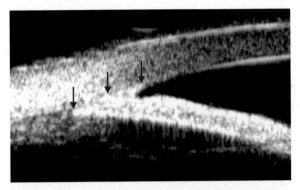

FIGURE 5-6. Peripheral anterior synechiae (*arrows*) (ultrasound biomicroscopy).

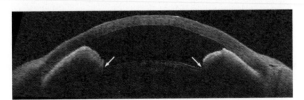

FIGURE 5-7. Iris configuration with absolute pupillary block (anterior segment optical coherence tomography). Extremely convex iris with absolute pupillary block caused by 360-degree posterior synechiae (*arrows*).

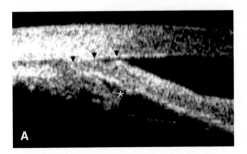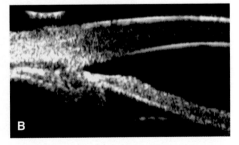

FIGURE 5-8. Plateau iris syndrome (ultrasound biomicroscopy). A. In plateau iris syndrome, the angle remains closed (*arrowhead*) after laser iridotomy because the ciliary processes are large and anteriorly positioned. The ciliary sulcus is absent (*asterisk*). **B.** Following peripheral iridoplasty, the appositional angle closure is relieved.

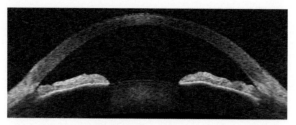

FIGURE 5-9. **Plateau iris syndrome (anterior segment optical coherence tomography).** Plateau configuration of the iris is prominent, although the ciliary body is not visualized.

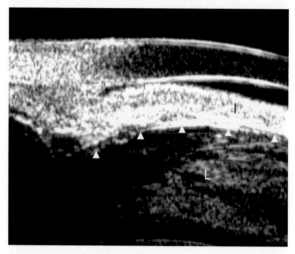

FIGURE 5-10. **Phacomorphic glaucoma (ultrasound biomicroscopy).** The intumescent lens (L and *arrowheads*) pushes the iris (I) and ciliary body into the angle.

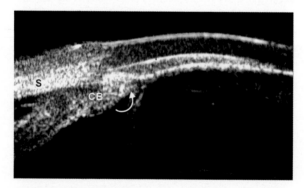

FIGURE 5-11. **Malignant glaucoma (ultrasound biomicroscopy).** Malignant glaucoma can result from aqueous misdirection or from annular ciliary body (CB) detachment. The CB is rotated anteriorly (*white arrow*). Fluid is visible in the supraciliary space. I, iris; S, sclera.

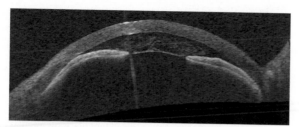

FIGURE 5-12. Malignant glaucoma (anterior segment optical coherence tomography). Anteriorly pushed iris and lens result in angle closure with a shallow anterior chamber. Ciliary body is not visualized.

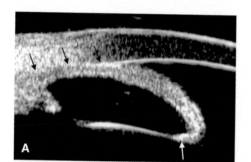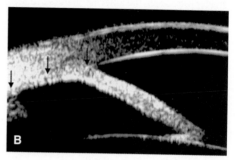

FIGURE 5-13. Pseudophakic pupillary block. A. This eye shows peripheral anterior (*black arrows*) and posterior synechiae (*white arrows*), resulting in an iris bombé configuration. **B.** After laser iridotomy, the iris configuration is flat while the peripheral anterior synechiae (*black arrows*) still hold the iris root to the trabecular meshwork.

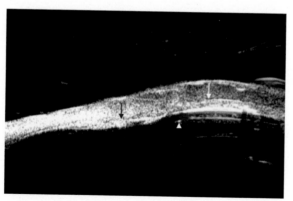

FIGURE 5-14. Pseudophakic malignant glaucoma. Peripheral iridocorneal touch (*white arrow*) with angle closure is visible (scleral spur at *black arrow*). The haptic is visible beneath the iris (*arrowhead*).

OPEN-ANGLE GLAUCOMA

Pigment Dispersion Syndrome and Pigmentary Glaucoma

The angle is widely open. The midperipheral iris characteristically assumes a concave configuration (reverse pupillary block), bringing the iris into contact with the anterior zonular bundles, and iridolenticular contact is greater than normal. The latter is thought to prevent equilibration of aqueous between the two chambers, leading to greater pressure in the anterior chamber than in the posterior chamber. The concave configuration is accentuated by accommodation.

When blinking is inhibited, the iris assumes a convex configuration which is immediately reversed upon blinking, suggesting that the act of blinking acts as a mechanical pump to push aqueous from the posterior to the anterior chamber. Laser iridotomy eliminates the pressure differential between the anterior and posterior chambers and relieves the iris concavity. The iris assumes a flat or planar configuration, and the extent of iridolenticular contact is decreased (Fig. 5-15).[8]

Exfoliation Syndrome

Exfoliation material may be detected clinically earliest on the ciliary processes and zonules. UBM can demonstrate various degrees of zonular disruption (Fig. 5-16).[9]

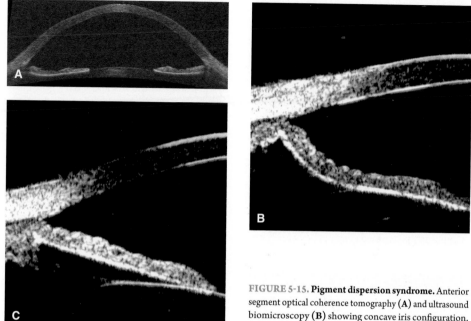

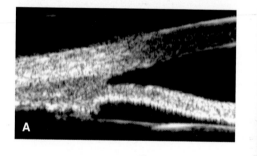

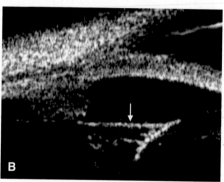

FIGURE 5-15. Pigment dispersion syndrome. Anterior segment optical coherence tomography (**A**) and ultrasound biomicroscopy (**B**) showing concave iris configuration. **C.** Planar iris configuration after laser iridotomy.

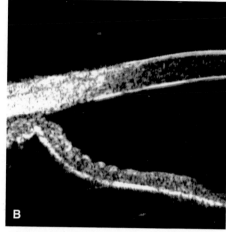

FIGURE 5-16. Exfoliation syndrome. A. Normal zonules. **B.** Deposited exfoliation material produces a diffuse patchy granular appearance to the zonules (*arrow*).

OTHER CONDITIONS

Cyclodialysis Cleft

Cyclodialysis is a separation of the longitudinal muscles of the ciliary body from the scleral spur. In blunt ocular trauma, UBM or AS-OCT should be kept in mind for evaluating any trauma-associated change in ocular anatomy. A cyclodialysis cleft is often accompanied by a supraciliary effusion (Fig. 5-17).

Iridociliary Cyst

A situation similar to plateau iris is often present, with the cysts functioning similarly to enlarged or anteriorly positioned ciliary processes. These

are easily diagnosed with UBM but poorly demarcated in AS-OCT images (Fig. 5-18).

Ciliary Body Tumors

UBM can be used to differentiate solid from cystic lesions of the iris and ciliary body. The dimensions of tumors can be measured and the extent to which they do or do not invade the iris root and ciliary face determined (Fig. 5-19). AS-OCT is rarely helpful in this condition.

Iridoschisis

Iridoschisis is a separation of the anterior and posterior iris stromal layers. Angle closure may occur (Fig. 5-20).

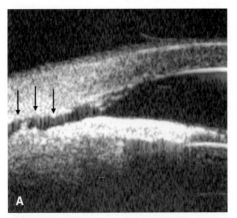
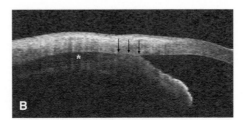

FIGURE 5-17. **Cyclodialysis cleft.** Ultrasound biomicroscopy (**A**) and anterior segment optical coherence tomography (**B**) reveal the separation between the longitudinal muscle of the ciliary body and the scleral spur (*arrows*). Note the supraciliary effusion (*asterisks*).

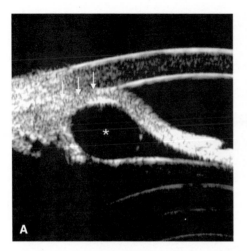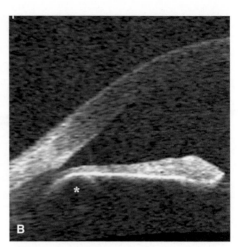

FIGURE 5-18. Iridociliary cysts. Iridociliary cysts (*asterisks*) in ultrasound biomicroscopy (**A**) and anterior segment optical coherence tomography (**B**) images are characterized by an echolucent lumen. The angle is focally closed (*arrows*).

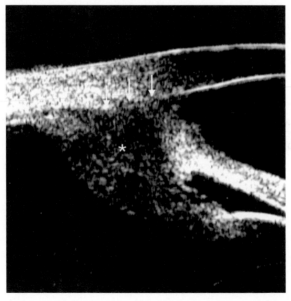

FIGURE 5-19. Ciliary body melanoma. In this eye with ciliary body melanoma (*asterisk*), the angle is focally closed (*arrows*).

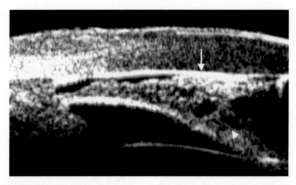

FIGURE 5-20. **Iridoschisis.** Extensive stromal separation (*arrowhead*) reaches the cornea and compromises aqueous outflow (*vertical arrow*).

SURGERY AND GLAUCOMA

Filtering Bleb

Successful blebs have a diffuse, spongy appearance. Blebs following surgery with adjunctive antimetabolites are often thin walled and cystic. Encapsulated blebs tend to be elevated and localized, with or without prominent vessels. Failed blebs are often flat and may be vascularized. The clinical appearance of a bleb, however, is not always an accurate predictor of functional status.

The UBM appearance of a functioning bleb shows a fluid track from the anterior chamber, through the internal ostium, beneath the scleral flap, and into the subconjunctival space (Fig. 5-21).[10] Accurate localization of the site of obstruction to fluid flow can be facilitated by UBM. Eyes with flat blebs have no evidence of subconjunctival filtration and demonstrate blockage to flow at the level of the episclera (Fig. 5-22). Tenon

cysts demonstrate a thick wall of conjunctiva and Tenon with or without a patent scleral flap (Fig. 5-23). Needling procedures may normalize IOP in eyes with encapsulated blebs.

The noncontact nature of AS-OCT provides a safer method to evaluate the filtering bleb morphology without distortion of bleb architecture or risk of infection, especially in the early postoperative period.[11] Owing to its higher resolution than UBM, AS-OCT can assess the superficial layers of the filtering bleb in more detail (Fig. 5-24).

Glaucoma Drainage Implants

The position, patency, and course of drainage tubes can be ascertained using UBM or AS-OCT (Fig. 5-25). UBM would be especially helpful in assessing the tube inserted into the ciliary sulcus. The anatomic relationships can be assessed, as can compression of the tube at the scleral entry site.

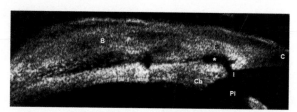

FIGURE 5-21. **Functioning filtering bleb.** The internal ostium (I), intrascleral fluid pathway (*asterisk*), and scleral flap (S) are seen. The bleb (B) is moderately elevated and homogeneously spongy with fluid-filled spaces. C, cornea; Cb, ciliary body; PI, peripheral iridectomy.

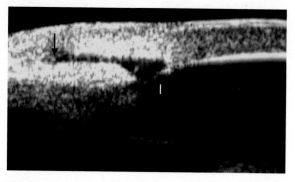

FIGURE 5-22. **Failed bleb.** The internal ostium (I) and intrascleral fluid pathway are patent, but the scleral pathway for aqueous is closed (*arrow*).

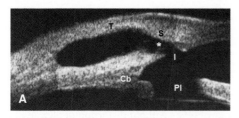 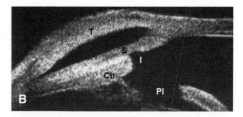

FIGURE 5-23. Bleb encapsulation. Tenon cyst wall (T) is thick because of fibroblastic proliferation. The intrascleral fluid pathway is patent (**A**, *asterisk*) or closed (**B**). Cb, ciliary body; I, internal ostium; PI, peripheral iridectomy; S, scleral flap.

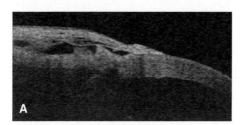 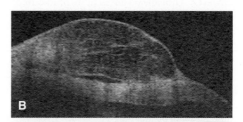

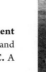

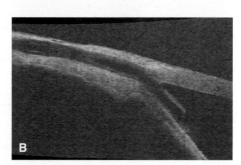

FIGURE 5-24. Filtering blebs (anterior segment optical coherence tomography). Moderately (**A**) and highly (**B**) elevated functioning filtering blebs. **C.** A failing filtering bleb with encapsulation.

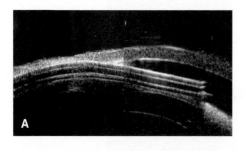

FIGURE 5-25. Glaucoma drainage implant. Ultrasound biomicroscopy (**A**) and anterior segment optical coherence tomography (**B**) showing the path of the tube from the anterior chamber.

AQUEOUS OUTFLOW PATHWAY

The conventional aqueous outflow pathway consists of the trabecular meshwork, Schlemm canal, collector channels, aqueous venous plexus, aqueous veins, and scleral/episcleral veins. Collector channels leave Schlemm canal diagonally or at right angles, exhibit various shapes and sizes, and vary in number, between 20 and 30, circumferentially around the globe. AS-OCT has been used to visualize microstructures of the trabecular aqueous outflow pathway.[12] More recently, higher quality images of the Schlemm canal and collector channels were obtained using enhanced-depth imaging spectral-domain OCT (**Fig. 5-26**).[13] This imaging method has also been used to evaluate the mechanisms of action of pharmacologic agents and laser procedure.[14–16] Topical pilocarpine administration resulted in expansion of the Schlemm canal increasing its cross-sectional area[14] and topical cyclopentolate administration caused shrinkage of the Schlemm canal decreasing its cross-sectional area (**Fig. 5-27**).[15] After selective laser trabeculoplasty in patients with primary open-angle glaucoma, Schlemm canal was expanded significantly and even more so with greater IOP reduction.[16]

REFERENCES

1. Ishikawa H, Liebmann JM, Ritch R. Quantitative assessment of the anterior segment using ultrasound biomicroscopy. *Curr Opin Ophthalmol.* 2000;11(2):133–139.
2. Radhakrishnan S, Rollins AM, Roth JE, et al. Real-time optical coherence tomography of the anterior segment at 1310 nm. *Arch Ophthalmol.* 2001;119(8):1179–1185.
3. Wirbelauer C, Karandish A, Häberle H, Pham DT. Noncontact goniometry with optical coherence tomography. *Arch Ophthalmol.* 2005;123(2):179–185.
4. Dada T, Sihota R, Gadia R, Aggarwal A, Mandal S, Gupta V. Comparison of anterior segment optical coherence tomography and ultrasound biomicroscopy for assessment of the anterior segment. *J Cataract Refract Surg.* 2007;33(5):837–840.
5. Prata TS, Dorairaj S, De Moraes CGV, Tello C, Liebmann JM, Ritch R. Indentation slit lamp-adapted optical coherence tomography technique for anterior chamber angle assessment. *Arch Ophthalmol.* 2010;128(5):646–647.
6. Ritch R. Argon laser peripheral iridoplasty: an overview. *J Glaucoma.* 1992;1:206–213.
7. Parc C, Laloum J, Bergès O. Comparison of optical coherence tomography and ultrasound biomicroscopy for detection of plateau iris. *J Fr Ophtalmol.* 2010;33(4):266.e1–266.e3.
8. Pavlin CJ, Macken P, Trope G, et al. Ultrasound biomicroscopic features of pigmentary glaucoma. *Can J Ophthalmol.* 1994;29(4):187–192.
9. Sbeity Z, Dorairaj SK, Reddy S, Tello C, Liebmann JM, Ritch R. Ultrasound biomicroscopy of zonular anatomy in unilateral exfoliation syndrome. *Acta Ophthalmol.* 2008;86:565–568.
10. Yamamoto T, Sakuma T, Kitazawa Y. An ultrasound biomicroscopic study of filtering blebs after mitomycin C trabeculectomy. *Ophthalmology.* 1995;102(12):1770–1776.
11. Leung CK, Yick DW, Kwong YY, et al. Analysis of bleb morphology after trabeculectomy with Visante anterior segment optical coherence tomography. *Br J Ophthalmol.* 2007;91(3):340–344.
12. Sarunic MV, Asrani S, Izatt JA. Imaging the ocular anterior segment with real-time, full-range Fourier-domain optical coherence tomography. *Arch Ophthalmol.* 2008;126(4):537–542.
13. Li P, Butt A, Chien JL, et al. Characteristics and variations of in vivo Schlemm's canal and collector channel microstructures in enhanced-depth imaging optical coherence tomography. *Br J Ophthalmol.* 2017;101(6):808–813.
14. Skaat A, Rosman MS, Chien JL, et al. Effect of pilocarpine hydrochloride on the Schlemm canal in healthy eyes and eyes with open-angle glaucoma. *JAMA Ophthalmol.* 2016;134(9):976–981.
15. Rosman MS, Skaat A, Chien JL, et al. Effect of cyclopentolate on in vivo Schlemm's canal microarchitecture in healthy subjects. *J Glaucoma.* 2017;26(2):133–137.
16. Skaat A, Rosman MS, Chien JL, et al. Microarchitecture of Schlemm's canal before and after selective laser trabeculoplasty. *J Glaucoma.* 2017;26(4):361–366.

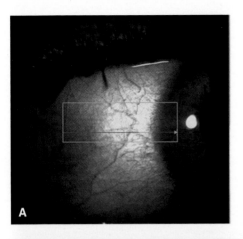

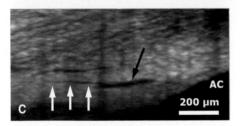

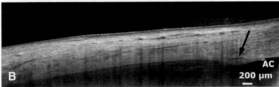

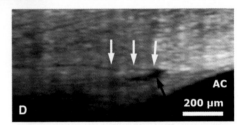

FIGURE 5-26. **Enhanced-depth spectral-domain OCT. A** and **B.** A horizontal enhanced-depth imaging spectral-domain optical coherence tomography scan covers the anterior chamber (AC), iridocorneal angle, corneoscleral limbus and sclera (*black arrow* = Schlemm canal). **C** and **D.** Schlemm canal (*black arrow*) and collector channels (*white arrow*) are clearly visualized in different scans.

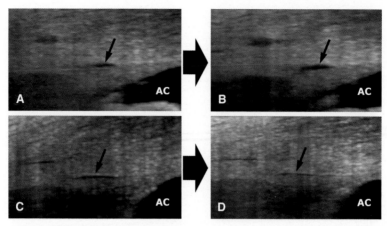

FIGURE 5-27. **Enhanced-depth spectral-domain OCT.** Representative enhanced-depth imaging optical coherence tomography B-scans of Schlemm canal (*black arrows*) before (**A**) and 1 hour after (**B**) 1% pilocarpine administration showing expansion of Schlemm canal, and before (**C**) and after (**D**) 1% cyclopentolate administration showing shrinkage of Schlemm canal. AC, anterior chamber.

Optic Nerve Imaging

Thomas D. Patrianakos and Michael C. Giovingo ■

INTRODUCTION

Making the diagnosis of glaucoma requires the presence of optic nerve head (ONH) damage and/or characteristic visual field changes. Although automated and static perimetry provides an excellent aid in documenting functional visual field loss from glaucoma, as much as 40% of the retinal nerve fiber layer (RNFL) may be lost before changes are detected on standard white-on-white visual field testing.[1] The need for more sensitive, reproducible, and accurate detection of glaucomatous damage has led to the development of various imaging devices for ONH and RNFL. To best utilize these new technologies, it is essential that physicians familiarize themselves with the information the tests provide and the strengths and weaknesses of each modality (**Table 6-1**).

REFERENCE

1. Quigley HA, Addicks EM, Green WR. Optic nerve damage in human glaucoma. *Arch Ophthalmol.* 1982;100:135.

TABLE 6-1. Principles and Clinical Parameters of Various Optic Nerve Imaging Devices

Device	Principles	Clinical Parameters Measured
Stereophotography	Simultaneous photographs taken with two cameras or two separate photographs of same nerve at different angles	Subjective interpretation of ONH and RNFL anatomy (pallor, disc hemorrhages, peripapillary atrophy)
HRT	CSLO	Optic disc tomography
GDx	SLP/birefringence	RNFL thickness
(TD, SD, SS)-OCT	Interferometry	Optic disc tomography and RNFL/macular thickness

CSLO, confocal scanning laser ophthalmoscopy; GDx, glaucoma diagnosis; HRT, Heidelberg retina tomography; OCT, optical coherence tomography; ONH, optic nerve head; RNFL, retinal nerve fiber layer; SD, spectral domain; SS, swept-source; SLP, scanning laser polarimetry; TD, time domain.

STEREOPHOTOGRAPHY

Assessment of changes in the ONH and RNFL over time can be evaluated using color stereophotographs (Fig. 6-1). This method is the most widely used imaging technique and is considered the gold standard for documentation of glaucomatous optic neuropathy (GON).[1]

Stereophotographs can be produced by taking two photographs in sequence, either by manually repositioning the camera or by using a sliding carriage adapter (Allen separator). Alternatively, they can be produced by taking two photographs simultaneously with two cameras that utilize the indirect ophthalmoscopic principle (Donaldson stereoscopic fundus camera) or a twin-prism separator. Simultaneous ONH photographs have demonstrated the best reproducibility over time.[2] Recently, alternation flicker of monoscopic optic disc images over time (digital stereochronoscopy) has also proved to be a sensitive method for detecting GON changes. Newer image processing and registration permits accurate alignment of optic nerve (ON) photographs and facilitates image comparison with detection of changes in vessel position, color, and other cues for contour change.[3] Digital stereochronoscopy may assist in optimizing the ability to detect structural changes and overcome some of the assessment variability between observers.[4]

The strengths of ONH stereophotographs include the ability to document parameters that cannot be quantified, such as disc hemorrhages, peripapillary atrophy, and pallor. They also allow the clinician to assess the impact of other nonglaucomatous processes that may influence functional testing. However, stereophotographs provide excellent documentation of the ONH, but their interpretation remains subjective and can therefore have increased variability and limited usefulness over time.[5] In addition, media opacities, such as cataracts, or a poorly focused photograph can inhibit optimal analysis.

REFERENCES

1. Fingeret M, Medeiros FA, Susanna R, et al. Five rules to evaluate the optic disc and retinal nerve fiber layer for glaucoma. *Optometry*. 2005;76:661–668.
2. Trobe JD, Glaser JS, Cassady J, et al. Nonglaucomatous excavation of the optic disc. *Arch Ophthalmol*. 1980;98:1046.
3. Berger JW, Patel TR, Stone RA, Herschler J, Anderson DR. Computerized stereochronoscopy and alternation flicker to detect optic nerve head contour change. *Ophthalmology*. 2000;107:1316–1320.
4. Syed ZA, Radcliffe NM, DeMorales LG. Detection of progressive glaucomatous optic neuropathy using automated alternation flicker with stereophotography. *Arch Ophthalmol*. 2011;129:512–526.
5. Takamoto T, Schwartz B. Reproducibility of photogrammetric optic disc cup measurements. *Invest Ophthalmol Vis Sci*. 1985;26:814.

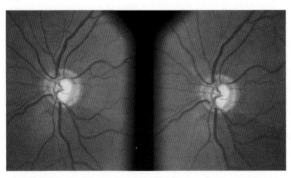

FIGURE 6-1. Stereophotography uses two simultaneous disc photographs. With the use of a special viewer, stereovision is achieved. Stereophotography is useful to assess optic nerve changes over time. (Courtesy of Tara A. Uhler, MD.)

CONFOCAL SCANNING LASER OPHTHALMOSCOPY

Heidelberg retina tomography (HRT; Heidelberg Engineering GmbH, Heidelberg, Germany) is a type of confocal scanning laser ophthalmoscopy used to provide a structural quantitative measurement of the ONH (Fig. 6-2A). A 670-nm diode laser is aimed through a pinhole onto the retina. The light reflected passes through a second pinhole into a detector, which transfers the maximum intensity of light at a given point to create an image. A series of 16 to 64 two-dimensional (2D) sequential scans, each measuring 384×384 pixels, is used to create a three-dimensional (3D) color-coded topographic image (Fig. 6-2B).

The reflectivity image (Fig. 6-2C) produced is used by the technician to draw a contour line around the inner border of the scleral ring, which is further separated into six sectors. This line remains standard for all future examinations and is used to calculate a series of parameters. The HRT 3.0 reduces technician dependence by producing automated results of the contour line as described by Swindale et al.[1] The graphic analysis (Fig. 6-2D) corresponds to all six sectors in the reflectivity image.

A reference plane defined as 50 μm below the surface of the retina along 6 degrees of the contour line in the temporal inferior region is designated as the cutoff between the neuroretinal rim (all structures above the reference plane) and the cup (all structures below the reference plane).

After the data are reconstructed, 12 stereometric parameters (Fig. 6-2E) are automatically obtained. According to univariate and multivariate analysis from the ocular hypertension treatment study, the most predictive parameters for glaucoma detection with the HRT were the ones independent of the reference plane (mean height contour, rim area, and mean cup depth).[2] Topography standard deviation is used as a measurement of image quality and reliability, with anything greater than 30 to 40 μm considered unreliable.

Moorfield's regression analysis (Fig. 6-2D) uses linear analysis between optic disc area and neuroretinal rim area in both global and localized segments to classify the nerve as "within normal limits," "borderline," or "outside normal limits" based on comparison to an age- and ethnicity-specific normative database.

Progression of GON on the HRT can be evaluated with event- or trend-type analysis software. Topographical change analysis (Fig. 6-3) is an event-type analysis that focuses on the difference between surface height measurements of follow-up images and those of a baseline image. Changes that are consistent are highlighted in a color-coded overlay on top of the reflectivity image, with red representing areas of statistically significant worsening. Trend-type analysis assesses the rate of change over time in one of the stereometric indices, such as rim area, to document progression.

Several studies have confirmed the ability of HRT to distinguish between healthy and glaucomatous eyes with a range of specificity from 75% to 95% and sensitivity from 51% to 97%.[3–5] Reproducibility is enhanced when at least three scans are combined.[6]

Among advantages of the HRT is the company's commitment to assure older software remains compatible with newer machines, thereby allowing for longer data series on individuals. Additional benefits include good image quality through undilated pupils and the capability to assess glaucomatous progression by comparing sequential scans, using either the glaucoma change probability analysis or topographic change analysis software.[7,8] A disadvantage of the older HRT 2.0 model is the requirement for an operator-dependent outline of the disc margin. An additional limitation is the standardized reference plane used to calculate many of the parameters because this may not accurately represent the true RNFL thickness in all individuals. These concerns have been addressed with the newer HRT 3.0 model. In addition, the HRT 3.0 software contains a larger ethnicity-specific normative database.[9]

REFERENCES

1. Swindale NV, Stjepanovic G, Chin A, Mikelberg FS. Automated analysis of normal and glaucomatous optic nerve head topography images. *Invest Ophthalmol Vis Sci.* 2000;41:1730–1742.

2. Zangwill LM, Weinreb RN, Beiser JA, et al. Baseline topographic optic disc measurements associated with the development of primary open-angle glaucoma: The Confocal Scanning Laser Ophthalmoscopy Ancillary Study to the Ocular Hypertension Treatment Study. *Arch Ophthalmol.* 2005;123(9):1188–1197.

3. Harasymowycz PJ, Papamatheakis DG, Fansi AK, Gresset J, Lesk MR. Validity of screening for glaucomatous optic nerve damage using confocal scanning laser ophthalmoscopy (Heidelberg Retina Tomograph II) in high-risk populations: A pilot study. *Ophthalmology.* 2007;112:2164–2171.

4. Reus NJ, de Graaf M, Lemij HG. Accuracy of GDx VCC, HRT I and clinical assessment of stereoscopic optic nerve head photographs for diagnosing glaucoma. *Br J Ophthalmol.* 2007;91:313.

5. Miglior S, Guareschi M, Albe E, Gomarasca S, Vavassori M, Orzalesi N. Detection of glaucomatous visual field changes using the Moorfields regression analysis of the Heidelberg retina tomography. *Am J Ophthalmol.* 2003;136:26–33.

6. Weinreb RN, Lusky M, Morsman D. Effect of repetitive imaging on topographic measurements of the optic nerve head. *Arch Ophthalmol.* 1993;111:636–638.

7. Chauhan BC, Blanchard JW, LeBlanc RP. Technique for detecting serial topographic changes in the optic disc and peripapillary retina using scanning laser tomography. *Invest Ophthalmol Vis Sci.* 2000;41:775–782.

8. Bowd C, Balasubramanian M, Weinreb RN. Performance of confocal scanning laser tomography Topographic Change Analysis (TCA) for assessing glaucomatous progression. *Invest Ophthalmol Vis Sci.* 2009;50:691–701.

9. Maslin JS, Mansouri K, Dorairaj SK. HRT for the diagnosis and detection of glaucoma progression. *Open Ophthalmol J.* 2015:58–67.

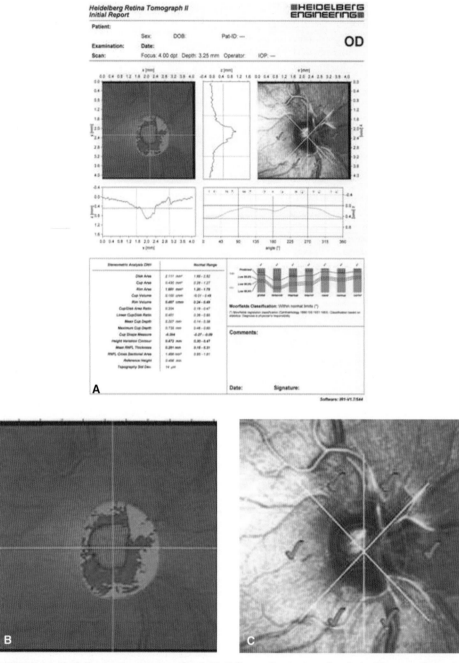

FIGURE 6-2. Heidelberg retina tomography. A. Heidelberg retina tomography of a healthy-appearing optic nerve (ON). **B.** Color-coded topographic image of a healthy-appearing ON. **C.** Reflectivity image separated into six sectors within a contour line.

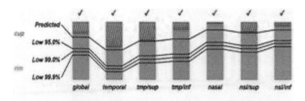

Moorfields Classification: Within normal limits (*)

(*) Moorfields regression classification (Ophthalmology 1998;105:1557-1563). Classification based on statistics. Diagnosis is physician's responsibility.

D

Stereometric analysis ONH		Normal range
Disc area	2.111 mm²	1.69–2.82
Cup area	0.430 mm²	0.26–1.27
Rim area	1.681 mm²	1.20–1.78
Cup volume	0.100 cmm	0.01–0.49
Rim volume	0.487 cmm	0.27–0.49
Cup/disk area ratio	0.204	0.16–0.47
Linear/disk area ratio	0.451	0.36–0.80
Mean cup death	0.207 mm	0.14–0.38
Maximum cup death	0.735 mm	0.46–0.90
Cup shape measure	-0.304	-0.27–-0.09
Height variation contour	0.472 mm	0.30–0.47
Mean RNFL thickness	0.291 mm	0.18–0.31
RNFL cross-sectional area	1.499 mm²	0.95–1.61
Reference height	0.486 mm	
Topography std dev.	14 μm	

E

FIGURE 6-2. (*continued*) **D.** Graphic analysis corresponding to all six sectors of the reflectivity image with Moorfield's regression analysis classification. **E.** Stereometric analysis parameters indicating an accurate scan with a topography standard deviation <40 μm. ONH, optic nerve head; RNFL, retinal nerve fiber layer. (Courtesy of David Hillman, MD.)

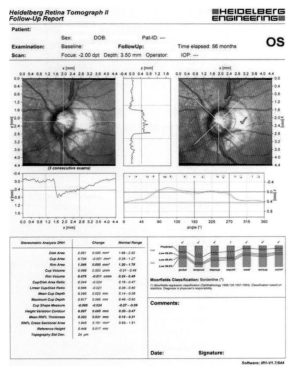

FIGURE 6-3. **Heidelberg retina tomography progression analysis** demonstrating worsening of glaucomatous optic neuropathy on topographic analysis with areas of red/yellow in the reflectivity image represents statistically significant worsening. Trend analysis of certain stereometric parameters over time additionally documents deterioration of the optic nerve head. (Courtesy of David Hillman, MD.)

SCANNING LASER POLARIMETRY

The glaucoma diagnosis (GDx) test (Laser Diagnostics Technologies, San Diego, CA) is the prototypical scanning laser polarimetry, which uses the birefringence properties of the RNFL to measure its thickness. A 780-nm diode laser passes through an orderly arrangement of axons and microtubules surrounding the ONH. As light passes through the RNFL, it undergoes a change in polarization referred to as retardation. The degree of change in polarization is proportional to the thickness of the RNFL and is detected by a built-in ellipsometer. These changes are then transformed to a topographic map of RNFL thickness measurements and given a numeric value by the GDx software using an assumed constant birefringence value.[1] However, birefringence is not constant around the ONH in all individuals, and thus, RNFL values may be falsely reported. In addition, the abundance of birefringent tissues in the eye can contaminate the actual values of the RNFL. Newer GDx models contain a variable corneal compensator (GDx-VCC) (Zeiss Meditec, Dublin, CA) (Fig. 6-4A) that eliminates the retardation contributed by the cornea. However, this is based on the macula as an internal reference and can be influenced by macular pathologies. The latest version of the instrument uses individualized anterior segment compensation for eyes with low signal-to-noise ratio called an enhanced corneal compensator (ECC).[2]

A fundus image (Fig. 6-4B) is used by the operator to manually define the ONH. A calculation circle with a fixed band measuring 0.4 mm wide (inner diameter 2.4 mm; outer diameter 3.2 mm) is automatically aligned around the disc based on illumination patterns and highlights the area where the RNFL measurements will be derived. Image quality and reliability of the test can be quantified by the appearance of the fundus image. Even illumination, good focus,

and proper disc/ellipse centration are essential for a reliable scan. In addition, each eye scanned is assigned a quality number or q value (scale 0 to 10; 10 = perfect scan), which can also be used to gauge the quality of the test. In general, anything with a q value ≥ 7 is acceptable for interpretation.

The RNFL thickness map (Fig. 6-4C) is a color-coded image corresponding to the thickness of the RNFL. Bright red or yellow colors represent areas of thick RNFL and are normally seen in an hourglass distribution superiorly and inferiorly. Blue colors relate to areas of thin RNFL and are normally seen nasally and temporally. GON is characterized by increasing blue colors of the superior/inferior portion of the ONH.

The deviation map (Fig. 6-4D) reveals the location and magnitude of RNFL defects over the entire thickness of the map and how much they deviate from the race- and age-matched normative database. These are color coded and assigned a relative statistical significance based on probability of normality.

The TSNIT (temporal, superior, nasal, inferior, temporal) graph (Fig. 6-4E) maps out the patient's RNFL modulation curve and superimposes it on a normative RNFL modulation curve. Normal RNFL modulation should follow a sinusoidal pattern (double hump at the superior and inferior portion) with flattening of the humps representing RNFL loss consistent with glaucoma.

The actual numeric values calculated to represent the RNFL thickness are listed in the TSNIT parameters (Fig. 6-4F). These values are also color coded and assigned a relative statistical significance based on the probability of normality. Studies have demonstrated that the nerve fiber indicator (NFI) correlates best with the existence of glaucoma.[3] It represents a global value based on the entire nerve fiber layer (NFL) thickness (range 1 [normal] to 100 [glaucoma]). Values ≥ 50 are highly suggestive of glaucoma. However, this number cannot be the sole determinant for the diagnosis of glaucoma because the NFI can be within the normal range when there is only a focal RNFL defect. In such cases, the deviation map would exhibit the color-coded local damage. Other important parameters include the inferior normalized area and the TSNIT average, both of which have been highly correlated with the detection of glaucoma.[4]

Progression in the GDx is documented using guided progression analysis (**Fig. 6-5**). This event analysis technique compares the retardation patterns of follow-up scans to a baseline and assesses the variability of the individual patient to that observed in a matched population.

The GDx-VCC has been shown to have good diagnostic accuracy, with an overall sensitivity ranging from 80% to 92% and specificity from 66% to 98%.[5-7]

Strengths of the GDx include a large race- and age-matched normative database and the ability to obtain rapid data on RNFL measurements through an undilated pupil. A limitation of older GDx devices, fixed corneal compensation, has been improved with the newer VCC. However, studies have found that even with VCC, atypical birefringence patterns can occur from artifact introduced by the device's attempt to compensate for poor noise-to-signal ratio.[8] The newer ECC model hopes to correct the shortcomings of the previous units.

REFERENCES

1. Sehi M, Guaqueta DC, Feuer WJ, et al. Scanning laser polarimetry with variable and enhanced corneal compensation in normal and glaucomatous eyes. *Am J Ophthalmol*. 2007;143:272–279.
2. Medeiros FA, Bowd C, Zangwill LM, et al. Detection of glaucoma using scanning laser polarimetry with enhanced corneal compensation. *Invest Ophthalmol Vis Sci*. 2007;48:3146–3153.
3. Medeiros FA, Zangwill LM, Bowd C, et al. Comparison of the GDx VCC scanning laser polarimeter, HRT II confocal scanning laser ophthalmoscope, and stratus OCT optical coherence tomograph for the detection of glaucoma. *Arch Ophthalmol*. 2004;122:827–837.
4. Funaki S, Shirakashi M, Yaoeda K, et al. Specificity and sensitivity of glaucoma detection in the Japanese population using scanning laser polarimetry. *Br J Ophthalmol*. 2002;86:70–74.
5. Colen TP, Lemij HG. Sensitivity and specificity of GDx: Clinical judgment of scanning laser polarimetric analysis of standard printouts versus the number. *J Glaucoma*. 2003;12:129–133.
6. Poinoosawmy D, Tan JCH, Bunce C, et al. The ability of the GDX nerve fiber analyser neural network to diagnose glaucoma. *Graefes Arch Clin Exp Ophthalmol*. 2001;239:122–127.
7. Medeiros FA, Zangwill LM, Bowd C, et al. Use of progressive glaucomatous optic disc changes as the reference standard for evaluation of diagnostic tests in glaucoma. *Am J Opthalmol*. 2005;139:1010–1018.
8. Bagga H, Greenfield DS, Feuer WJ, et al. Quantitative assessment of atypical birefringence images using scanning laser polarimetry with variable corneal compensation. *Am J Ophthalmol*. 2005;139:437–446.

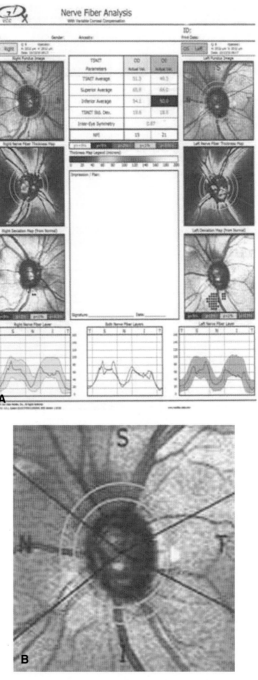

FIGURE 6-4. Scanning laser polarimetry. A. Glaucoma diagnosis with variable corneal compensator of a glaucoma suspect demonstrating slight inferior retinal nerve fiber layer (RNFL) loss in the left eye. **B.** Fundus image with the calculation circle.

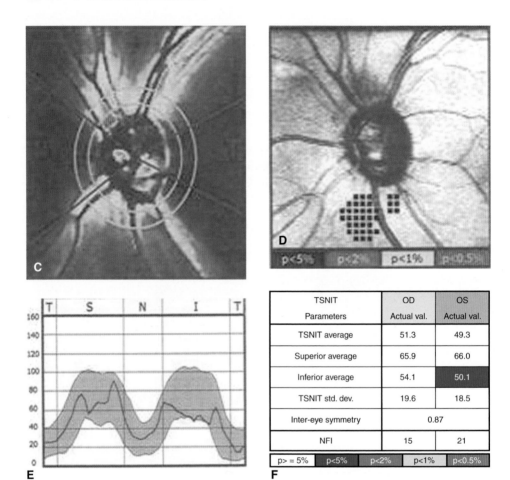

TSNIT Parameters	OD Actual val.	OS Actual val.
TSNIT average	51.3	49.3
Superior average	65.9	66.0
Inferior average	54.1	50.1
TSNIT std. dev.	19.6	18.5
Inter-eye symmetry	0.87	
NFI	15	21

FIGURE 6-4. (*continued*) C. RNFL thickness map demonstrating bright red or yellow colors representing areas of thick RNFL normally seen in an hourglass distribution superiorly and inferiorly. D. Deviation map with color-coded areas exemplifying RNFL deviation from a race- and age-matched normative database. E. TSNIT (temporal, superior, nasal, inferior, temporal) graph showing slight inferior RNFL thinning superimposed on a normative RNFL modulation curve. F. TSNIT parameters that are color coded and assigned a relative statistical significance based on the probability of normality. NFI, nerve fiber indicator.

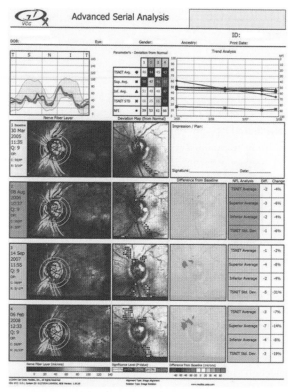

FIGURE 6-5. **Progression of glaucomatous optic neuropathy** with glaucoma diagnosis–guided progression and trend analysis comparing follow-up scans to a baseline scan. The deviation map shows focal thinning of the superior and inferior retinal nerve fiber layer (RNFL), which is further exemplified by color-coded difference from baseline scans. Temporal, superior, nasal, inferior, temporal (TSNIT) parameters also demonstrate worsening of glaucoma by increasing nerve fiber indicator values and decreasing RNFL values over time.

OPTICAL COHERENCE TOMOGRAPHY

Optical coherence tomography (OCT) is a noninvasive diagnostic technique that provides high-resolution, real-time, cross-sectional imaging of the retina and ONH. It splits a low-coherence, near-infrared 810-nm diode laser into two arms, with one beam aimed at the retina and the other at a reference mirror. The echo time delay and intensity of back-reflected light from the retina create an interference pattern, which is analyzed by a photodetector. The differences in retinal layers are illustrated in an image because of the unique time delay of the reflections from various tissue components.

The OCT is unique among ONH analysis equipment in that it contains a variety of quantitative analysis protocols used to evaluate both ON and retinal pathology. Its ability to provide high-resolution scans of multiple anatomic areas has made it a very popular method of ancillary testing. Glaucoma detection can be monitored with the RNFL analysis, ONH analysis, and ganglion cell analysis scans; however, studies have shown that RNFL analysis provides the best discrimination between normal and glaucomatous eyes.[1,2] There are currently three main methods of OCT: time-domain OCT (TD-OCT), spectral-domain OCT (SD-OCT), and swept-source OCT (SS-OCT) (Table 6-2).

TD-OCT was the first commercially available form of OCT. Carl Zeiss Meditec (Dublin, CA) produced the most commonly used TD-OCT, the third-generation Stratus OCT. It scans at an average rate of 400 axial scans per second and provides a 10-μm axial image resolution. Peripapillary RNFL analysis scanning (Fig. 6-6) involves the acquisition of three circular scans with a 3.4-mm diameter centered on the ONH. Characteristic changes in reflectivity observed at the inner and outer retinal boundaries are automatically converted to quantitative NFL thickness data by a computer algorithm. The TSNIT image provides comparison of the patient's NFL thickness (black line) to an age-related normative database. This is further displayed as a circular diagram of 12 clock-hour sections, 30 degrees each, and color coded to match a normative database. Various measurements are then listed in the Tabular Data Section. The most significant of which for glaucoma are Smax/Imax (maximum thickness of superior/inferior quadrant), Smax/Tavg or Imax/Tavg (maximum thickness of superior or inferior/average thickness of temp quadrant), Smax, Imax, and Tavg.[2,3] Finally, scan image and video image of ONH help determine the accuracy of the test. In general, signal strengths of 7 or higher are considered acceptable for interpretation. The TD-OCT has been shown to have good diagnostic accuracy in detecting GON, with an overall sensitivity ranging from 61% to 84% and specificity from 85% to 100%.[4,5]

More recently, SD-OCT has become the most commonly used OCT because of better axial resolution and increased scanning speed. The implementation of broadband light sources into SD-OCT systems improved the axial resolution from approximately 10 μm to as high as 2 μm in tissue.[6] Acquisition speed has improved considerably by detecting backscattering signals in the frequency domain, which means backscattered depth information at a given location can be collected without the movement of a reference mirror.[7] The higher speed and higher resolution scans allow for the creation of 3D datasets, which permit registration of scan from session to session to ensure the same measurement location. Similar glaucoma discriminating ability has been demonstrated when comparing equal parameters between TD-OCT and SD-OCT.[8] The use of landmarks within the 3D volume in SD-OCT, however, assures that the scan is being consistently placed in the same location and allows for higher reproducibility than in conventional TD-OCT.[9]

Currently, there are several commercially available SD-OCTs, each offering its own unique benefits. The two most commonly used SD-OCTs are the Cirrus OCT (Carl Zeiss Meditec) and the Spectralis OCT (Heidelberg Engineering). The fourth-generation Cirrus OCT is an SD-OCT with an axial resolution of 5 μm and an A-scan acquisition rate of 27 kHz. The ONH and RNFL analysis scan (Fig. 6-7) generates information on ONH topography and RNFL parameters from a 6 × 6 mm cubed area at a diameter of 3.4 mm centered on the ONH. Changes in reflectivity are used to detect the anterior surface of the RNFL and the retinal pigment epithelium (RPE). These markers are then used to measure all features of disc anatomy. Several studies have shown that the highest performing ONH parameters, such as the cup-to-disc ratio and integrated rim volume, have diagnostic accuracies equivalent to the best RNFL parameters.[10-12] Macular thickness analysis scan (Fig. 6-8) detects the RNFL and RPE of the macula with a cube scan. A color-coded map is created, illustrating the retinal thickness for specific regions of the macula. Images obtained provide information about tissue structures in all layers of the retina.

The Spectralis OCT is very similar to the Cirrus in terms of imaging capabilities (Fig. 6-9). Additional features of the Spectralis include eye tracking, fluorescein angiography, indocyanine green angiography, and autofluorescence. Also, the axial resolution is increased to 4 μm, which aids in obtaining higher resolution photographs.

Both types of SD-OCTs contain trend analysis software to assess progression (Fig. 6-10A and B) by plotting a linear regression of RNFL thickness against age. The Cirrus SD-OCT also uses event-based guided progression analysis to compare the RNFL thickness patterns of follow-up scans to a baseline scan and indicates thinning as possible loss (yellow) or likely loss (red).

The latest advance in OCT technology has been the SS-OCT. This technology obtains real-time encoded spectral information by sweeping a narrow bandwidth laser through a broad optical spectrum. Backscattered intensity is detected with a photodetector, and thus, there is no signal drop-off with depth. This, in combination with deeper penetration from longer wavelengths, allows for imaging through denser media and improved delineation of anatomic structures (Fig. 6-11).[13] The clinical applicability of SS-OCT in glaucoma is still in the research phase, but it is showing promise because it renders even higher quality images than the previous technology.

Additional advantages of OCT to other ON imaging devices include its ability for anterior segment OCT. Current technology allows for analysis of the angle structures/iris configuration (Fig. 6-12) and corneal thickness (Fig. 6-13).

REFERENCES

1. Medeiros FA, Zangwill LM, Bowd C, et al. Evaluation of retinal nerve fiber layer, optic nerve head, and macular thickness measurements for glaucoma detection using optical coherence tomography. *Am J Ophthalmol.* 2005;139:44–55.
2. Wollstein G, Ishikawa H, Wang J, Beaton SA, Schuman JS. Comparison of three optical coherence tomography scanning areas for detection of glaucomatous damage. *Am J Ophthalmol.* 2005;139:39–43.
3. Bourne RR, Medeiros FA, Bowd C, Jahanbakhsh K, Zangwill LM, Weinreb RN. Comparability of retinal nerve fiber layer thickness measurements of optical coherence tomography instruments. *Invest Ophthalmol Vis Sci.* 2005;46:1280–1285.
4. Chang RT, O'Rese KJ, Dudenz DL, et al. Sensitivity and specificity of time-domain versus spectral-domain optical coherence tomography in diagnosing early to moderate glaucoma. *Ophthalmology.* 2009;116:2294–2299.
5. Budenz DL, Michael A, Katz J, et al. Sensitivity and specificity of the Stratus OCT for perimetric glaucoma. *Ophthalmology.* 2005;112:3–9.
6. Drexler W, Morgner U, Ghanta RK, Kartner FX, Schuman JS, Fujimoto JG. Ultrahigh-resolution ophthalmic optical coherence tomography. *Nat Med.* 2001;7:502–507.
7. Gabriele ML, Wollstein G, Schuman JS, et al. Optical coherence tomography: history current status and laboratory work. *Invest Ophthalmol Vis Sci.* 2011;52(5):2425–2436.
8. Schuman JS. Spectral domain optical coherence tomography for glaucoma (an AOS thesis). *Trans Am Ophthalmol Soc.* 2008;106:426–458.

9. Kim JS, Ishikawa H, Sung KR. Retinal nerve fibre layer thickness measurement reproducibility improved with spectral domain optical coherence tomography. *Br J Ophthalmol.* 2009;93:1057–1063.

10. Leung CK, Chan WM, Hui YL, et al. Analysis of retinal nerve fiber layer and optic nerve head in glaucoma with different reference plane offsets, using optical coherence tomography. *Invest Ophthalmol Vis Sci.* 2005;46:891–899.

11. Leung CK, Chan WM, Hui YL, et al. Comparison of macular and peripapillary measurements for the detection of glaucoma: An optical coherence tomography study. *Ophthalmology.* 2005;112:391–400.

12. Manassakorn A, Nouri-Mahdavi K, Caprioli J, et al. Comparison of retinal nerve fiber layer thickness and optic disc algorithms with optical coherence tomography to detect glaucoma. *Am J Ophthalmol.* 2006;141:105–115.

13. Zhang J, Rao B, Chen Z. Swept source based Fourier domain functional optical coherence tomography. *Conf Proc IEEE Eng Med Biol Soc.* 2005;7:7230–7233.

TABLE 6-2. Comparison of Time Domain, Spectral Domain, Swept-source-OCT Devices

	Light Source	Advantages	Disadvantages
TD-OCT	Broadband width	Intensity information acquired in time domain Cheaper cost	Moving reference mirror limits acquisition rate Variability between scans
SD-OCT	Broadband width	Higher sensitivity than TD-OCT (3D datasets) Higher scanning speed and axial resolution	Signal drop-off with depth because of camera-based detection
SS-OCT	Narrow band swept through broad range	Same advantages as SD-OCT Higher scanning speeds and resolution No signal drop-off with depth May improve AS-OCT images	Increased cost of light source Not commercially available

AS, anterior segment; OCT, optical coherence tomography; SD, spectral-domain; SS, swept-source.

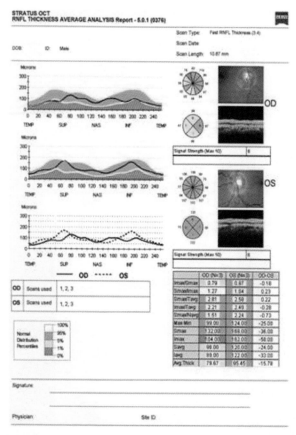

FIGURE 6-6. Stratus time-domain optical coherence tomography retinal nerve fiber layer (RNFL) analysis scan demonstrating RNFL thinning consistent with glaucoma in the right eye and a normal-appearing left eye.

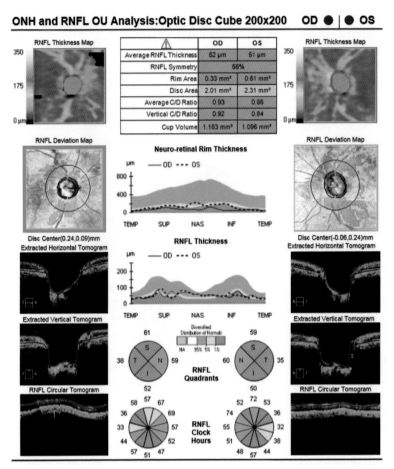

FIGURE 6-7. **Cirrus spectral-domain optical coherence tomography** optic nerve head and retinal nerve fiber layer (RNFL) imaging scan of a patient with advanced glaucoma demonstrating classic thinning of the inferior and superior RNFL in both eyes. ONH, optic nerve head. INF, inferior; NAS, nasal; OU, both eyes; SUP, superior; TEMP, temporal.

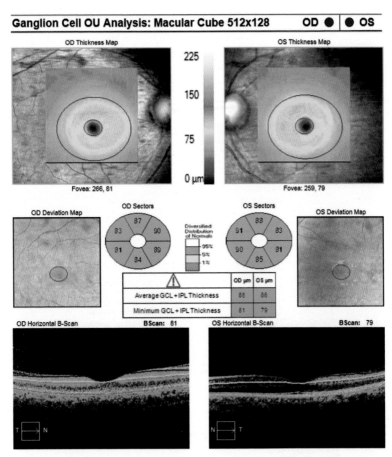

FIGURE 6-8. Cirrus spectral-domain optical coherence tomography macular thickness analysis scan demonstrating the retinal nerve fiber layer and retinal pigment epithelium of the macula (ganglion cell analysis). GCL, ganglion cell layer; IPL, inner plexiform layer.

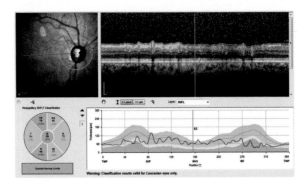

FIGURE 6-9. Spectralis spectral-domain optical coherence tomography retinal nerve fiber layer demonstrating a physiologic healthy optic nerve with enlarged cup-to-disc ratio.

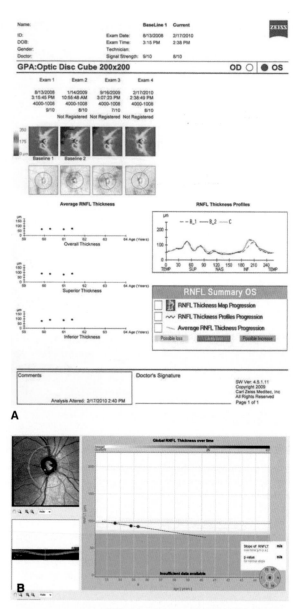

FIGURE 6-10. A. Cirrus spectral-domain optical coherence tomography (SD-OCT) progression analysis software demonstrating no evidence of progression over time on both event- and trend-based analysis. INF, inferior; NAS, nasal; OU, both eyes; SUP, superior; TEMP, temporal. **B.** Spectralis SD-OCT progression analysis showing loss of global retinal nerve fiber layer over time, indicative of worsening glaucoma.

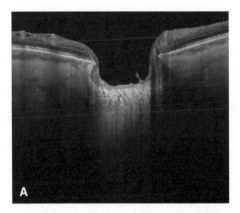 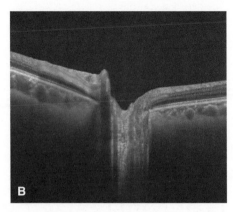

FIGURE 6-11 Swept-source optical coherence tomography. A and **B.** Glaucomatous nerve viewed with swept-source optical coherence tomography. (Courtesy of Louis Pasquale, MD and Lucy Shen, MD.)

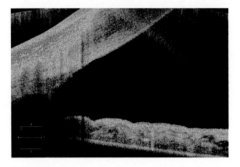 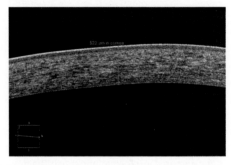

FIGURE 6-12. Anterior segment optical coherence tomography imaging of the angle.

FIGURE 6-13. Corneal optical coherence tomography with pachymetry measurement.

Glaucoma Imaging: Optic Nerve Head, Peripapillary, and Macular Regions

Zinaria Y. W. Liu, Fabio Lavinsky, Gadi Wollstein, Kimberly V. Miller, and Joel S. Schuman ∎

INTRODUCTION

Glaucoma is the leading cause of irreversible blindness globally. It is estimated that the prevalence of glaucoma will increase to over 110 million in 2040.[1] It may occur in any age group, but is common especially after 40 years of age. Elevated intraocular pressure is the most important causal risk factor for glaucoma, but high intraocular pressure is not necessary for glaucomatous damage to occur. The physical impact of glaucomatous optic neuropathy includes an irreversible loss of retinal ganglion cells that is clinically manifested as optic nerve head (ONH) cupping and localized or diffuse defects of the retinal nerve fiber layer (RNFL). Because glaucomatous damage is irreversible but largely preventable, early and accurate diagnosis and progression detection are important.

REFERENCE

1. Tham YC, Li X, Wong TY, Quigley HA, Aung T, Cheng CY. Global prevalence of glaucoma and projections of glaucoma burden through 2040: a systematic review and meta-analysis.. *Ophthalmology*. 2014;121:2081–2090.

FUNCTIONAL TESTS

Evaluation of the optic nerve and nerve fiber layer includes examinations that test their structure and function. Glaucomatous retinal ganglion cell loss results structurally in RNFL and optic nerve defects, and functionally in visual field changes that can be assessed by automated perimetry and electrophysiology testing. Glaucomatous visual field defects include nasal steps, arcuate defects, localized paracentral scotomas, and, more uncommonly, temporal defects (**Fig. 7-1**). The most common location of visual field defects related to glaucoma is within an arcuate area commonly referred to as Bjerrum's region, which extends from the blind spot to the median raphe.

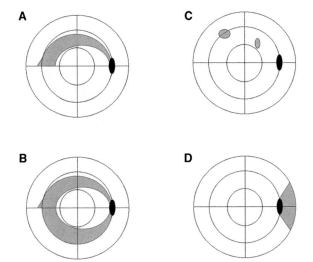

FIGURE 7-1. **Visual field defects. A.** Arcuate defect in Bjerrum's region. **B.** Double arcuate defect. **C.** Paracentral scotomas. **D.** Temporal wedge defect. (Adapted with permission from Epstein DL. *Chandler and Grant's Glaucoma.* 4th ed. Baltimore, MD: Williams & Wilkins; 1997.)

AUTOMATED PERIMETRY

Standard automated perimeters (SAPs) test the visual field by presenting static stimuli of constant size and varying light intensity at specific locations for a short period of time while recording the patient's response at each location. The Humphrey field analyzer 24–2 standard achromatic examination (Humphrey Systems, Dublin, CA) uses a white stimulus with white background illumination; similar programs are present on other automated perimeters. Standard achromatic automated perimetry, along with clinical examination, has been the gold standard for following glaucoma; however, this automated testing strategy is time consuming, often resulting in patient fatigue and patient errors with high short-term and long-term variability. Advances in automated perimetry have aimed at reducing testing time and at developing strategies for earlier detection of visual damage in glaucoma. The SAP provides global indexes, such as the mean deviation, pattern standard deviation, and visual field index that are commonly used for diagnosis and monitoring disease progression. Glaucoma hemifield test is a parameter that compares specified regions of the visual field above and below the horizontal midline[1] (Fig. 7-2). These parameters are present in most automated perimeters.

The most commonly used test strategy is the Swedish interactive threshold algorithms (SITAs; Figs. 7-3 and 7-4). SITA uses information gained throughout the program to determine the threshold strategy for adjacent points. This allowed shortening the test duration in comparison with earlier iteration of the test without scarifying test reliability.[2,3]

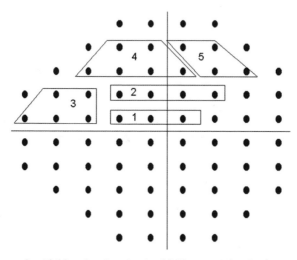

FIGURE 7-2. **Glaucoma hemifield testing.** Superior visual field zones used in the glaucoma hemifield test. Each zone is compared with its mirror zone below the horizontal meridian. Numbers 1 to 5 refers to the zones of the GHT. (Adapted with permission from Epstein DL. *Chandler and Grant's Glaucoma.* 4th ed. Baltimore, MD: Williams & Wilkins; 1997.)

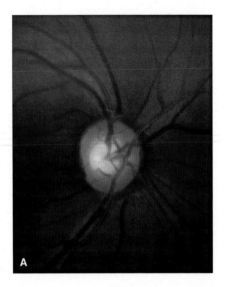

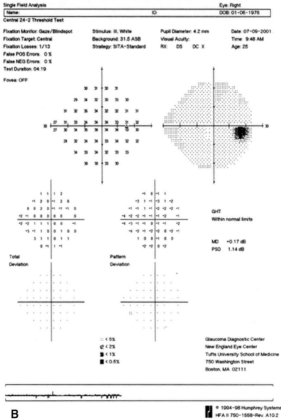

FIGURE 7-3. Healthy eye. A. Optic nerve head photograph. **B.** Normal Swedish interactive threshold algorithm visual field.

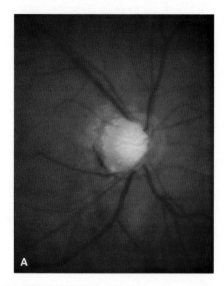

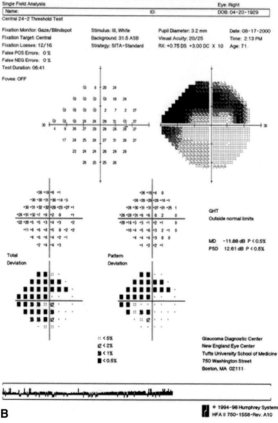

FIGURE 7-4. Glaucomatous eye. A. Optic nerve head photograph of an eye with glaucoma. **B.** Swedish interactive threshold algorithm visual field showing a superior arcuate scotoma and an inferior nasal step.

REFERENCES

1. Asman P, Heijl A. Glaucoma hemifield test. Automated visual field evaluation. *Arch Ophthalmol.* 1992;110:812–819.
2. Bengtsson B, Olsson J, Heijl A, Rootzen H. A new generation of algorithms for computerized threshold perimetry, SITA. *Acta Ophthalmol Scand.* 1997;75:368–375.
3. Bengtsson B, Heijl A, Olsson J. Evaluation of a new threshold visual field strategy, SITA, in normal subjects. Swedish interactive thresholding algorithm. *Acta Ophthalmol Scand.* 1998;76:165–169.

ACKNOWLEDGMENTS

Supported in part by NIH R01-EY13178.

GLAUCOMA PROGRESSION ANALYSIS

Guided progression analysis (GPA) is progression analysis technique available in the Humphrey visual field report.[1,2] GPA includes both event- and trend-based analysis to identify progression (**Fig. 7-5**). Event-based analysis identifies a point as progressing when it changed from the level at the baseline tests beyond the change that was detected in the population. Trend analysis is using linear regression to determine if the slope at any visit exceeds the no progression rate. When the change occurs in the same location over two consecutive tests, the GPA flags "possible progression." "Likely progression" is flagged when change is detected in three consecutive tests.

When to Use Guided Progression Analysis

• GPA is useful for longitudinal evaluation of subjects with glaucoma and glaucoma suspects.

Limitations

• Points that are depressed beyond the range of the GPA analysis software are identified with an "x." Such points are not used in the analysis and if progression is occurring at an "x"-labeled point, GPA will not demonstrate it.

REFERENCES

1. Bengtsson B, Heijl A. A visual field index for calculation of glaucoma rate of progression. *Am J Ophthalmol.* 2008;145:343–353.
2. De Moraes CG, Liebmann JM, Levin LA. Detection and measurement of clinically meaningful visual field progression in clinical trials for glaucoma. *Prog Retin Eye Res.* 2017;56:107–147.

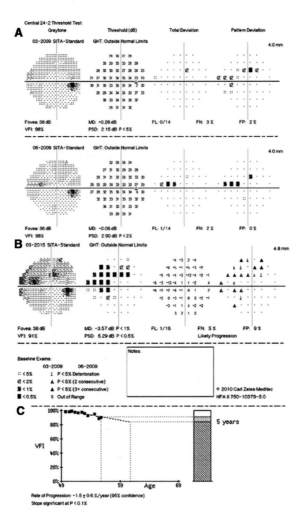

FIGURE 7-5. Guided progression analysis of a glaucomatous eye showing likely progression at the last visit (**B**) when compared with the baseline examinations (**A**). Trend analysis (**C**) showing a significant slope of progression over time and projected progression.

ELECTROPHYSIOLOGY TESTS

The functional evaluation of glaucoma is prone to important limitations, such as subjectivity and marked variability. Electrophysiology tests eliminate most of these shortcomings and provide an objective testing. Devices such as pattern electroretinogram can assess the ganglion cell layer and inner retina; electroretinogram assesses the retinal function and visual evoked potential of the entire visual pathway[1-3] (Figs. 7-6 and 7-7). Glaucoma is predominantly a disease of localized damage; thus, multifocal electrophysiology modalities that evaluate specific areas in the retina offer a better potential for correspondence with structural evaluation of the retina. To this date, despite the high diagnostic potential, no electrophysiology examination has been incorporated into the standard clinical practice of glaucoma.[4]

REFERENCES

1. Hood DC. Objective measurement of visual function in glaucoma. *Curr Opin Ophthalmol.* 2003;14:78–82.
2. Parisi V, Manni G, Centofanti M, et al. Correlation between optical coherence tomography, pattern electroretinogram and visual evoked potentials in open-angle glaucoma. *Ophthalmology.* 2001;108:905–912.
3. Bach M, Poloscheck CM. Electrophysiology and glaucoma: current status and future challenges. *Cell Tissue Res.* 2013;353:287–296.
4. Lucy KA, Wollstein G. Structural and functional evaluations for the early detection of glaucoma. *Expert Rev Ophthalmol.* 2016;11:367–376.

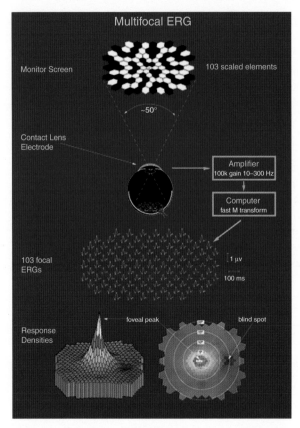

FIGURE 7-6. Multifocal electroretinogram (mfERG). Schematic display of the mfERG showing stimulus array, the response trace array, and three- and two-dimensional plots. (Courtesy of Erich Sutter, PhD, Electro-Diagnostic Imaging, San Mateo, CA.)

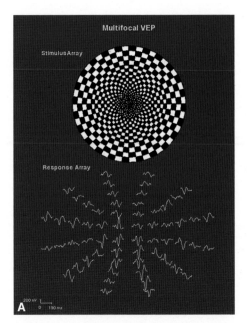

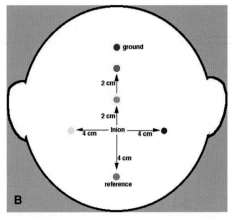

FIGURE 7-7. **Multifocal visual evoked potential (mf VEP). A.** Stimulus and response array of a normal mf VEP. **B.** Diagram of electrode placements above and lateral to the inion. (**A** and **B**, Courtesy of Erich Sutter, PhD, Electro-Diagnostic Imaging, San Mateo, CA.)

STRUCTURAL TESTS

Glaucoma is evaluated structurally by assessing the ONH cupping, RNFL defects, and macular thickness including the measurement of the ganglion cell layer/inner plexiform layer. The constant evolution of advanced ocular imaging technologies that provide noninvasive, objective techniques and novel parameters that evaluate the optic nerve and retinal structures aids in clinical decisions and management of subjects with glaucoma.

PHOTOGRAPHY

Stereoscopic ONH photography is one of the most common imaging methods of the posterior pole. This method allows documenting the ONH and its surrounding region for subjective evaluation and for assessing changes occurring over time. The glaucomatous features usually seen are neural tissue loss with global or localized thinning of the neuroretinal rim with corresponding enlargement of the cup. Changes in blood vessels with baring of the circumlinear vessels as well as splinter hemorrhages can also be appreciated. Peripapillary atrophy with the alpha (peripheral area of hypo- and hyperpigmentation) and beta (closer to the disc area of atrophy of the retinal pigment epithelium and the choriocapillaris) zones is also seen in glaucoma. RNFL photography, more difficult and less frequently used than ONH photography, permits extended evaluation of the RNFL following a patient examination. Specific retinal abnormalities associated with glaucoma include focal and diffuse RNFL thinning. RNFL losses in glaucoma are associated with visual field abnormalities.

How Stereoscopic Photography Works

• Stereo images can be produced using sequential (consecutive) or simultaneous photographic techniques.

• Sequential stereoscopic photography captures two consecutive images using a manual shift of the camera joystick.

• Simultaneous stereoscopic photography captures instantaneous stereo images with a single exposure to produce a split-frame image of two images on one or two frames depending on the system used (Fig. 7-8).

• Several conventional smartphone applications also allow acquisition of ONH images.

• The images can be viewed stereoscopically using a specialized viewing apparatus.

When to Use Stereoscopic Photography

• Stereoscopic ONH photography should be used to evaluate and document the findings in subjects with glaucoma and glaucoma suspects.

Limitations

• Stereoscopic ONH photography requires qualitative evaluation and does not offer a quantitative system for interpretation of the optic nerve.

How Retinal Nerve Fiber Layer Photography Works

• The RNFL is composed of the axons from the ganglion cells, neuroglia, and astrocytes. Axons of the ganglion cells travel toward the optic nerve in an organized manner (Fig. 7-9).

• The RNFL is best observed using a red-free, blue, or green light. Green or blue wavelengths are highly absorbed by the retinal pigment epithelium and choroid, whereas the axon bundles reflect the light and appear as silvery striations (Figs. 7-10 and 7-11).

When to Use Retinal Nerve Fiber Layer Photography

• RNFL examination is useful in the differential diagnosis between glaucoma suspects and true glaucoma damage.

- Defects in the RNFL may precede ONH and visual field changes. Therefore, correlating RNFL appearance with the corresponding area of presumed loss in the visual fields is an objective way to demonstrate structural-functional damage.

Limitations

- Media opacities, such as cataract, poorly focused photographs, and poor contrast because of a lightly pigmented fundus, are among the factors that can cause difficulty in evaluating or photographing the RNFL.

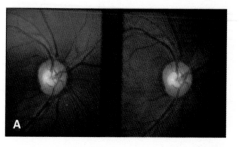 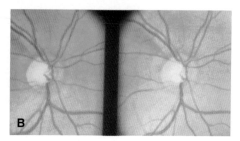

FIGURE 7-8. **Stereoscopic photography. A.** Stereo photograph of healthy eye. **B.** Stereo photograph of an optic nerve with a superonasal retinal nerve fiber layer defect.

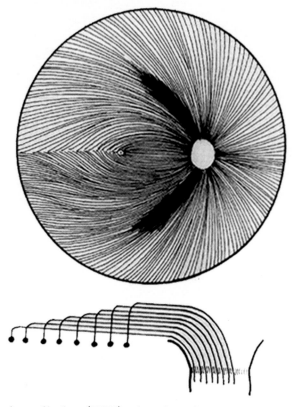

FIGURE 7-9. **Retinal nerve fiber layer (RNFL) pathway.** Lower drawing represents the topography of the RNFL where the distal ganglion cell axons project to the peripheral area of the optic disc rim. (Reprinted with permission from Schuman JS. *Imaging in Glaucoma*. Thorofare, NJ: SLACK; 1997.)

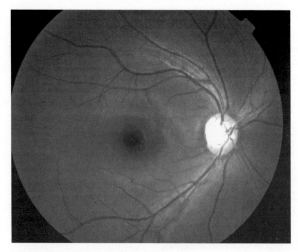

FIGURE 7-10. **Retinal nerve fiber layer photograph,** healthy eye.

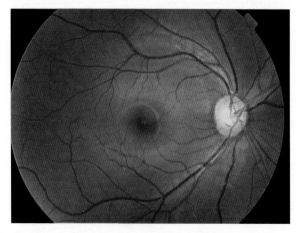

FIGURE 7-11. **Color retinal nerve fiber layer photograph,** healthy eye.

CONFOCAL SCANNING LASER OPHTHALMOSCOPY

Confocal scanning laser ophthalmoscopy (CSLO) is a method for acquiring and analyzing real-time three-dimensional topographic images of the ONH.

How Confocal Scanning Laser Ophthalmoscopy Works

- The Heidelberg retina tomograph (HRT; Heidelberg Engineering GmbH, Heidelberg, Germany) is the only commercially available confocal scanning laser ophthalmoscope.

- It uses a confocal scanning system based on the principle of spot illumination and spot detection. In this system, one spot on the retina or ONH is illuminated at a time, allowing only light originating from the illuminated area to pass through the aperture whereas scattered light and tissue planes that are out of focus do not. Thus, areas that do not lie close to the plane of focus are not illuminated and are not seen. This allows for high-contrast images.

- HRT uses a diode laser of 670 nm to scan the posterior segment. A three-dimensional image is obtained from a series of optical sections at consecutive focal planes. The information is displayed in two images—a topographic image and a reflectivity image.

- The optical transverse resolution is approximately 10 μm, whereas the axial resolution is about 300 μm.

- Moorfield's regression analysis, provided as part of the test report, compares both global and sectoral ONH parameters with normative data aiding to identify glaucomatous structural abnormalities (Fig. 7-12).[1] A second way of analyzing ONH measurements is the glaucoma probability score, which has the advantage of being independent of an operator-drawn contour line.[2]

- Topographic change analysis provides progression analysis capabilities with the confocal scanning laser. Locations where change from baseline exceed the variability recorded between the two baseline scans are marked (Fig. 7-13).

When to Use Confocal Scanning Laser Ophthalmoscopy

- CSLO is useful in detecting glaucoma and following its progression.

Limitations

- The user is required to define the ONH margin in order for the machine to generate the quantitative analysis. This adds a major source of variability in the measurements. However, this contour line can be automatically aligned to all subsequent tests, reducing this source of variability for longitudinal analysis.

- An automatically defined reference plane is needed for the software to calculate many of the ONH parameters. This reference plane might change over time, especially in subjects with glaucoma who have changing topography.[3] This variation increases the uncertainty in identifying changes.

- The software cannot differentiate between vascular and neuroretinal tissue and often overestimating the rim size, giving the impression of a healthier ONH than it is in reality.

REFERENCES

1. Wollstein G, Garway-Heath DF, Hitchings RA. Identification of early glaucoma cases with the scanning laser ophthalmoscope. *Ophthalmology.* 1998;105:1557–1563.
2. Alencar LM, Bowd C, Weinreb RN, et al. Comparison of HRT-3 glaucoma probability score and subjective stereophotograph assessment for prediction of progression in glaucoma. *Invest Ophthalmol Vis Sci.* 2008;49:1898–1906.
3. Mikelberg F, Wijsman K, Schulzer M. Reproducibility of topographic parameters obtained with the Heidelberg retina tomograph. *J Glaucoma.* 1993;2:101–103.

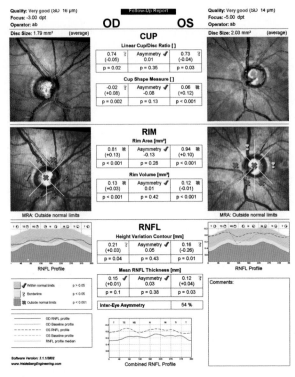

FIGURE 7-12. Moorfield's regression analysis (MRA) print out, glaucomatous eye. Signal strength and disc size described at top of page. MRA outcome represented as red X, yellow "!" and green check mark, corresponding with abnormal, borderline, and within normal limits, respectively. Contour line represented by green line circumferential to optic nerve. RNFL, retinal nerve fiber layer.

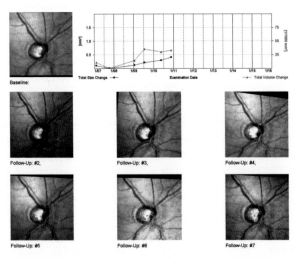

FIGURE 7-13. Topographic change analysis. Progression shown by increasing area of red signal in the infero-temporal neuroretinal rim.

OPTICAL COHERENCE TOMOGRAPHY

Optical coherence tomography (OCT) is a noninvasive technology that provides real-time high-resolution "optical biopsy-like" cross-sections of the scanned regions of interest.[1] The OCT technology is steadily evolving and the current U.S. Food and Drug Administration approved commercially available iteration of OCT in the United States is the spectral-domain OCT (SD-OCT). The peripapillary RNFL is the most commonly used OCT parameter to diagnose and monitor glaucoma. Other parameters that were demonstrated to be useful in glaucoma management include macular ganglion cell/inner plexiform layer and ONH parameters, such as rim area, minimal rim width (minimal distance between Bruch membrane opening and ONH surface), cup volume, and cup-to-disc (C/D) ratio.[2,3] Several machines now include progression analysis of ONH and macular parameters as part of their operating software.[4]

How Optical Coherence Tomography Works

• SD-OCT is using a wideband width light source that projects a near infrared light into the eye and to a stationary reference arm. Depth-resolved information from the scanned area is encoded in the magnitude and delay of the backreflected light from the eye. This information is matched with the corresponding pattern from the reference arm, using the low coherence principle, to resolve the tissue structure. The axial resolution of commercial SD-OCT ranges between 5 and 7 μm in the eye with transverse resolution of approximately 20 μm. Scan speed varies between 25,000 and 100,000 axial scans/second among the different devices. The scan depth is approximately 2 mm (Fig. 7-14). Automated segmentation of the retina and ONH region is provided by all commercial devices (Figs. 7-15 through 7-18).

• Swept-source OCT (SS-OCT) is a newer iteration available for clinical use, at the time of this writing, in several countries but not yet approved in the United States. This iteration of the technology uses a short cavity swept laser (center wavelength of 1,050 nm) with faster scanning speed (over 100,000 axial scans/second) and deeper penetration into the tissue, allowing detailed visualization of structures, such as the lamina cribrosa and choroid[5] (Figs. 7-19 and 7-20).

• Common scan patterns used in glaucoma management include circumpapillary scan encompassing all retinal ganglion cells axons on their way to the ONH, and radial or raster scans centered on the ONH or macula.

• This segmentation enables quantification of ocular structures with high reproducibility.[6] These parameters have been shown to allow detection of glaucomatous damage with high sensitivity. SD-OCT software also provide disease progression of trend- and event-based analysis that varies between the devices (Figs. 7-21 and 7-22).

• OCT angiography (OCTA) is a recently introduced iteration of the OCT technology that allows visualization of different levels of the vasculature without using contrast. OCTA can demonstrate the radial peripapillary capillaries network that is involved in the perfusion of the RNFL. To date, the utility of this system in glaucoma practice, including ways to quantify the microvascular structure, is under research with encouraging initial results[7,8] (Fig. 7-23).

• Additional OCT systems being studied are the polarization-sensitive OCT that generates images with tissue-specific characteristics that alter its polarization state; the visible-light OCT that uses a wideband width light source that enables in vivo oximetry and spectrometry; and the adaptive optics systems that correct optical aberrations of the eye using wave-front sensing and deformable mirrors to improve the transverse resolution. Adaptive optics can be coupled with scanning laser ophthalmoscopy or OCT and enhance visualization of structures, such as the lamina cribrosa microstructures (pores and beams) and RNFL bundles[9] (**Fig. 7-24**).

When to Use Optical Coherence Tomography

• OCT is useful in detecting glaucoma and following its progression. OCT can be used to assess the relationship between structure and function. Several devices include in their report a composite image of both ONH and macula scans with an overlay of the visual field. Corresponding abnormalities with both structure and function enhance the clinician certainty in making informed decision.

Limitations

• Media opacities may limit the ability to perform OCT.[10] Flowing blood within blood vessels obliterates the OCT signal behind them, causing shadows. This can interfere with the automated segmentation of the retina and limit visibility of the lamina cribrosa.

REFERENCES

1. Huang D, Swanson EA, Lin CP, et al. Optical coherence tomography. *Science.* 1991;254:1178–1181.
2. Tan O, Chopra V, Lu AT, et al. Detection of macular ganglion cell loss in glaucoma by Fourier-domain optical coherence tomography. *Ophthalmology.* 2009;116:2305–2314.
3. Dong ZM, Wollstein G, Schuman JS. Clinical utility of optical coherence tomography in glaucoma. *Invest Ophthalmol Vis Sci.* 2016;57:OCT556–OCT567.
4. Leung CK. Diagnosing glaucoma progression with optical coherence tomography. *Curr Opin Ophthalmol.* 2014;25:104–111.
5. Kostanyan T, Wollstein G, Schuman JS. New developments in optical coherence tomography. *Curr Opin Ophthalmol.* 2015;26:110–115.
6. Schuman JS. Spectral domain optical coherence tomography for glaucoma (an AOS thesis). *Trans Am Ophthalmol Soc.* 2008;106:426–458.
7. Liu L, Jia L, Takusagawa HL, et al. Optical coherence tomography angiography of the peripapillary retina in glaucoma. *JAMA Ophthalmol.* 2015;133:1045–1052.
8. Mase T, Ishibazawa A, Nagaoka T, et al. Radial peripapillary capillar network visualized using wide-field montage optical coherence tomography angiography. *Invest Ophthalmol Vis Sci.* 2016;57:OCT504–OCT510.
9. Dong ZM, Wollstein G, Wang B, Schuman JS. Adaptive optics optical coherence tomography in glaucoma. *Prog Retin Eye Res.* 2017;57:76–88.
10. Swanson EA, Izatt JA, Hee MR, et al. In vivo retinal imaging by optical coherence tomography. *Opt Lett.* 1993;18:1864–1866.

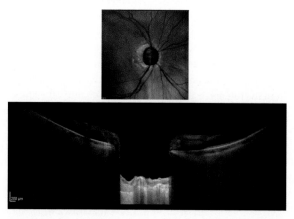

FIGURE 7-14. Spectral-domain optical coherence tomography enhanced-depth imaging. Vertical cross-section of the optic nerve head showing a prominent cupping and the deep optic nerve head structures including the lamina cribrosa and the prelaminar tissue.

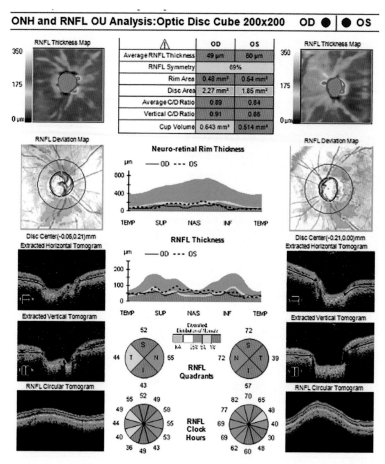

FIGURE 7-15. Spectral-domain optical coherence tomography optic nerve head report. Advanced glaucomatous damage showing in both eyes with marked thinning of the retinal nerve fiber layer (RNFL). The neural rim area, the average and vertical cup-to-disc ratio, and the cup volume are all outside normal limits. INF, inferior; NAS, nasal; OU, both eyes, SUP- superior.

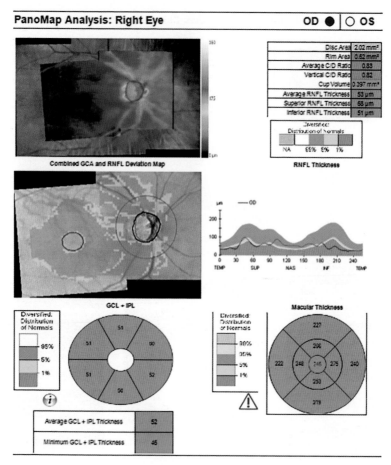

FIGURE 7-16. **Spectral-domain optical coherence tomography PanoMap report.** This report provides a campsite of the retinal nerve fiber layer (RNFL) deviation map in the peripapillary region and the macular ganglion cell/inner plexiform layer thickness. This subject is demonstrating advanced glaucomatous damage in both peripapillary and macular regions. GCA, ganglion cel analysis; IPL, inner plexiform layer.

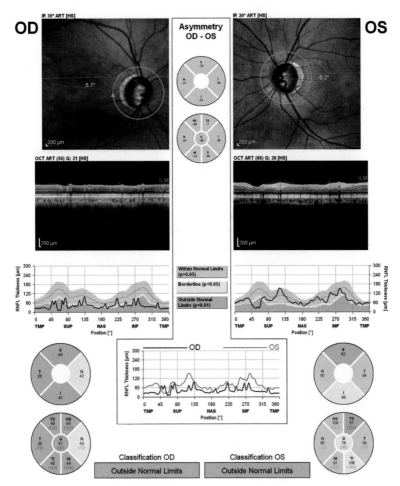

FIGURE 7-17. Spectral-domain optical coherence tomography (OCT), glaucomatous eye. OCT of peripapillary retinal nerve fiber layer (RNFL) showing widespread damage in the right eye and a focal superior defect in the left eye. INF, inferior; NAS, nasal; SUP, superior; TEMP, temporal.

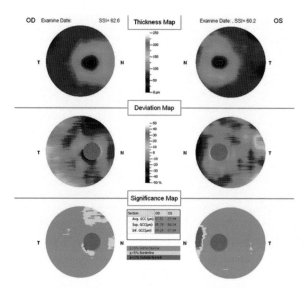

FIGURE 7-18. Spectral-domain optical coherence tomography (OCT), glaucomatous eye. OCT of macular ganglion cell complex in glaucomatous eye showing focal thinning in the superonasal region in the right eye.

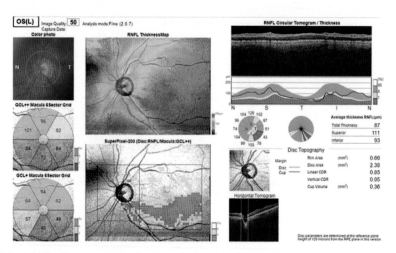

FIGURE 7-19. Wide glaucoma report of swept-source optical coherence tomography. An inferotemporal wedge defect extending from the disc margin to the macular region. The optic nerve photography (**upper left**) is showing thinning of the inferior rim. (Courtesy of Prof. D. Lavinsky, MD.)

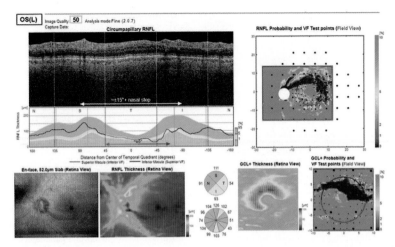

FIGURE 7-20. Wide glaucoma report of swept-source optical coherence tomography. The thickness map is rotated to match the overlay visual filed testing points to highlight locations with expected visual field abnormality (**upper right and lower right**). RNFL, retinal nerve fiber layer. GCL, ganglion cell layer; SS, swept source; VF, visual field. (Courtesy of Prof. D. Lavinsky, MD.)

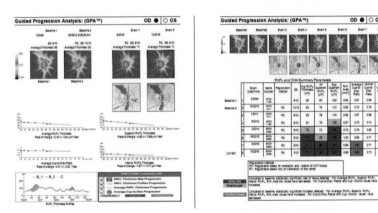

FIGURE 7-21. Guided progression analysis of the optic nerve head (ONH). Wedge defects are gradually evident in both superior and inferior regions. Both trend and event analysis showing likely progression. The second page of the report (**right**) shows the deviation maps of the retinal nerve fiber layer (RNFL) of each visit and a table with the measurements of the ONH parameters at each visit. OCT, optical coherence tomography.

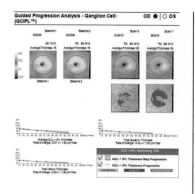
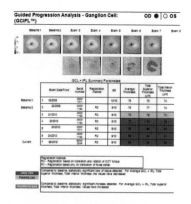

FIGURE 7-22. Guided progression analysis of the macular ganglion cell–inner plexiform layer (GCIPL). Significant slopes of progression of average, inferior, and superior GCIPL. The second page of the report (**right**) shows the deviation maps of each visit and a table with the measurements of the macular parameters at each visit. OCT, optical coherence tomography. GCL, ganglion cell layer; SS, swept source; VF, visual field.

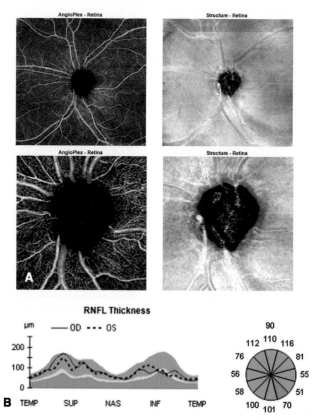

FIGURE 7-23. Optical coherence tomography angiography and corresponding retinal thickness report. (**left**) angiography maps demonstrating a temporal inferior wedge of vascular drop off. (**right**) corresponding retinal nerve fiber layer (RNFL) thinning is noticeable. GCL, ganglion cell layer; INF, inferior; NAS, nasal; SS, swept source; SUP, superior; TEMP, temporal; VF, visual field.

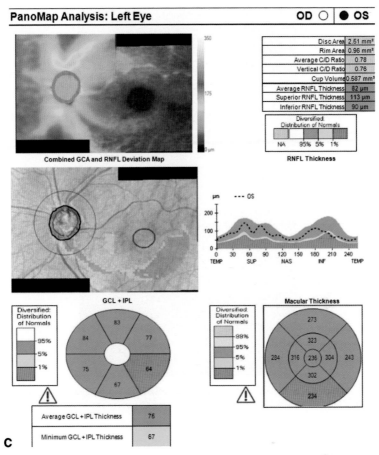

FIGURE 7-23. (*continued*) **C.** PanoMap demonstrating extension of the affected region into the macula.

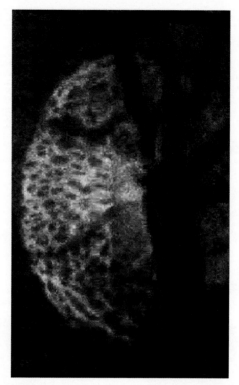

FIGURE 7-24. Adaptive optics spectral-domain optical coherence tomography. Incorporation of adaptive optics technology improves the transverse resolution allowing to resolve the lamina cribrosa microstructure showing pores and beams.

Psychophysical Testing

Douglas J. Rhee, Tara A. Uhler, and L. Jay Katz ∎

INTRODUCTION

The goal of this chapter is to show representative visual field patterns for glaucoma rather than provide a comprehensive discussion of perimetry. There are several texts dedicated solely to the extended description of perimetry and atlases dedicated to just perimetric findings.

The broad term *psychophysical testing* refers to the subjective testing of vision of an eye. In clinical terms for the glaucoma patient, this involves perimetry to assess the peripheral vision of an eye. Because the pathophysiology of glaucoma affects the paracentral and peripheral vision before affecting central acuity, there are both diagnostic and therapeutic benefits to assessing the patient's visual field. It is important to note that usage of the term *peripheral* vision does not necessarily mean far periphery. In fact, most glaucomatous visual field defects occur paracentrally (within 24 degrees of fixation). Our use of the term *peripheral* refers to anything beyond central fixation (i.e., greater than the central 5 to 10 degrees).

Contrast sensitivity is not routinely tested in glaucoma patients. Contrast sensitivity is affected in even early glaucoma (but not ocular hypertension, that is, an elevated intraocular pressure [IOP] without the presence of optic nerve damage), and progressively worsens with continued optic nerve damage. Contrast sensitivity highly correlates to the perceived visual problems in patients with glaucoma (Fig. 8-1A). The Pelli Robson chart is the most commonly used (Fig. 8-1B and C), but other charts have been developed. When testing, it is important to use standard illumination.

Ishihara color plates are not generally affected in glaucoma until very advanced stages of disease. Even patients with very small central islands have minimal defects on color plate testing. Using techniques with more refined color discrimination, patients with even early glaucoma can have decreases primarily in the blue-yellow axis which is exploited by the short-wave automated perimetry (SWAP) test.

BIBLIOGRAPHY

Anderson AJ, Sainer MJ. A control experiment for studies that show improved visual sensitivity with intraocular pressure lowering in glaucoma. *Ophthalmology.* 2014;121:2028–2032.

Anderson DR, Patella VM. *Automated Static Perimetry.* 2nd ed. St. Louis, MO: Mosby; 1999.

Aulhorn E, Harms H. Early visual field defects in glaucoma. In: Leydhecker W, ed. Glaucoma Symposium, Tutzing Castle, August 1966, held in Connection with the 20th International Congress of Ophthalmology, Munich. Basel, Switzerland: S. Karger; 1967:151–186.

Bambo MP, Ferrandez B, Guerri N, et al. Evaluation of contrast sensitivity, chromatic vision, and reading ability in patients with primary open-angle glaucoma. *J Ophthalmol.* 2016;2016:7074016.

Budenz DL. *Atlas of Visual Fields.* Philadelphia, PA: Lippincott-Raven; 1997.

Drance SM, Wheeler C, Patullo M. The use of static perimetry in the early detection of glaucoma. *Can J Ophthalmol.* 1967;2:249–258.

Ekici F, Loh R, Waisbourd M, et al. Relationships between measures of the ability to perform vision-related activities, vision-related quality of life, and clinical findings in patients with glaucoma. *JAMA Ophthalmol.* 2015;1333:1377–1385.

Fatehi N, Nowroozizadeh S, Henry S, Coleman AL, Caprioli J, Nouri-Mahdavi K. Association of structural and functional measures with contrast sensitivity in glaucoma. *Am J Ophthalmol.* 2017;178:129–139.

Harwerth RS, Carter-Dawson L, Shen F, et al. Ganglion cell losses underlying visual field defects from experimental glaucoma. *Invest Ophthalmol Vis Sci.* 1999;40:2242–2250.

Heijl A. Automatic perimetry in glaucoma visual field screening. A clinical study. *Graefes Arch Clin Exp Ophthalmol.* 1976;200:21–37.

Heijl A, Lundqvist L. The location of earliest glaucomatous visual field defected documented by automatic perimetry. *Doc Ophthalmol Proceed Series.* 1983;35:153–158.

Katz J, Tielsch JM, Quigley HA, et al. Automated perimetry detects visual field loss before manual Goldmann perimetry. *Ophthalmology.* 1995;102:21–26.

Lynn JR. Examination of the visual field in glaucoma. *Invest Ophthalmol.* 1969;8:76–84.

Nuzzi R, Bellan A, Boles-Careenini B. Glaucoma, lighting and color vision. An investigation into their relationship. *Ophthlamologica.* 1997;211:25–31.

Quigley HA, Dunlelberger GR, Green WR. Retinal ganglion cell atrophy correlated with automated perimetry in human eyes with glaucoma. *Am J Ophthalmol.* 1989;107:453–464.

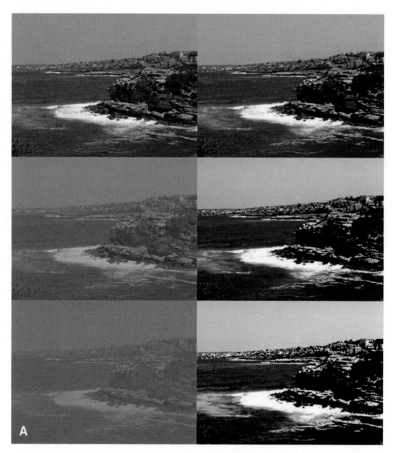

FIGURE 8-1. Contrast sensitivity. A. Photoshop simulation of the effect of worsening levels of contrast. The original image without manipulation is the top left. Down the left-hand column is decreasing contrast by 50% (**middle left**) and 75% (**bottom left**). The right-hand column increasing contrast by 25% (**top right**), 50% (**middle right**), and 75% (**bottom right**). (Figure from: https://commons.wikimedia.org/w/index.php?curid=750555.) Pelli Robson Contrast Sensitivity Chart (**B**) letters in triplet with decreasing contrast as one moves from left to right and down each row. The testing distance is 1 m using an illumination of 85 cd/mm². The score of the test is recorded by the faintest triplet, out of which at least two letters are correctly identified. The log CS value for this triplet is given by the number on the scoring pad.

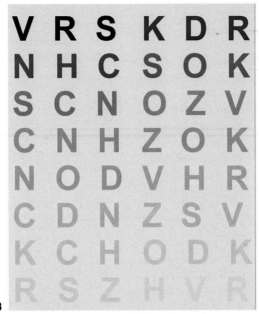

B

PELLI-ROBSON

0.00	H S Z	D S N	0.15
0.30	C K R	Z V R	0.45
0.60	N D C	O S K	0.75
0.90	O Z K	V H Z	1.05
1.20	N H O	N R D	1.35
1.50	V R C	O V H	1.65
1.80	C D S	N D C	1.95
2.10	K V Z	O H R	2.25

C

FIGURE 8-1 (*continued*) **C.** Shows sample letters (different from **A**) without fading and the log values next to the triplet. Grossly, normal contrast perception is being able to see 6 to 7 lines (12–14 triplets), moderate loss is seeing 4 to 5 lines, severe loss is being able to see 2 to 3 lines, and profound loss would be to only see 1 line.

PURPOSE OF TEST

Diagnosis

• As part of the initial evaluation of a patient suspected of having glaucoma, automated monochromatic visual field testing is an important aspect of the diagnostic determination of glaucomatous optic nerve damage. Visual field abnormalities have localizing value for lesions along the entire visual tract, which extends from the retina to the occipital lobes. Glaucomatous visual field defects are those that are typically found with lesions localizing to the optic nerve.

• It is important to note that the presence of a so-called optic nerve field (i.e., defects that localize to the optic nerve) is not solely diagnostic of glaucoma. This must occur in the presence of a characteristic optic nerve appearance (covered in Chapter 6) and history.

• Other findings, such as IOP, gonioscopic appearance, and anterior segment findings, may help categorize the specific type of glaucoma. All optic neuropathies (e.g., anterior ischemic optic neuropathies, compressive optic neuropathies, etc.) demonstrate "optic nerve" visual fields.

• It is also critical to note that the absence of an optic nerve field does not exclude the diagnosis of glaucoma. Although in the year 2002, automated achromatic static visual field (AASVF) testing was the gold standard for the evaluation of optic nerve function, its threshold of sensitivity to detect ganglion cell loss is still limited. Clinicopathologic and experimental evidence indicates that the earliest visual field defect detectable by AASVF corresponds to approximately 40% ganglion cell loss.

Management

• AASVF testing along with serial optic nerve evaluations remains the gold standard for the monitoring of glaucoma.

• The goal (or target) IOP is the therapeutic range at which we modify the ocular physiology in an attempt to protect the optic nerve from further barotraumas. However, the determination of the target pressure is empirical, meaning that we estimate what the goal should be. AASVF and serial optic nerve evaluations are the ways in which we determine whether that empirically derived pressure range is actually effective at protecting the optic nerve.

DESCRIPTION

• Perimetric testing attempts to determine the visual threshold at a particular location in the visual field. The visual threshold is defined as the minimum level of light that can be perceived at a given location in the visual field; this concept is also termed *retinal sensitivity*.

• This is a different concept from the lowest level of photic energy that will stimulate a photoreceptor cell or area of the retina. Perimetric testing relies on the patient to subjectively determine what he or she can see. Therefore, the visual threshold is subject to some level of cognitive and intraretinal processing, hence the name psychophysical testing.

• The visual threshold is highest in the fovea, which is defined as the center of the visual field. As the field extends peripherally, the sensitivity decreases. The three-dimensional representation of this is often called the "hill of vision" (**Fig. 8-2**). The visual field for one eye extends 60 degrees superiorly, 60 degrees nasally, 75 degrees inferiorly, and 100 degrees temporally.

• There are two main methods of perimetry: static and kinetic (**Fig. 8-3**).

   ▪ Historically, various forms of kinetic testing were developed first, and these are generally performed manually. Briefly, a visual stimulus of known size and intensity is brought from the far periphery, where it would not be expected to be perceived, toward the center. At some point, it will move into an area where it is perceived; this is the visual threshold at that location. This process is continued with varying stimuli of size and intensities to give a topographic map of the hill of vision. The Goldmann visual field attempts to map the entire visual field (Fig. 8-4).

▪ Static visual field testing presents visual stimuli in varying sizes and intensities at fixed locations. Although there are many different strategies for determining the visual threshold, most use the following basic principle.

 ▶ The examiner begins by presenting stimuli of higher intensity and, in measured steps, presents stimuli of lower intensity until the patient no longer perceives the stimulus. Then, the test

is usually rechecked by presenting a gradually increasing intensity of stimulus in smaller increments until the patient again can perceive the stimulus. That intensity of light is defined as the visual threshold in that region of the visual field. Generally, static visual field testing is automated and presents white-colored stimuli on a white background, hence the name AASVF testing.

 ▶ There are many makers of AASVF machines; among them are Humphrey (Allergan, Irvine, CA), Octopus (Fig. 8-5), and Dicon.

● Various testing algorithms have been developed, such as full threshold, FASTPAC, STATPAC, and Swedish interactive threshold algorithm (SITA), among others. They vary with regard to length of test time and slightly with regard to depth of field defect.

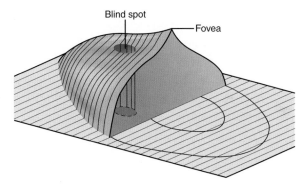

FIGURE 8-2. The "hill of vision." A three-dimensional representation of the visual threshold in various locations within the visual field of a normal eye. (From Haley MJ, ed. *The Field Analyzer Primer*. 2nd ed. San Leandro, CA: Humphrey Instruments; 1987:4. Fig. 1.)

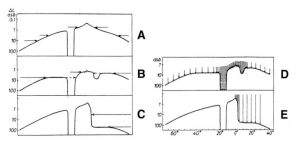

FIGURE 8-3. Comparison of static and kinetic perimetry. Slopes and scotomas are shown better by static than by kinetic perimetry. **A.** Although the normal visual field with its gradual slope and absence of abnormal scotomas is well outlined by kinetic testing, the presence of field defects makes this method less precise than static testing. **B.** The flat temporal slope might yield a response at any point between 40 and 12 degrees if the test object was optimum for testing that zone. Nasally, the best-chosen kinetic test might be reported anywhere between 25 and 7 degrees, and it would miss the relative scotoma between 7 and 12 degrees. **C.** When the slope is steep, kinetic perimetry usually outlines the defect well with a few well-chosen test objects, but the choice is often arbitrary and may fail to reveal the actual steepness of the slope. Static tests elucidate well the flat slopes and small scotomas in **D** and both kinds of slope in **E.** (From Leydhecker W. *Glaucoma Symposium, Tutzing Castle, August 1966, held in Connection with the 20th International Congress of Ophthalmology, Munich.* Basel, Switzerland: S. Karger; 1967:151–186. With permission from S. Karger AG, Basel, Switzerland.)

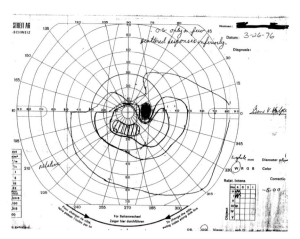

FIGURE 8-4. Goldmann visual field testing. Goldmann visual field test of the right eye showing superior nasal step and arcuate defect.

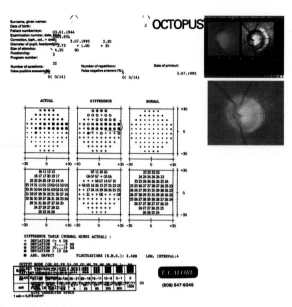

FIGURE 8-5. **Octopus AASVF test** with corresponding optic nerve photograph and Heidelberg retinal tomography scan.

COMMON OPTIC NERVE VISUAL FIELDS FOUND IN PATIENTS WITH GLAUCOMA

- The anatomic location of the defect in glaucoma is in the optic nerve, with focal spots within the lamina cribrosa. On the field test, the visual defects manifest in relatively specific patterns because of the anatomy of the retinal nerve fiber layer (RNFL). The RNFL is composed primarily of the axons from the ganglion cells projecting through the optic nerve to the lateral geniculate nucleus (Fig. 8-6).

- Axons from ganglion cells located nasal to the optic disc travel straight into optic disc; defects in the optic nerve affecting fibers from this region produce a temporal wedge defect (Fig. 8-7).

  - Axons from ganglion cells located temporal to the optic nerve arc into the optic nerve. A line that intersects the fovea and the optic nerve defines the horizontal raphe. Ganglion cells located superiorly to the horizontal raphe arc superiorly and deliver their fibers to the superotemporal aspect of the optic nerve.

  - The converse is true for ganglion cells located temporal to the optic nerve and inferior to the horizontal raphe.

- Defects in the optic nerve affecting fibers from the area temporal to the optic nerve produce both nasal step defects and arcuate defects.

  - The nasal step defect (Figs. 8-8 and 8-9) gets its name not only from the nasal location of the field defect but also from the fact that the defect respects the horizontal median. The horizontal raphe is the anatomic basis for this appearance.

  - The arcuate defect gets its name from the appearance of the defect (Fig. 8-10). Nasal step and arcuate defects are far more common than temporal wedge defects.

  - As glaucoma progresses, multiple defects can present (Fig. 8-11) in a single eye (Fig. 8-12).

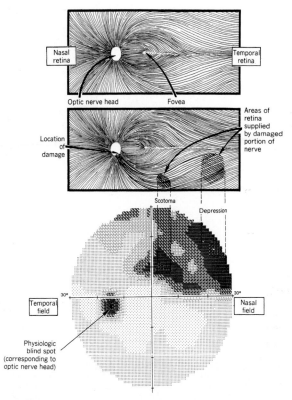

FIGURE 8-6. Glaucomatous damage to nerve bundles and location of resulting visual abnormalities. Damage at the lower pole of the optic disc causes abnormalities in the visual field as shown (left eye). (From Anderson DR, Patella VM. *Automated Static Perimetry.* 2nd ed. St. Louis, MO: Mosby; 1999:51. Fig. 4-4.)

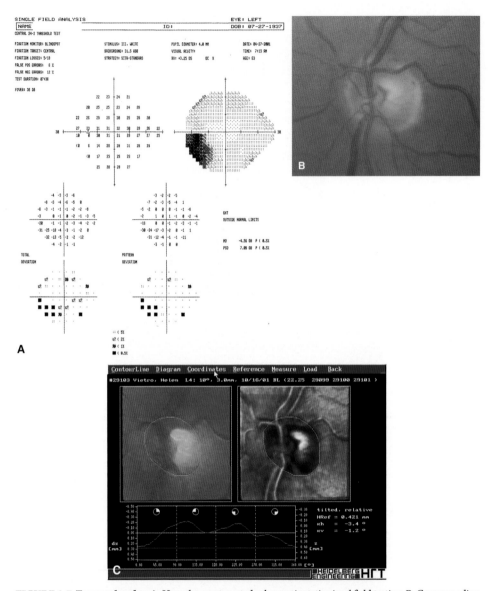

FIGURE 8-7. Temporal wedge. A. Humphrey automated achromatic static visual field testing. **B.** Corresponding optic nerve photograph showing some nasal thinning. **C.** Corresponding Heidelberg retinal tomography scan.

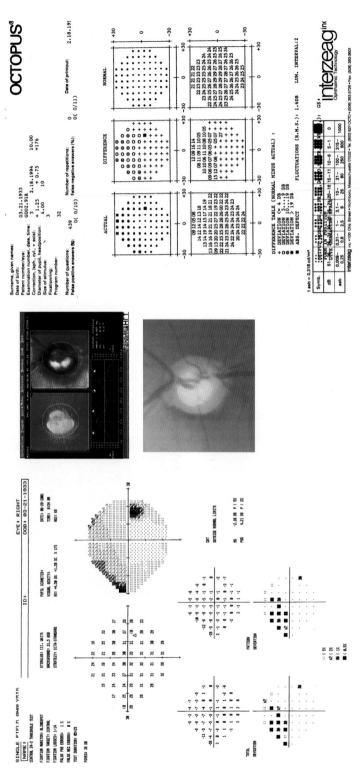

FIGURE 8-8. **Early superior nasal step defect.** This patient has had both Humphrey and Octopus automated achromatic static visual field testing. The corresponding optic nerve photograph and Heidelberg retinal tomography scan showing early inferotemporal thinning are also provided. Although the Humphrey and Octopus fields are separated by many years, this patient had no clinical progression of disease, so the fields are roughly comparable.

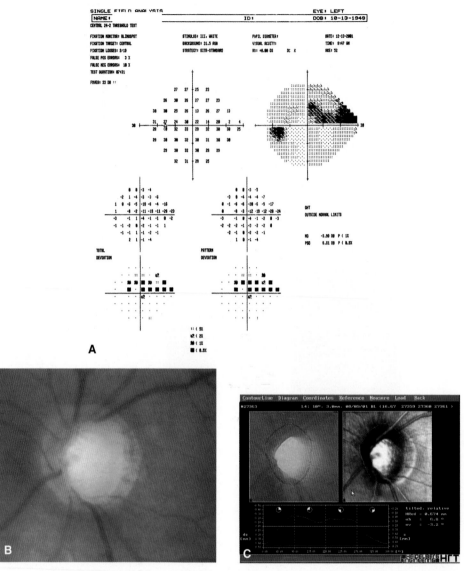

FIGURE 8-9. More advanced superior nasal step defect. A. Humphrey automated achromatic static visual field testing. **B.** Corresponding optic nerve photograph showing more advanced inferotemporal thinning. **C.** Corresponding Heidelberg retinal tomography scan.

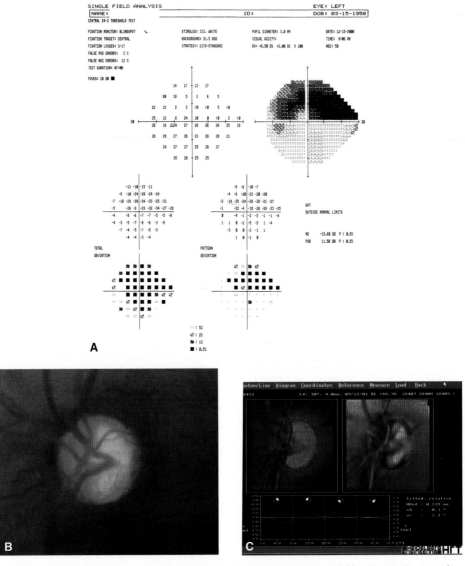

FIGURE 8-10. Arcuate defect. A. Humphrey automated achromatic static visual field testing. **B.** Corresponding optic nerve photograph showing some nasal thinning. **C.** Corresponding Heidelberg retinal tomography I scan.

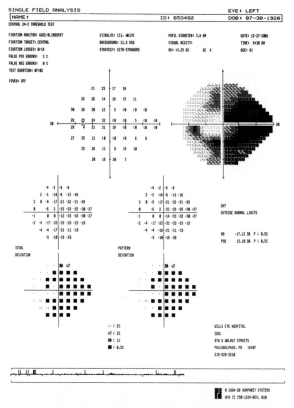

FIGURE 8-11. **Automated achromatic static visual field test** from a Humphrey machine demonstrating a combination of defects. There are both superior and inferior nasal steps with both inferior and superior arcuate defects. The inferior arcuate is more prominent than the superior arcuate.

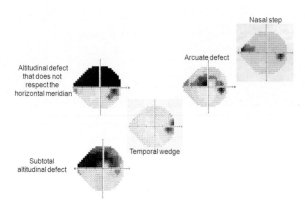

FIGURE 8-12. **Summary of characteristic glaucomatous visual field defects** that localize to the retinal nerve fiber layer.

NEWER PSYCHOPHYSICAL TESTING: FREQUENCY-DOUBLING PERIMETRY AND SHORT-WAVE AUTOMATED PERIMETRY

- Both frequency-doubling perimetry (FDP) and SWAP rely on isolating a subpopulation of ganglion cells.

- FDP isolates a subset of large-diameter ganglion cells, called M_y cells, that are thought to project to the magnocellular layers of the lateral geniculate nucleus, whereas SWAP isolates bistratified blue-yellow ganglion cells sensitive to blue stimuli that are thought to project to the parvocellular layers of the lateral geniculate nucleus.

- These have an increased sensitivity of detection that may be related by isolating a subpopulation of ganglion cells; there is a decreased functional reserve (Figs. 8-13 to 8-15).

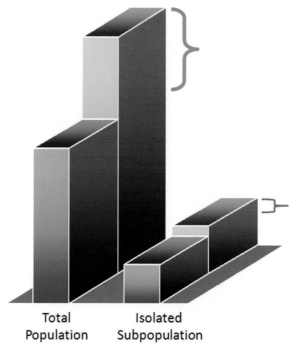

Total Population   Isolated Subpopulation

FIGURE 8-13. **Schematic of functional reserve.** *Yellow bar* schematically represents the full undamaged number of ganglion cells. The *blue bars* schematically represent the level of ganglion cells in which symptomatic dysfunction would occur. Thus, the differences as represented by the *red* and *green brackets* represent the functional reserve.

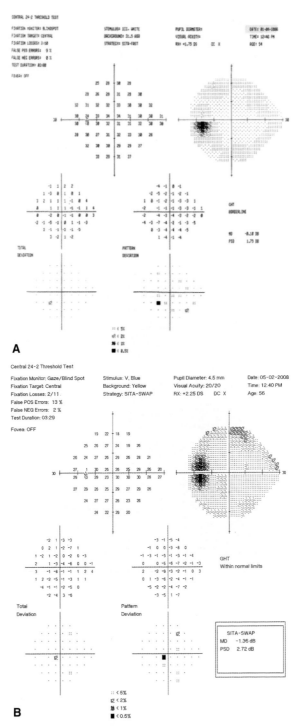

FIGURE 8-14. Visual fields from the same patient using the 24–2 testing strategies of the Humphrey field analyzer (Zeiss) with the SITA-FAST strategy (**A**), 24–2 SITA SWAP (**B**), and 24–2 frequency-doubling perimetry (**C**).

LEFT EYE

Test Duration: 04:24 min

Threshold (dB)

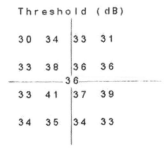

```
30  34 │33  31

33  38 │36  36
──────36──────────
33  41 │37  39

34  35 │34  33
```

Deviation

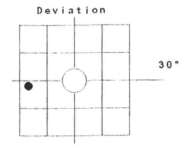

30°

MD   +2.56 dB
PSD   +3.19 dB

FIXATION ERRS: 0/6
FALSE POS ERRS: 0/6
FALSE NEG ERRS: 0/3

Probability Symbols

Symbol	Probability
☐	P >= 5%
⋯	P < 5%
▨	P < 2%
▨	P < 1%
▥	P < 0.5%

C

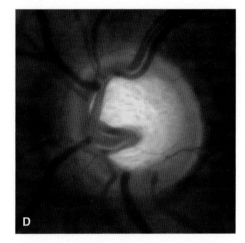

D

FIGURE 8-14. (*continued*) **D.** The corresponding optic nerve. SITA, Swedish interactive threshold algorithm; SWAP, short-wave automated perimetry.

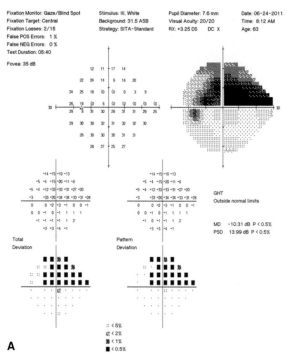

FIGURE 8-15. Example of abnormal Humphrey visual field and frequency-doubling perimetry. Corresponding achromatic visual field (**A**), FDP visual field (**B**), and corresponding optic nerve (**C**).

LEFT EYE

Test Duration: 04:21 min

Threshold (dB)

```
20   13 |  2    2

21    6 |  1    0
————————30—————————
29   30 |23   23

29   22 |29   27
```

Total Deviation

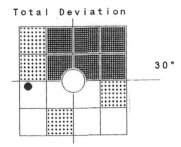

30°

Pattern Deviation

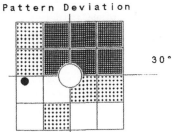

30°

MD   -7.17 dB   P < 0.5%
PSD   +13.20 dB   P < 0.5%

FIXATION   ERRS: 0/6
FALSE POS ERRS: 0/6
FALSE NEG ERRS: 0/3

Probability Symbols
    P >= 5%
    P < 5%
    P < 2%
    P < 1%
    P < 0.5%

B

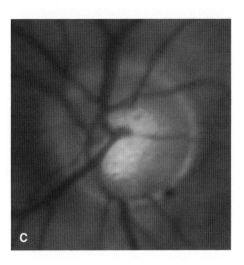

FIGURE 8-15. (*continued*)

Blood Flow in Glaucoma

Brent Siesky, Alon Harris, Katie Hutchins, and Josh Gross ■

INTRODUCTION

Glaucoma is a multifactorial and progressive optic neuropathy with strong evidence of vascular influences in many individuals. Numerous cross-sectional and longitudinal studies have identified low ocular perfusion pressure (calculated from blood pressure − intraocular pressure [IOP]) is an independent risk factor for the prevalence, incidence, and progression of glaucoma. Important anatomic vascular beds of interest in glaucoma include the retrobulbar vessels, peripapillary choroid, pre- and intra-laminar optic nerve head, and the capillary plexus of the superficial retinal nerve fiber layer (RNFL). Recent longitudinal studies have identified vascular factors as predictors of open-angle glaucoma (OAG) progression. In addition, ocular vascular health may be a more influential contributing factor in the pathophysiology of OAG in patients of African descent compared to European descent.

Advancements in imaging modalities of ocular blood flow have increased the understanding of ocular vascular dynamics, and have helped describe its role in glaucoma pathophysiology. Historically, evaluation of ocular and optic nerve blood flow in glaucoma has presented many challenges, and, therefore, many techniques focus on vascular regions accessible by ultrasound, laser, or other principles. It is important to acknowledge that no single technology is capable of assessing all significant vascular beds. Herein, clinically impactful and emerging ocular blood flow measurement techniques are presented and discussed (**Fig. 9-1**).

BIBLIOGRAPHY

Abegao Pinto L, Willekens K, Van Keer K, et al. Ocular blood flow in glaucoma—the Leuven Eye Study. *Acta Ophthalmol*. 2016;94(6):592–598.

Costa VP, Harris A, Anderson D, et al. Ocular perfusion pressure in glaucoma. *Acta Ophthalmol*. 2014;92(4):e252–e266.

Kanakamedala P, Harris A, Siesky B, et al. Optic nerve head morphology in glaucoma patients of African descent is strongly correlated to retinal blood flow. *Br J Ophthalmol*. 2014;98(11):1551–1554.

Moore NA, Harris A, Wentz S, et al. Baseline retrobulbar blood flow is associated with both functional and structural glaucomatous progression after 4 years. *Br J Ophthalmol*. 2017;101(3):305–308.

Siesky B, Harris A, Carr J, et al. Reductions in retrobulbar and retinal capillary blood flow strongly correlate with changes in optic nerve head and retinal morphology over 4 years in open-angle glaucoma patients of African descent compared with patients of European descent. *J Glaucoma*. 2016;25(9):750–757.

Tobe LA, Harris A, Hussain RM, et al. The role of retrobulbar and retinal circulation on optic nerve head and retinal nerve fibre layer structure in patients with open-angle glaucoma over an 18-month period. *Br J Ophthalmol*. 2015;99(5):609–612.

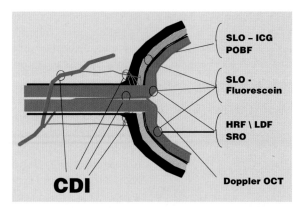

FIGURE 9-1. Instruments used to measure hemodynamics. Different technologies measure hemodynamics in specific ocular tissue beds. In addition, newly emerging technologies such as optical coherence tomography angiography (OCT-A) and spectral retinal oximetry measure capillary vessel density within and surrounding the optic nerve, as well as retinal vessel oxygen content, respectively. CDI, color Doppler imaging; HRF, Heidelberg retinal flowmeter; ICG, Indocyanine green; LDF, laser doppler flowmetry; POBF, pulsatile ocular blood flow; SLO, scanning laser ophthalmoscope; SRO, spectral retinal oximetry.

OPTICAL COHERENCE TOMOGRAPHY ANGIOGRAPHY

Purpose

● Evaluation of retinal, optic nerve, and choroidal hemodynamics

Description

Optical coherence tomography angiography (OCT-A) is a novel and noninvasive imaging modality that builds on existing OCT technology and offers the promise of highly specialized outcomes of optic nerve vascularity. OCT-A utilizes the differences in amplitude between subsequent beams of reflected infrared light to analyze both cross-sectional structural information and compute the quantity of retinal and choroidal blood flow (dimensionless units), providing vessel density percentage in the retina and optic nerve in 3 to 4 seconds. Two algorithms, split-spectrum amplitude-decorrelation angiography (SSADA) and optical microangiography (OMAG), have been widely used in research and are commercially available for clinical application. The SSADA algorithm utilizes the reflected amplitude of an infrared laser to find the decorrelation between consecutive B-scans (Fig. 9-2). OMAG utilizes a Hilbert transformation to assess scattering light reflections as either static or in motion. These calculations are used to generate high-resolution 3D (18 μm in coronal plane) images of the optic disc vasculature with segmentation of vascular layers (Fig. 9-3), including deep into the lamina cribrosa (2- to 3-mm penetration depth), and provide simultaneous structural and vascular assessments.

● Specialized angiography SSADA algorithm provides a reduction of artifacts from saccadic eye movements, high signal-to-noise ratio and vessel continuity, as well as vessel quantification in terms of density and flow index. OMAG allows for highly sensitive capillary images, and detection of blood flow as slow as 4 μm/s[3].

● Vessel density (%) demonstrated similar diagnostic accuracy compared to RNFL thickness measurement for differentiating between healthy subjects and those with glaucoma (Fig. 9-4).

● Current cross-sectional studies in glaucoma patients show correlations between lower peripapillary vessel density and visual field defects, and correlation of visual field deficits to be stronger with vessel density deficits than with RNFL thinning (Fig. 9-5).

● Current limitations include difficulty imaging deep vasculature of the optic disc because of shadow interference from the larger and overlying central retinal vessels, flow index of the optic disc may include retinal microvasculature, difficulty distinguishing between decreased vascularity because of tissue loss versus ischemia, vascular leakage cannot be assessed, and no longitudinal studies of glaucoma progression have been performed, thus resulting in unknown prognostic ability.

● It does not provide a comprehensive assessment of all significant vascular beds in glaucoma; therefore, reductions in vascularity may represent a consequence of decreased upstream blood flow.

BIBLIOGRAPHY

Koustenis A, Harris A, Gross J, et al. Optical coherence tomography angiography: an overview of the technology and an assessment of applications for clinical research. *Br J Ophthalmol.* 2017;101(1):16–20.

Yarmohammadi A, Zangwill LM, Diniz-Filho A, et al. Optical coherence tomography angiography vessel density in healthy, glaucoma suspects, and glaucoma eyes. *Invest Ophthalmol Vis Sci.* 2016;57(9):OCT451–OCT459.

Yarmohammadi A, Zangwill LM, Diniz-Filho A, et al. Relationship between optical coherence tomography angiography vessel density and severity of visual field loss in glaucoma. *Ophthalmology.* 2016;123(12):2498–2508.

Zhang A, Zhang Q, Chen CL, et al. Methods and algorithms for optical coherence tomography-based angiography: a review and comparison. *J Biomed Opt.* 2015;20(10):100901.

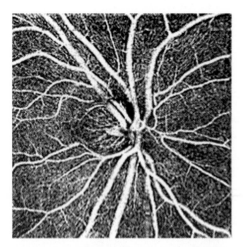

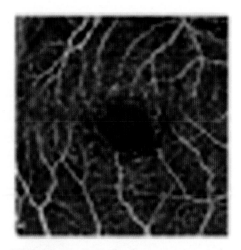

FIGURE 9-2. Optical coherence tomography angiography split-spectrum amplitude-decorrelation angiography in a healthy subject. (Courtesy of Optovue Inc., Fremont, CA.)

FIGURE 9-3. Optical coherence tomography angiography split-spectrum amplitude-decorrelation angiography showing en face colorization that quickly identifies retinal layers. *White*, superficial capillary plexus; *Purple*, deep capillary plexus. (Courtesy of Optovue Inc., Fremont, CA.)

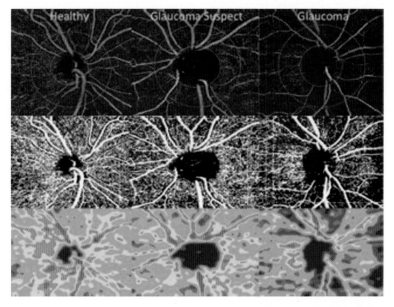

FIGURE 9-4. Optical coherence tomography angiography vessel density demonstrated similar diagnostic accuracy to retinal nerve fiber layer measurements for differentiating between healthy and glaucoma. (From Yarmohammadi A, Zangwill LM, Diniz-Filho A, et al. Optical coherence tomography angiography vessel density in healthy, glaucoma suspects, and glaucoma eyes. *Invest Ophthalmol Vis Sci.* 2016;57(9):OCT451–OCT49.)

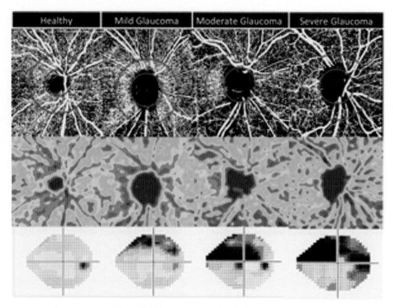

FIGURE 9-5. Optical coherence tomography angiography (OCT-A) glaucoma disease severity with corresponding visual fields: Correlation between vessel densities measured with OCT-A and visual field results, in both healthy controls and glaucomatous patients. Glaucomatous patients of differing disease severity have progressive peripapillary vessel deficits that correspond to greater relative visual field loss. This demonstrates a relationship between structural changes and functional changes. (Yarmohammadi A, Zangwill LM, Diniz-Filho A, et al. Relationship between optical coherence tomography angiography vessel density and severity of visual field loss in glaucoma. *Ophthalmology.* 2016;123(12):2498–2508.)

SPECTRAL RETINAL OXIMETRY

Purpose

- Evaluate ocular tension in the retina and optic nerve head

Description

Measurement of ocular blood flow aims to provide inferential information about tissue metabolic status and possible ischemic affects. However, retinal oximetry is a highly reproducible technique that provides an assessment of ocular tissue metabolic status by measuring light absorption in the retinal vessels and calculating oxygen saturation, and is a step toward understanding the true impact of ischemia on retinal cellular pathophysiology. A standard digital fundus photograph is performed, and four equivalent images are recorded and filtered to isolate particular frequencies. The frequencies of interest include the frequency at which oxygenated and deoxygenated hemoglobin reflect identically, and the frequency at which oxygenated hemoglobin reflection is maximized when compared with deoxygenated hemoglobin reflection. The optical density, or absorbance of light, is then determined for the retinal vasculature using an algorithm that follows the path of reflected light along vessels. A ratio between the optical densities of two of the images is used to determine the oxygen saturation (Fig. 9-6).

- Studies of glaucoma (open-angle, normal pressure) patients demonstrated higher baseline mean SO_2 in retinal veins and decreased arteriovenous SO_2 difference compared to healthy subjects.

- In glaucoma patients, correlations were found between worsening rim area, RNFL thickness, and visual field defects with increased SO_2 in retinal venules and decreased arteriovenous SO_2 difference.

- Higher venous oxygen saturation has been found in glaucoma patients of African descent compared to European descent (Fig. 9-7).

- Current limitations include lack of longitudinal studies, thereby limiting the understanding of oxygen utilization in glaucoma conversion and progression.

BIBLIOGRAPHY

Abegao Pinto L, Willekens K. Van Keer K, et al. Ocular blood flow in glaucoma—the Leuven Eye Study. *Acta Ophthalmol.* 2016;94(6):592–598.

Goharian I, Iverson SM, Ruiz RC, Kishor K, Greenfield DS, Sehi M. Reproducibility of retinal oxygen saturation in normal and treated glaucomatous eyes. *Br J Ophthalmol.* 2015;99(3):318–322.

Ramm L, Jentsch S, Peters S, Augsten R, Hammer M. Investigation of blood flow regulation and oxygen saturation of the retinal vessels in primary open-angle glaucoma. *Graefes Arch Clin Exp Ophthalmol.* 2014;252(11):1803–1810.

Siesky BA, Harris A, Racette L, et al. *Retinal Oximetry in Primary Open-Angle Glaucoma: Differences in Patients of African and European Descent* [Abstract 4471]. Rockville, MD: Association for Research in Vision and Ophthalmology; 2013.

Tobe LA, Harris A, Scroeder A, et al. Retinal oxygen saturation and metabolism: how does it pertain to glaucoma? An update on the application of retinal oximetry in glaucoma. *Eur J Ophthalmol.* 2013;23(4):465–472.

Vandewalle E, Abegao Pinto L, Olafsdottir OB, et al. Oximetry in glaucoma: correlation of metabolic change with structural and functional damage. *Acta Ophthalmol.* 2014;92(2):105–110.

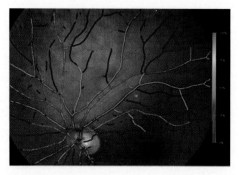

FIGURE 9-6. **Spectral retinal oximetry.** Healthy individual demonstrating normal oxygen saturation in the retinal arteries (*red*) and veins (*green*). (Courtesy of Glaucoma Research and Diagnostic Center.)

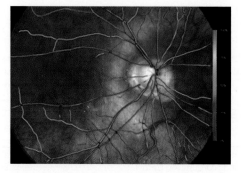

FIGURE 9-7. **Spectral retinal oximetry.** Glaucoma patient of African descent with elevated oxygen saturation in the retinal veins. (Courtesy of Glaucoma Research and Diagnostic Center.)

DOPPLER OPTICAL COHERENCE TOMOGRAPHY

Purpose

• To assess volumetric blood flow in retinal vessels

Description

• This methodology couples a measurement of Doppler frequency shift of light reflecting from moving red blood cells with optical coherence tomography (OCT) to provide volumetric blood flow measurement in absolute units.

• The OCT obtains cross-sectional images of a given blood vessel, and a Doppler analysis provides the velocity of blood flow in the vessel. The area and velocity measurements are combined to derive the blood flow in that vessel. By analyzing the blood flow in each of the major vessels, total retinal blood flow, as well as blood flow in a single quadrant or hemisphere, can be determined.

• Studies in glaucoma patients have shown reduced total retinal blood flow associated with disease progression and visual field loss.

• The major advantages of this method are that it measures retinal blood flow in absolute units and that it is noninvasive. Limitations include sensitivity to anatomic artifacts, such as eye movements, and that it has not yet been sufficiently validated.

BIBLIOGRAPHY

Mohindroo C, Ichhpujani P, Kumar S. Current imaging modalities for assessing ocular blood flow in glaucoma. *J Curr Glaucoma Pract.* 2016;10(3):104–112.

Wang Y, Lu A, Gil-Flamer J, Tan O, Izatt JA, Huang D. Measurement of total blood flow in the normal human retina using Doppler Fourier-domain optical coherence tomography. *Br J Ophthalmol.* 2009;93:634–637.

CONFOCAL SCANNING LASER DOPPLER FLOWMETRY

Purpose

- To assess capillary perfusion in the retina, optic nerve head, and choroid

Description

- Confocal scanning laser Doppler flowmetry (CSLDF) uses an infrared laser to evaluate retinal capillary blood flow. By combining a laser Doppler device with a scanning laser tomograph, CSLDF enhances the ability of the system to exclude choroidal blood flow when measuring retinal capillaries.

- The Heidelberg retinal flowmeter (HRF) is a commonly utilized CSLDF device (Fig. 9-8) that employs a 790-nm laser to scan each pixel within the targeted area of the retina. Using this method, volumetric blood flow can then be calculated using the frequencies in the Doppler-shifted spectra (which signify the velocities of blood cells) together with the signal amplitude at each frequency (which signify the proportion of the blood cells at each velocity) (Fig. 9-9).

- Studies have shown lower blood flow velocities in and around the optic nerve head in glaucoma patients. In addition, a recent study found strong correlations between retinal blood blow and structural changes in glaucoma patients of African descent.

- A significant limitation of CSLDF is that volumetric blood flow is measured in relative, not absolute, units. In addition, these imaging systems are no longer in commercial production.

BIBLIOGRAPHY

Logan JF, Rankin SJ, Jackson AJ. Retinal blood flow measurements and neuroretinal rim damage in glaucoma. *Br J Ophthalmol.* 2004;88(8):1049–1054.

Siesky B, Harris A, Carr J, et al. Reductions in retrobulbar and retinal capillary blood flow strongly correlate with changes in optic nerve head and retinal morphology over 4 years in open-angle glaucoma patients of African descent compared with patients of European descent. *J Glaucoma.* 2016;25(9):750–757.

Zion IB, Harris A, Moore D, et al. Interobserver repeatability of Heidelberg retinal flowmetry using pixel-by-pixel analysis. *J Glaucoma.* 2009;18:280–283.

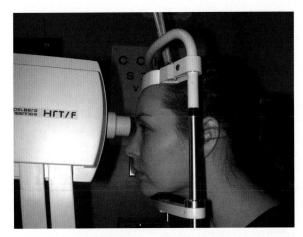

FIGURE 9-8. Heidelberg retinal flowmeter (HRF). The HRF combines a laser Doppler device with a scanning laser tomograph to measure retinal capillary blood flow, velocity, and volume.

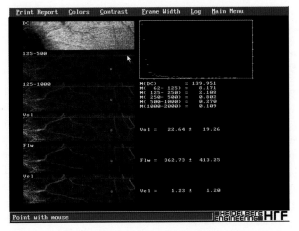

FIGURE 9-9. Heidelberg retinal flowmeter. The amplitudes of Doppler-shifted frequencies caused by moving blood cells are used to create a flow map of the peripapillary retina and optic disc.

SCANNING LASER OPHTHALMOSCOPE ANGIOGRAPHY

Scanning laser ophthalmoscope angiography builds upon fluorescein angiography and uses a low-power argon laser beam to achieve better penetration through lens and corneal opacities (Fig. 9-10) than do traditional photographic or video angiography techniques. The laser frequency, which is chosen according to properties of the injected dye, is reflected off the dye and exits the pupil where a detector measures the intensity of the light in real time and is then analyzed off-line to obtain measurements such as arteriovenous passage (AVP) time and mean dye velocity.

Fluorescein Scanning Laser Ophthalmoscope Angiography

Purpose

- Evaluation of retinal hemodynamics

Description

- High clarity allows isolation of individual retinal vessels in both the superior and inferior retina (Fig. 9-11). AVP represents the amount of time between the first appearance of dye in a retinal artery and its appearance in the associated vein that allows localization of measurements to a specific retinal quadrant,

and it has been shown to be sensitive to small changes in retinal blood flow (Fig. 9-12). Mean dye velocity evaluates the average speed of blood flowing through large retinal vessels by measuring the amount of time the dye takes to travel between two locations on the same retinal artery.

Indocyanine Green Scanning Laser Ophthalmoscope Angiography

Purpose

- Evaluation of choroidal hemodynamics

Description

- Indocyanine green (ICG) dye is used in conjunction with a higher penetrating laser beam frequency than that of the fluorescein dye to optimize visualization of the choroidal vasculature (Fig. 9-13). ICG has an increased affinity for plasma proteins, reducing leakage of the dye from choroidal vessels into surrounding tissue.

- Area dilution analysis (Fig. 9-14) measures the brightness of six areas in the optic disc and macula to determine the time required to reach predefined levels of brightness (10% and 63%). The six areas are then compared to each other to determine their relative brightness. Relative comparisons are possible because all data are collected through an identical optical system with all six areas filmed simultaneously.

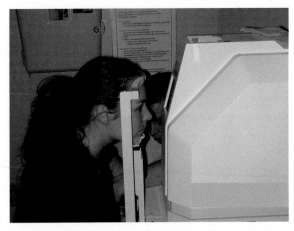

FIGURE 9-10. **Scanning laser ophthalmoscope (SLO) angiography.** The SLO can use either fluorescein or Indocyanine green dye to analyze retinal or choroidal vessels.

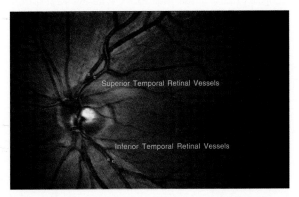

FIGURE 9-11. **Fluorescein scanning laser ophthalmoscope (SLO) angiography.** Fluorescein SLO angiography provides high-clarity visualization of retinal vessels.

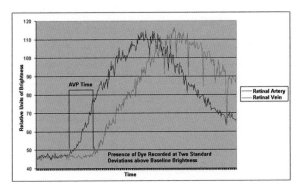

FIGURE 9-12. **Arteriovenous passage (AVP) time.** AVP time equals the time differences in dye arrival between the isolated retinal artery and adjacent retinal vein.

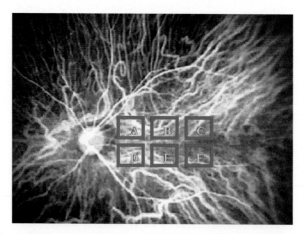

FIGURE 9-13. Indocyanine green scanning laser ophthalmoscope (SLO) angiography. Indocyanine green SLO angiography allows analysis of six areas of the choroid: two areas near the optic disc, and four areas centered around the macula. **A.** Superior temporal peripapillary area. **B.** Superior nasal macula. **C.** Superior temporal macula. **D.** Inferior temporal peripapillary area. **E.** Inferior nasal macula. **F.** Inferior temporal macula.

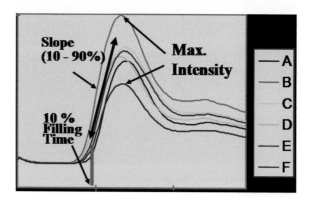

FIGURE 9-14. Area dilution analysis. Area dilution analysis measures the brightness of an area to determine the time required to reach predefined levels of brightness (10% and 63%). It also allows relative brightness comparisons to be made between the six areas.

COLOR DOPPLER IMAGING

Purpose

- Evaluation of retrobulbar vessels, specifically the ophthalmic, central retinal, and nasal and temporal short posterior ciliary arteries.

Description

- Color Doppler imaging (CDI) is a noninvasive ultrasound technique that combines two-dimensional structural ultrasound imaging (B-scan) with superimposed color-coded Doppler to measure blood flow velocity. Measurements are generally taken with the patient in a reclined position using a multifunctional probe (**Fig. 9-15**). The velocity data are graphed against time, and the peak and trough are identified as the peak systolic velocity (PSV) and end diastolic velocity (EDV) (**Fig. 9-16**). Pourcelot resistive index (RI) is a measure of downstream resistance that is calculated as PSV – EDV/PSV.

- CDI has been shown to be reliable and reproducible, and several longitudinal studies have shown predictive properties of its parameters in glaucoma progression, especially in patients of African descent.

- Limitations of CDI include the inability to assess volumetric blood flow due to lack of vessel diameter.

BIBLIOGRAPHY

Ehrlich R, Harris A, Siesky BA, et al. Repeatability of retrobulbar blood flow velocity measured using color Doppler imaging in the Indianapolis glaucoma progression study. *J Glaucoma.* 2011;20(9):540–547.

Moore NA, Harris A, Wentz S, et al. Baseline retrobulbar blood flow is associated with both functional and structural glaucomatous progression after 4 years. *Br J Ophthalmol.* 2017;101(3):305–308.

Siesky B, Harris A, Carr J, et al. Reductions in retrobulbar and retinal capillary blood flow strongly correlate with changes in optic nerve head and retinal morphology over 4 years in open-angle glaucoma patients of African descent compared with patients of European descent. *J Glaucoma.* 2016;25(9):750–757.

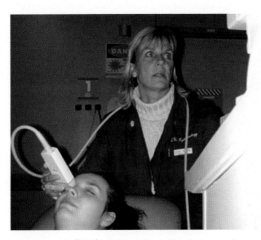

FIGURE 9-15. **Color Doppler imaging (CDI).** CDI is performed by placing a probe over the closed eye with coupling gel.

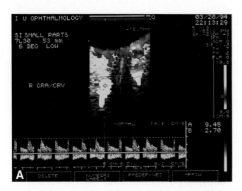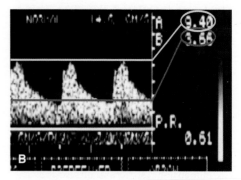

FIGURE 9-16. Color Doppler imaging (CDI). A. Specific retrobulbar vessels can be chosen with CDI. These include the ophthalmic, central retinal, and nasal and temporal short posterior ciliary arteries. **B.** Peak systolic velocity (PSV) and end diastolic velocity (EDV) are taken from the peak and trough of the velocity plot, and Pourcelot RI can then be calculated as PSV – EDV/PSV.

MEASUREMENT OF OCULAR PULSATION (PULSATILE OCULAR BLOOD FLOW)

Purpose

● Estimation of choroidal blood flow

Description

● Pulsatile ocular blood flow is a nonimaging modality that measures ocular pulse amplitude (peak to trough of IOP), and provides an estimate of total orbital pulse, which has been (unconfirmed) used to estimate choroidal blood flow.

BIBLIOGRAPHY

Zion IB, Harris A, Siesky B, et al. Pulsatile ocular blood flow: Relationship with flow velocities in vessels supplying the retina and choroid. *Br J Ophthalmol.* 2007;91:882–884.

DISCLOSURES

There are no conflicts of interest. Dr. Alon Harris would like to disclose that he receives remuneration from AdOM and SHIRE and CIPLA for serving as a consultant. Dr. Harris also holds an ownership interest in AdOM, Nano Retina, and Oxymap. All relationships listed above are pursuant to Indiana University's policy on outside activities.

Section II ■ Clinical Syndromes

Introduction to Clinical Syndromes

Douglas J. Rhee ■

The glaucoma syndromes are divided into two main groups: primary and secondary. The primary glaucomas are those for which the cause of increased resistance to outflow and elevated intraocular pressure (IOP) is unknown. The secondary glaucomas are associated with known ocular or systemic conditions responsible for the elevated IOP and resistance to outflow.

Primary open-angle glaucoma is the most common form of glaucoma in the United States. It constitutes about two-thirds of all cases of glaucoma. This particular disease is probably the final common pathway for a variety of yet undistinguished separate pathophysiologic processes. As our understanding of the genetic and pathophysiologic components continues to expand, I predict that we will eventually distinguish several other conditions with these characteristic optic nerve and visual field defects.

To date, our best understanding is that the damage and functional loss from glaucoma are caused by some combination of a sensitivity to barotrauma of retinal ganglion cell axons at the lamina cribrosa and a relative elevation of IOP, for example, a relative IOP increase as a result of aging and senescence of the drainage system— (1) children never have ocular hypertension (adjusted for central corneal thickness–induced measurement artifact) as a normal state and (2) even in low-tension glaucoma, the lowering of IOP reduces the progression of optic nerve and visual field damage.

Since the late 1950s, it has been understood that primary pathophysiology of all high IOP glaucomas is inhibited aqueous drainage. In primary open-angle glaucoma, the pathophysiology is an alteration and accumulation of extracellular matrix in the juxtacanalicular trabecular meshwork (TM); other mechanisms, such as increased cell and tissue rigidity within the juxtacanalicular region and a decreased number of TM cells, are being elucidated. To date, there have been no pathologic findings within the uveoscleral outflow pathway or aqueous hypersecretion. Our understanding of the molecular mechanisms responsible for this pathophysiology improves as molecular biologic and genetic studies continue.

In secondary open-angle glaucomas, the pathophysiologic mechanisms still affect the drainage system such as deposition of pseudoexfoliative material in the juxtacanalicular region (i.e., pseudoexfoliative glaucoma), loss of TM cells leading to fusion of TM beams (i.e., pigmentary and open-angle inflammatory glaucomas), and so on. Steroid-induced glaucoma leads to accumulations of aberrant extracellular matrix in the juxtacanalicular region through several different mechanisms.

The chapters in this section include representative photographs and briefly describe the major glaucoma syndromes:

- Congenital glaucomas
- Primary open-angle glaucoma
- Secondary open-angle glaucoma
- Inflammatory glaucomas
- Lens-associated glaucomas
- Uveitic glaucomas
- Primary angle-closure glaucoma
- Secondary angle-closure glaucoma

Childhood Glaucomas (Congenital Glaucomas)

Oscar V. Beaujon-Balbi, Oscar Beaujon-Rubin, Claudia L. Pabon, and Douglas J. Rhee ■

INTRODUCTION

The World Glaucoma Association defines Childhood Glaucoma as a related intraocular pressure damage to the eye. This definition was adopted as a result of a consensus made in 2013. Developmental glaucomas are a group of conditions characterized by a developmental abnormality of the aqueous outflow system of the eye. This group includes the following:

● Congenital glaucoma, in which the developmental abnormality of the anterior chamber angle is not associated with other ocular or systemic anomalies

● Developmental glaucomas with associated anomalies, in which ocular or systemic anomalies are present

● Secondary glaucomas of childhood, in which other ocular pathologies are the cause of the impairment of the aqueous outflow

Several different systems are used to classify developmental glaucomas. The most common are the Shaffer–Weiss and the Hoskin anatomic classifications. The former divides congenital glaucoma into three major groups:

■ Primary congenital glaucoma (PCG)

■ Glaucoma associated with congenital anomalies

■ Secondary glaucomas of childhood

The latter defines the actual developmental disorder clinically evident at the time of examination and also includes three groups:

● Isolated trabeculodysgenesis with malformation of the trabecular meshwork in the absence of iris or corneal anomalies

● Iridotrabeculodysgenesis that includes angle and iris anomalies

● Corneotrabeculodysgenesis, usually associated with iris anomalies

The identification of anatomic defects can be useful in determining the appropriate therapy and prognostic factors. The world Glaucoma Association, as a result of consensus made in 2013, classifies childhood glaucoma as primary and secondary glaucomas. The latest are subdivided according to whether the condition is present at birth or is acquired after birth. Nonacquired glaucomas are then classified as associated to ocular or systemic signs.

PRIMARY CONGENITAL GLAUCOMA

PCG is the most common form of infantile glaucoma, representing 50% of all cases of congenital glaucoma. It is characterized by a trabecular meshwork anomaly and is not associated with other ocular or systemic diseases. Seventy-five percent of PCG cases occur bilaterally.

Epidemiology

• The incidence is 1 in 5,000 to 10,000 live births. More than 80% of cases present before 1 year of age: 40% at birth, 70% between 1 and 6 months, and 80% before 1 year.

• The disorder is more common in males (70% males, 30% females), and 90% of cases are sporadic, without a family history.

• Although an autosomal-recessive model with variable penetrance has been suggested, it is thought that most of the cases are the result of multifactorial inheritance with nongenetic factors involved (e.g., environmental factors).

History

• Epiphora, photophobia, and blepharospasm form the classic triad.

• Usually, children with congenital glaucoma prefer dimly lit places and avoid exposure to intense light. The caregiver may describe an excessive amount of tearing.

• In unilateral cases, the mother may note an asymmetry between eyes, referring to an enlarged (affected side) or decreased (normal side) eye size (Fig. 11-1).

Clinical Examination

Initial evaluation is usually done at the office. The child may have at least one of the symptoms as photophobia, tearing, and blepharospasm. Sometimes big eyes or bupthalmos are the main complaint. The physician may evaluate visual acuity according to age, as pupil contraction at light stimulus at birth, light fixation around 3 months of age. Inspection for systemic and facial associations and evaluation at the slit lamp, to evaluate cornea transparency, anterior chamber configuration, iris, and crystalline lens. Intraocular pressure can be measured at the office using the Tono-Pen and recently the use of rebound tonometry, which does not require fluorescein nor topical anesthesic drops (Fig. 11-2).

If posible, an ultrasound evaluation can be performed to determine axial length. If the axial length is higher than expected for age, glaucoma is one potential cause. An evaluation under anesthesia must be performed in children who cannot be fully evaluated in the office. This is often followed by a surgical intervention to treat the glaucoma at the same session (Fig. 11-3).

• The normal horizontal corneal diameter in a full-term newborn is 10 to 10.5 mm. This increases to the adult diameter of approximately 11.5 to 12 mm by 2 years of age. A diameter greater than 12 mm in an infant is highly suggestive of congenital glaucoma.

• Measurements of the cornea are made in the horizontal meridian with calipers. Other findings include corneal cloudiness, tears in the Descemet membrane (Haab striae), deep anterior chamber, intraocular pressure greater than 21 mm Hg, iris stroma hypoplasia, isolated trabeculodysgenesis on gonioscopy, and increased optic nerve cupping. Haab striae may be single or multiple and are characteristically oriented horizontally or concentrically to the limbus (Figs. 11-4 and 11-5).

• Optic nerve evaluation is a very important part of the glaucoma evaluation. Glaucomatous disc changes occur more rapidly in infants and at lower pressures than in older children or adults. Cup-to-disc ratios greater than 0.3 are rare in normal infants and must be considered suspicious for glaucoma. Asymmetry of optic nerve cupping is also suggestive of glaucoma, particularly differences of greater than 0.2 between the two eyes. The glaucomatous cupping may be oval in configuration but is more often round and central (Fig. 11-6). Reversal of optic nerve cupping has been observed after normalization of intraocular pressure.

- Evaluation of the anterior chamber angle is essential for an accurate diagnosis and treatment. The developmental anomalies can present in two major forms: (1) flat iris insertion, in which the iris inserts directly or anterior to the trabecular meshwork with iris processes that can overcome the scleral spur (Fig. 11-7A) and (2) concave iris insertion, in which the iris is observed behind the trabecular meshwork but is covered with a dense abnormal tissue (Fig. 11-7B). For comparison, a gonioscopic photograph of a normal anterior chamber angle from an infant is also presented (Fig. 11-8).

- Elevation of the intraocular pressure causes rapid enlargement of the globe with progressive enlargement of the cornea in children younger than 3 years. As the cornea enlarges, stretching leads to ruptures in Descemet membrane, epithelial and stromal edema, and corneal clouding. The iris is stretched so that the stroma appears thinned. The scleral canal through which the optic nerve passes also enlarges with elevated intraocular pressure. This results in rapid cupping of the optic nerve, which can quickly reverse if the intraocular pressure is normalized.

  ▪ This dramatic reversal in cupping is not seen in adult eyes and is probably related to the greater elasticity of the optic nerve head connective tissue in the infant. If the intraocular pressure is not controlled, a buphthalmos can develop (Fig. 11-9; see also Fig. 11-1).

Differential Diagnosis

- Other causes of corneal changes include megalocornea, metabolic diseases, corneal dystrophies, obstetric trauma, and keratitis.

- Epiphora or photophobia may occur in nasolacrimal duct obstruction, dacryocystitis, and iritis.

- Optic nerve anomalies simulating a glaucomatous nerve include optic pits, colobomas, and hypoplasia.

Management

- The treatment of congenital glaucoma is surgical. Medical treatment can be used for a limited time while the surgery is being scheduled.

- Procedures that involve trabecular incisions are the choice in this condition.

  ▪ Goniotomy requires a clear cornea for visualization of the angle.

  ▪ Trabeculectomy with an external approach to Schlemm canal does not require corneal transparency.

- The goniotomy is performed using a goniotome and direct gonioscopy lens. Traditionally, a Barkan goniolens is preferred. An incision is made in the dense abnormal tissue at the trabecular meshwork for an extension of 90 to 180 degrees using the goniotome through clear cornea (Figs. 11-10 and 11-11).

- Alternatively, a modified Swan-Jacob lens can be used with a sharp blade, for example, MVR blade, Wheeler knife, or even a 30-gauge needle. The advantage of a flat blade is that it will create less distortion of the corneal wound and allow the wound to be closed more easily (Fig. 11-12).

- For a patient with cloudy or opacified corneas, trabeculotomy is indicated. A scleral flap is made and Schlemm canal must be found to perform the procedure. The trabecular meshwork is broken using a trabeculotome (Fig. 11-13) or by using a suture (usually propylene) through Schlemm canal (Lynch procedure). An alternative to suture trabeculotomy is to use a fiberoptic catheter (iCath, iScience), which has the advantage of an illuminated tip that identifies the location of the catheter (Fig. 11-14). At present, we perform a surgical technique similar to canaloplasty. We have found it to be effective to perform a scleral flap of 3 × 3 mm at 50% thickness and a second deeper flap of 2 mm extending to the clear cornea. The Sclemm canal is found and viscodilated to pass the illuminated catheter in 360 grades and pulled

through to incise the trabecular meshwork all around (Fig. 11-15). The deeper flap is excised and the first flap is tightly closed (Figs. 11-15 and 11-16).

● In cases where Schlemm canal is not found, trabeculectomy is performed. Another choice is the placement of a valved or nonvalved glaucoma-filtering device (Fig. 11-17).

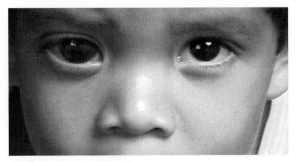

FIGURE 11-1. **Unilateral primary congenital glaucoma.** This photograph demonstrates a cloudy cornea and buphthalmos.

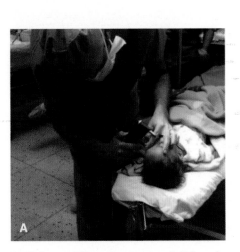

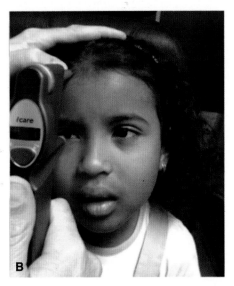

FIGURE 11-2. **Rebound tonometry. A.** Rebound tonometry during the induction before general anesthetics. **B.** Using the rebound tonometer at the office.

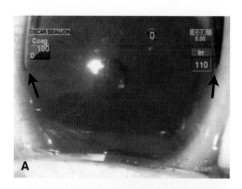

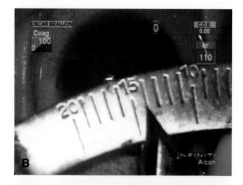

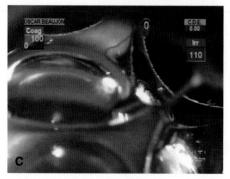

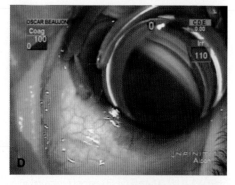

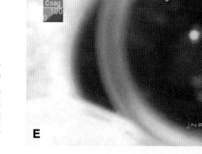

FIGURE 11-3. Evaluation under anesthesia. A and **B.** Measuring corneal diameter with caliper (*black arrows* identify the tips of the caliper). **C.** Gonioscopy with a four-mirror lens. **D.** Gonioscopy with a Transcend Volk Goniolens (TVG) surgical goniolens. **E.** Optic disc and retina observation using a handheld lens and the operating room (OR) microscope.

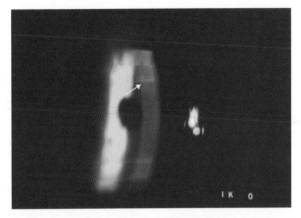

FIGURE 11-4. **Haab striae.** *Arrow* indicates break in Descemet membrane.

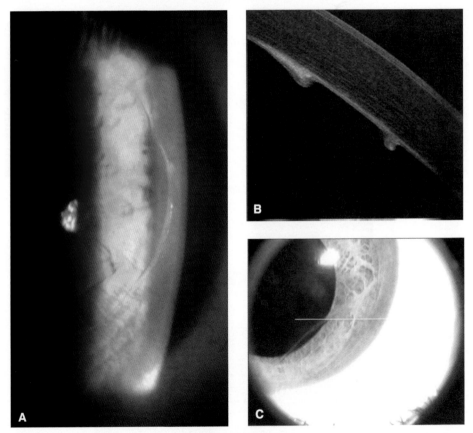

FIGURE 11-5. **Haab striae. A.** Haab striae concentrically to the limbus. **B.** Optical coherent tomography of striae with Descemet scrolls at both borders. **C.** Area evaluated by the cross section showed on **B.**

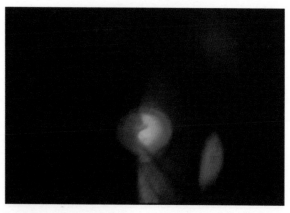

FIGURE 11-6. **Round cupping.** Round cupping in congenital glaucoma.

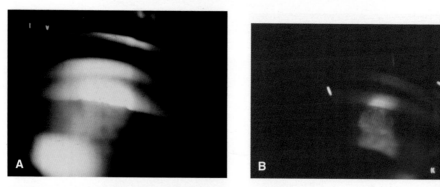

FIGURE 11-7. **Gonioscopy. A.** Flat iris insertion. **B.** Concave iris insertion.

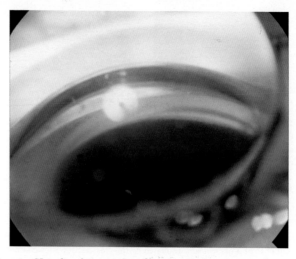

FIGURE 11-8. **Gonioscopy.** Note the relative paucity of anterior chamber pigment of a normal anterior chamber angle in an infant.

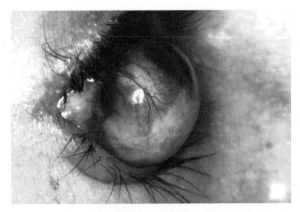

FIGURE 11-9. Buphthalmos. An extreme example of buphthalmos with corneal and scleral thinning.

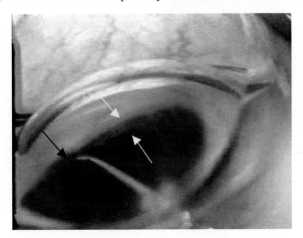

FIGURE 11-10. Congenital glaucoma during goniotomy. Note the difference in angle configuration between the goniotomy-treated portion of trabecular meshwork (*white arrows*) and the nontreated portion (*black arrow*).

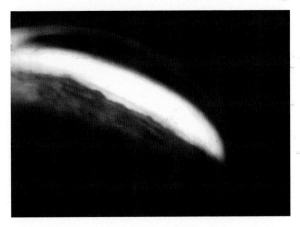

FIGURE 11-11. Angle visualization. Visualization of the angle after goniotomy.

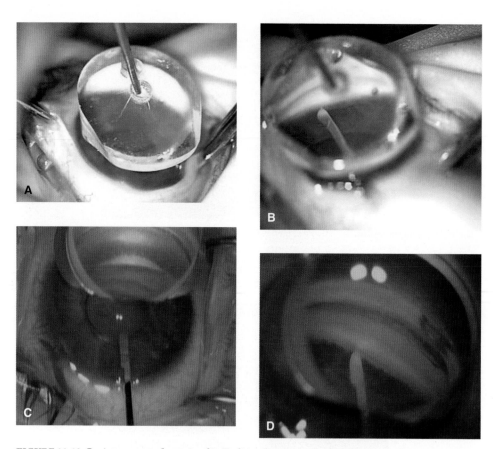

FIGURE 11-12. Goniotomy procedures. A and **B.** Traditional goniotomy performed with a Barkan lens, goniotome knife, with fixation of the superior and inferior rectus muscles using locking toothed forceps. This technique relies on an assistant to fixate the forceps and rotate the eye to allow the surgeon access to a wider portion of the angle. **C** and **D.** Alternative method that does not require an assistant using a modified Swan lens and goniotome knife.

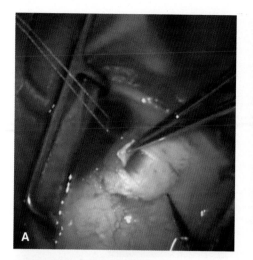

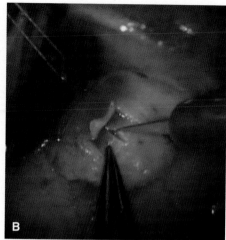

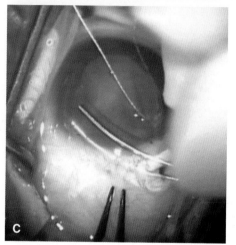

FIGURE 11-13. Mechanical trabeculectomy. A. Partial-thickness dissection over the limbus. **B.** Sharp cut down to Schlemm canal. **C.** Harms trabeculotome is cannulated through into Schlemm canal, then gently passed into the anterior chamber to allow a communication between the anterior chamber and collecting channels.

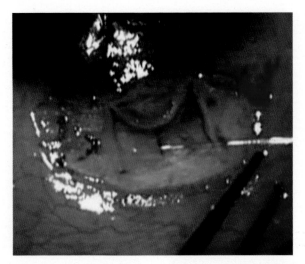

FIGURE 11-14. **Suture trabeculectomy with iTrack.** The red illuminated tip helps identify the location of the catheter.

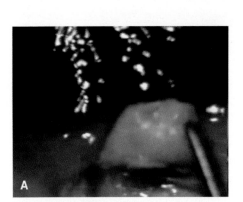

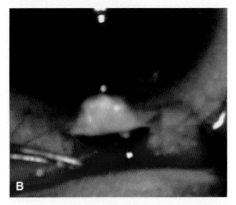

FIGURE 11-15. **360 Degrees Trabeculotomy. A.** The Schlemm canal is viscodilated and the illuminated catheter introduced after excising a deep sclera flap. **B.** Both extremes of the catheter are pulled out excising the trabecular meshwoirk in 360 degrees.

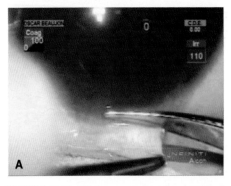

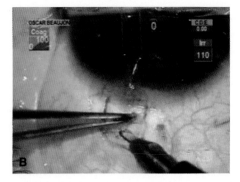

FIGURE 11-16. **360 Degrees trabeculotomy. Surgical technique. A.** Conjunctival incision. **B.** 3 × 3 mm scleral flap at 50% deep.

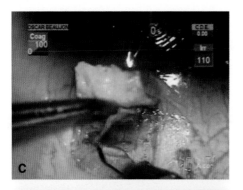

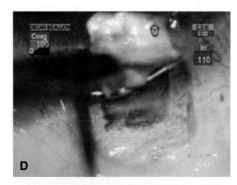

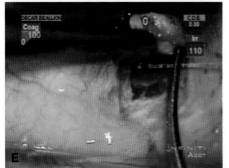

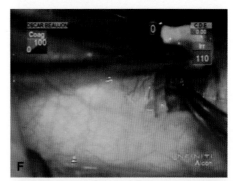

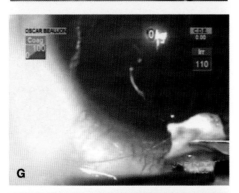

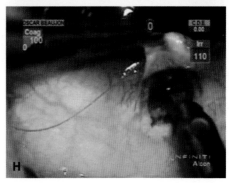

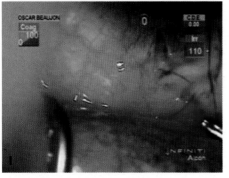

FIGURE 11-16. (*continued*) **C.** 2 × 2 mm deeper scleral flap. **D.** Canalization and viscodilation of Schlemm canal. **E** and **F.** Canalization with illuminated tip in 360 degrees. **G.** Deeper flap excision. **H.** Corneal incision of 1 mm. **I.** Scleral flap closure.

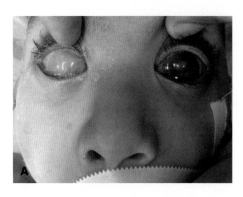

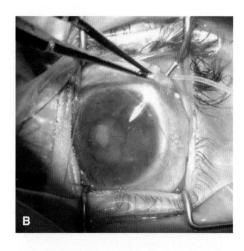

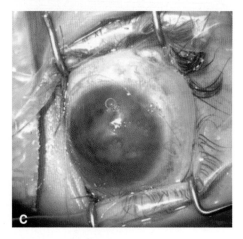

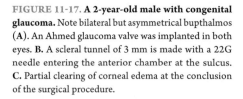

FIGURE 11-17. A 2-year-old male with congenital glaucoma. Note bilateral but asymmetrical bupthalmos (**A**). An Ahmed glaucoma valve was implanted in both eyes. **B.** A scleral tunnel of 3 mm is made with a 22G needle entering the anterior chamber at the sulcus. **C.** Partial clearing of corneal edema at the conclusion of the surgical procedure.

GLAUCOMA ASSOCIATED WITH CONGENITAL ANOMALIES

ANIRIDIA

- Aniridia is a bilateral congenital anomaly in which the iris is markedly underdeveloped, but there is generally a rudimentary iris stump of variable extent visible on examination of the angle (Fig. 11-18).

- Two-thirds of cases are dominantly transmitted with a high-degree penetrance. Twenty percent of the cases are associated with Wilms tumor.

- A deletion of the short arm of chromosome 11 has been associated with Wilms tumor and sporadic aniridia.

- Poor visual acuity is common because of foveal and optic nerve hypoplasia. Other associated ocular conditions include keratopathy, cataract (60% to 80%), and ectopia lentis (Fig. 11-19). Photophobia, nystagmus, decreased vision, and strabismus are common manifestations in aniridia. Progressive corneal opacification and pannus usually occur circumferentially in the periphery (Fig. 11-20).

- Glaucoma associated with aniridia does not usually develop until late childhood or early adulthood. It may be the result of trabeculodysgenesis or of progressive closure of the trabecular meshwork by the residual iris stump. If it develops during infancy, a goniotomy or trabeculectomy may be indicated.

- It has been suggested that early goniotomy may prevent the progressive adherence of the residual peripheral iris to the trabecular meshwork.

- In older children, medical therapy to control intraocular pressure should first be attempted. Any form of surgery has the risk of injuring the unprotected lens and zonules, and filtering procedures have an increased risk of vitreous incarceration. Cyclodestructive procedures may be necessary in certain patients with uncontrolled advanced glaucoma.

AXENFELD ANOMALY

- Axenfeld anomaly is characterized by peripheral cornea, anterior chamber angle, and iris anomalies. A prominent Schwalbe line, referred to as *posterior embryotoxon*, is a peripheral cornea alteration in these patients. Iris strands attaching to the posterior embryotoxon and hypoplasia of the anterior iris stroma may be present.

- The disease is usually bilateral and has an autosomal-dominant inheritance (Fig. 11-21).

- Axenfeld syndrome includes glaucoma and occurs in 50% of patients with the anomaly. If glaucoma occurs in infancy, goniotomy or trabeculectomy is often successful. If glaucoma occurs later, medical therapy should be tried initially, and filtering surgery should be used if needed.

RIEGER ANOMALY

- Rieger anomaly represents a more advanced degree of angle dysgenesis. Besides the clinical aspect observed in Axenfeld anomaly, a marked iris hypoplasia is observed with polycoria and corectopia.

- It is usually bilateral and inherited in an autosomal-dominant pattern, although the anomaly can be present sporadically.

- Glaucoma develops in more than half of cases, often requiring surgery.

RIEGER SYNDROME

- When the findings of Rieger anomaly are associated with systemic malformations, the term *Rieger syndrome* is preferred.

- The most commonly associated systemic anomalies are developmental defects of the teeth and facial bones. Dental abnormalities include a reduction of crown size (microdontia), a decreased but evenly spaced number of teeth, and a focal absence of teeth (commonly the anterior maxillary primary and permanent central incisors; Figs. 11-22 and 11-23).

• Because of the similarity of anterior chamber angle abnormalities in these entities, it has been proposed that they represent a spectrum of developmental disorders that have been named *anterior chamber cleavage syndrome* and *mesodermal dysgenesis of cornea and iris.* They are also referred to as Axenfeld-Rieger syndrome.

PETERS ANOMALY

• Peters anomaly represents a major degree of anterior chamber developmental disorder. A corneal opacity associated with a posterior

stromal defect is present, also known as von Hippel corneal ulcer. The iris is adherent to the cornea at the collarette. The lens can be included on these adhesions with an absent corneal endothelium.

• Peters anomaly is bilateral and frequently associated with glaucoma and cataract.

• Corneal transplant with cataract removal to improve visual acuity has a guarded prognosis. In these cases, a trabeculectomy or glaucoma drainage implant devices are required for glaucoma control (Figs. 11-24 and 11-25).

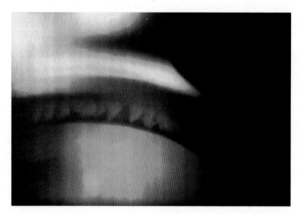

FIGURE 11-18. Aniridia. Gonioscopic photograph showing an iris remnant with ciliary processes below.

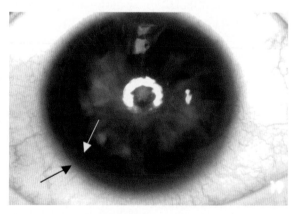

FIGURE 11-19. Aniridia and cataract. *Arrows* indicate the remnant portion of the iris.

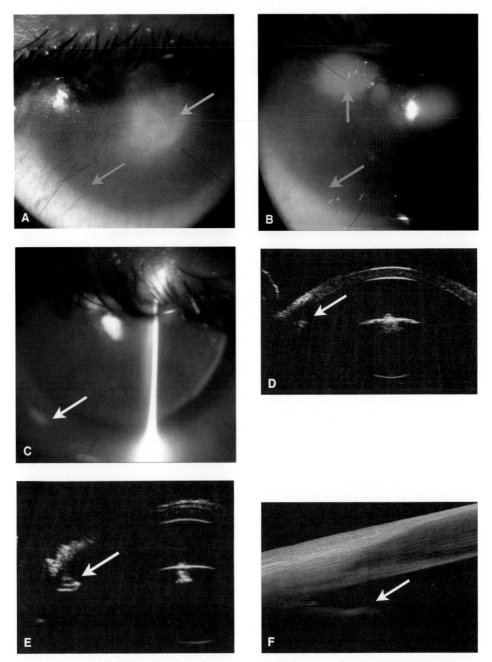

FIGURE 11-20. Patient with aniridia. A and **B.** Images of right and left eye. Pannus (*green arrows*) with leukomas (*blue arrows*). **C.** Aniridia with some remanent iris tissue (*white arrow*). **D** and **E.** Ultrasound biomicroscopy images and optical coherence tomography image (**F**) of the angle with aniridia. **D.** An anterior polar cataract is present. **F.** An iris remnant can be seen.

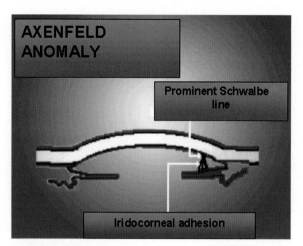

FIGURE 11-21. Axenfeld anomaly diagram.

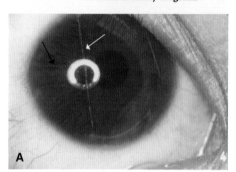 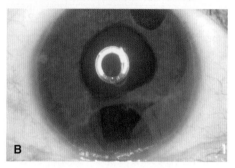

FIGURE 11-22. **Rieger syndrome. A.** Notice prominent anterior embryotoxon (*white arrow*) and iris hypoplasia (*black arrow*). **B.** The mother of the patient in **A** showing prominent anterior embryotoxon, corectopia, and polycoria.

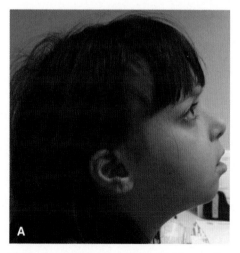 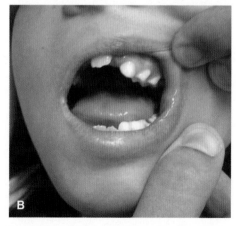

FIGURE 11-23. **Rieger syndrome.** Facial anomalies, maxillary hypoplasia (**left**). Dental anomalies, hypodontia, and anodontia (**right**). (Courtesy of Dr. Adael Soares, Escola Paulista de Medicina, UNIFESP, São Paulo, Brazil.)

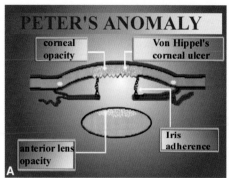
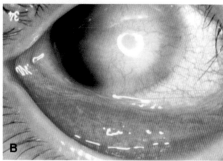

FIGURE 11-24. **Peters anomaly. A.** Diagram of anomaly. **B.** Note the corneal opacity (leukoma), along with corneal pannus.

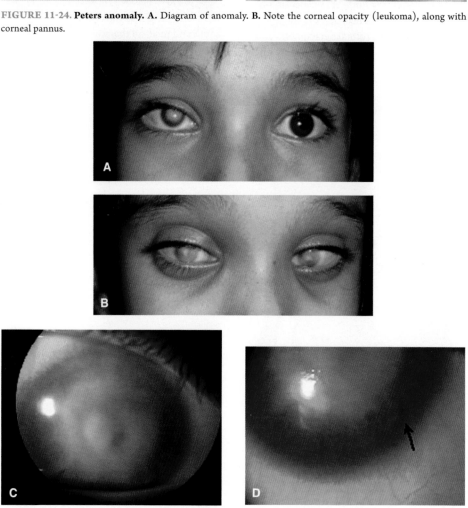

FIGURE 11-25. **Peters anomaly present in fraternal twin female. A.** Unilateral corneal involvement. **B.** Bilateral total corneal opacities. **C.** Central corneal opacification with a relative clear peripheral cornea. **D.** Iris anomalies seen peripherally. **C** and **D** are from the unilateral case in frame **A.**

MARFAN SYNDROME

• Marfan syndrome is characterized by musculoskeletal abnormalities, such as arachnodactyly, excessive height, long extremities, hyperextensive joints, and scoliosis, cardiovascular disease, and ocular abnormalities.

• Transmission is autosomal dominant with high penetrance, although approximately 15% of cases are sporadic (Fig. 11-26).

• Ocular features include ectopia lentis, microphakia, megalocornea, myopia, keratoconus, iris hypoplasia, retinal detachment, and glaucoma (Fig. 11-27). The zonules are often attenuated and broken, leading to upward subluxation of the lens (the lens may also become dislocated into the pupil or anterior chamber, leading to lens-induced glaucoma).

• Open-angle glaucoma may also develop, frequently in childhood or adolescence, and is associated with congenital abnormalities of the anterior chamber angle. Dense iris processes bridge the angle recess, inserting anterior to the scleral spur. Iris tissue sweeping across the recess may have a concave configuration.

• Usually the glaucoma occurs in older childhood, and medical therapy should first be attempted.

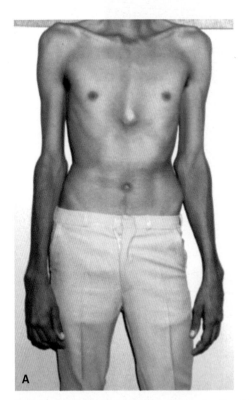

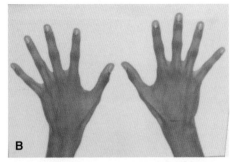

FIGURE 11-26. **Marfan syndrome. A.** Note the tall and thin body habitus; this patient also has pectus excavatum. **B.** Arachnodactyly.

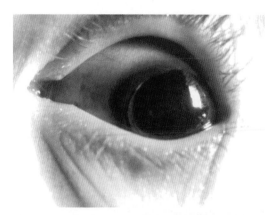

FIGURE 11-27. **Marfan syndrome.** Anterior ectopia lentis. In this eye, the crystalline lens has dislocated anteriorly.

MICROSPHEROPHAKIA

● Microspherophakia may occur as an isolated disorder that is inherited as an autosomal-recessive or -dominant trait or it may be associated with Weill-Marchesani syndrome. This syndrome is characterized by short stature, brachydactyly, brachycephaly, and microspherophakia.

● The lens is small and spherical and may move anteriorly, resulting in pupillary-block glaucoma (Fig. 11-28).

● Angle-closure glaucoma can be treated using mydriatics, iridectomy, or lens extraction.

● Glaucoma usually occurs in late childhood or early adulthood.

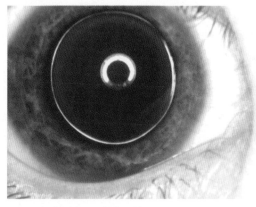

FIGURE 11-28. **Microspherophakia.** The small, round lens can be visualized within the aperture of the dilated pupil.

STURGE-WEBER SYNDROME (ENCEPHALOTRIGEMINAL ANGIOMATOSIS)

- Patients with Sturge-Weber syndrome have a facial hemangioma following the distribution of the trigeminal nerve. The facial hemangioma is usually unilateral but may be bilateral. Conjunctival, episcleral, and choroidal hemangiomas are also common abnormalities. Diffuse uveal involvement has been termed the "tomato-catsup" fundus.

- No clear hereditary pattern has been established.

- Glaucoma more often occurs when the ipsilateral facial hemangioma involves the lids and conjunctiva.

- Glaucoma may occur in infancy, late childhood, or young adulthood. The glaucoma that occurs in infancy looks and behaves like glaucoma associated with isolated trabeculodysgenesis and responds well to goniotomy. The glaucoma that appears later in life is probably related to elevated episcleral venous pressure from arteriovenous fistulas.

- In older children, medical therapy should be attempted first. However, if this is not successful, trabeculectomy should be considered.

- Filtering surgery has an increased risk of choroidal hemorrhage, resulting in shallowing or flattening of the anterior chamber related to the diminution of the intraocular pressure at the moment of surgery. This probably occurs when the intraocular pressure level falls below that of arterial blood pressure and results in effusion of choroidal fluid into surrounding tissues (**Figs. 11-29** and **11-30**).

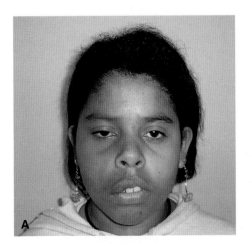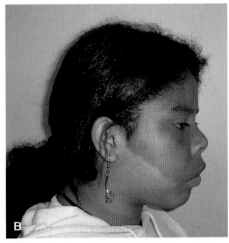

FIGURE 11-29. **A** and **B.** Sturge-Weber syndrome. Note unilateral frontal and maxillary distribution. (Courtesy of Dr. Claudia Pabon Bejarano, Escola Paulista de Medicina, UNIFESP, São Paulo, Brazil.)

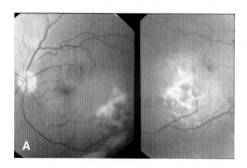

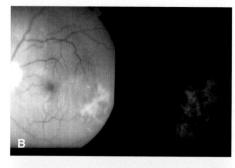

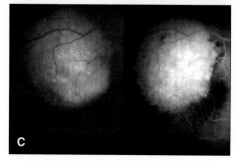

FIGURE 11-30. **Sturge-Weber syndrome. A–C.** Choroid hemangioma. (Courtesy of Dr. Dario Fuenmayor, Caracas, Venezuela.)

NEUROFIBROMATOSIS (VON RECKLINGHAUSEN DISEASE AND BILATERAL ACOUSTIC NEUROFIBROMATOSIS)

- Neurofibromatosis is an inherited disorder of the neuroectodermal system that results in hamartomas of the skin, eyes, and nervous system. The syndrome primarily affects tissue derived from the neural crest, particularly the sensitive nerves, Schwann cells, and melanocytes.

- Neurofibromatosis has two forms: NF-1, or classic von Recklinghausen neurofibromatosis, and NF-2, or bilateral acoustic neurofibromatosis.

  - NF-1 is the most common form and includes involvement of skin with café-au-lait spots and cutaneous neurofibromas, iris hamartomas called Lisch nodules, and optic nerve gliomas (**Fig. 11-31**). NF-1 occurs in an estimated 0.05% of population and has a prevalence of 1 in 30,000. It is inherited in an autosomal-dominant pattern with complete penetrance.

  - NF-2 is less common, with an estimated prevalence of 1 in 50,000.

- Cutaneous involvement includes café-au-lait spots, which appear as hyperpigmented macules on any part of the body and tend to increase in age, and multiple neurofibromas, which are benign tumors of nerve connective tissue and vary from tiny, isolated nodules to huge pedunculus soft-tissue masses.

- Ophthalmic involvement includes the following:

  - Iris hamartomas, clinically observed as bilateral, raised, smooth-surfaced, dome-shaped lesions

  - Plexiform neurofibromas of the upper lid, which appear clinically as an area of thickening of the lid margin with ptosis and an S-shaped deformity

  - Retinal tumors, most commonly astrocytic hamartomas

  - Optic nerve gliomas, which manifest as unilateral decreased visual acuity or strabismus and have been observed in 25% of cases

- Ipsilateral glaucoma is also occasionally seen and is usually associated with plexiform neurofibroma of the upper lid.

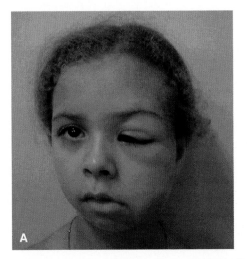
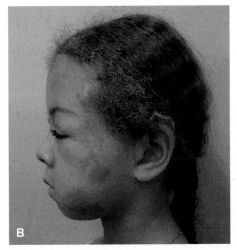

FIGURE 11-31. **Neurofibromatosis. A** and **B.** Note café-au-lait spots and plexiform neurofibroma of the upper lid. (Courtesy of Dr. Claudia Pabon Bejarano, Escola Paulista de Medicina, UNIFESP, São Paulo, Brazil.)

CONGENITAL ANTERIOR STAPHYLOMA AND KERATECTASIA

- Congenital anterior staphyloma and keratectasia are rare, congenital, and usually unilateral conditions resulting in severe corneal protrusion through the eye lids. It's etiology is attributed to intrauterine keratitis. Typically, it present as a progressive central opacity at birth that increases in size, height, and becomes vascularized and secondary keratinized over the following months (Fig. 11-32). Histologically, there is keratinized stratified squamous epithelium, the stroma is highly vascularized and Descemet and endothelium absent with adherence of uveal tissue because of secondary closure glaucoma. The posterior segment is usually normal. A glaucoma device could be placed to control the secondary glaucoma and a penetrating keratoplasty may be attempted to restore corneal structure and transparency.

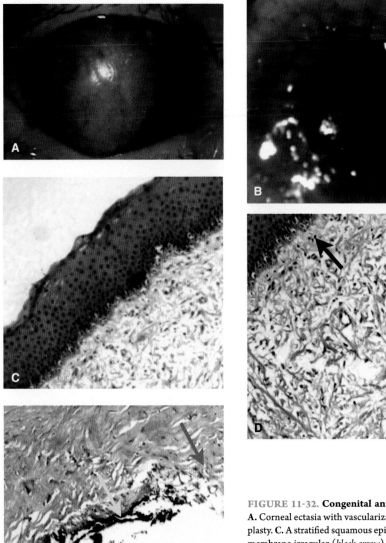

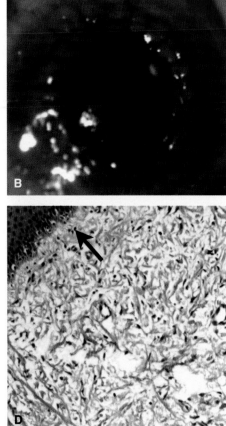

FIGURE 11-32. **Congenital anterior staphyloma.**
A. Corneal ectasia with vascularization. **B.** Postkerato-plasty. **C.** A stratified squamous epithelium. **D.** Bowman membrane irregular (*black arrow*), and vascularization and inflammation of stroma. **E.** Iris and uveal tissue adherence to posterior cornea (*yellow arrow*) and absence of Descemet membrane and endothelium (*red arrow*).

SCLEROCORNEA

● Sclerocornea is a rare, congenital, and usually bilateral nonprogressive, noninflamatory condition. It can be partial or complete, its etiology is unknown, and most cases are sporadic. It clinically manifests with opacification and vascularization of the peripheral cornea; in some cases, the entire cornea can be affected. It is often associated with cornea plana and may have associated glaucoma and anterior segment dysgenesis. The treatment is oriented to controlling the glaucoma. Penetrating keratoplasty could be attempted in bilateral cases but generally has a poor prognosis (Fig. 11-33).

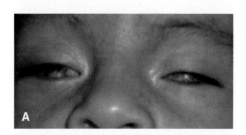 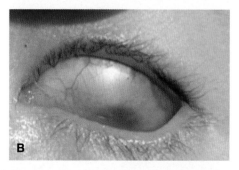

FIGURE 11-33. Sclerocornea. A. Bilateral sclerocornea. **B.** Vascularization of peripheral cornea. (Courtesy of Dr. Pedro Mattar UOCA, Caracas, Venezuela.)

ECTOPIA LENTIS AND ECTOPIA LENTIS ET PUPILLAE

- Ectopia lentis is a displacement of the lens that may be congenital, developmental, or acquired. The lens can be subluxated to where its dislocation to the anterior chamber or pupil may cause pupillary-block and angle-closure glaucoma. It is commonly associated with Marfan syndrome, homocystenuria, aniridia, and congenital glaucoma. It may occur as an isolated anomaly, usually inherited as an autosomal-dominant manner; but could be associated with pupillary abnormalities in ectopia lentis et pupillae, which is an autosomal-recessive disorder where the lens and the pupils are displaced in opposite directions. The pupil is irregular, oval, and displaced from the normal position, usually bilateral but asymmetrical (**Fig. 11-34**).

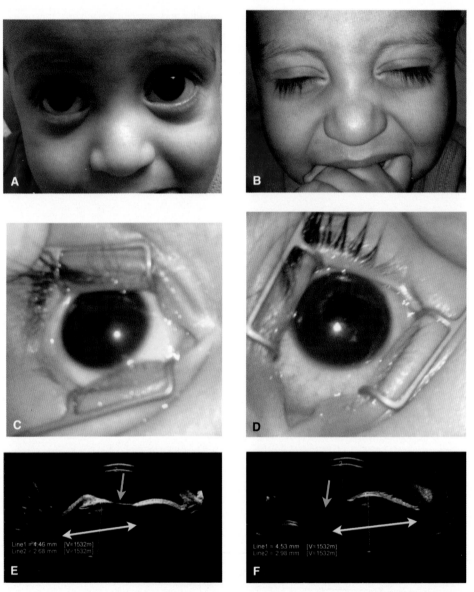

FIGURE 11-34. A 1-year-old male with ectopia lentis et pupillae. A. Fixating on the camera. **B.** Photophobia when the flash is on. Pupils are dislocated superotemporally OD and OS (**C** and **D**), respectively. UBM OD (**E**) and UBM OS (**F**), in both eyes, the crystalline lens (*double-ended yellow arrows*) and pupil (noted by the *green arrows*) are dislocated in the opposite direction. UBM, ultrasound biomicroscopy. OD, right eye; OS, left eye.

Primary Open-Angle Glaucoma

George L. Spaeth and Daniel Lee ■

INTRODUCTION

Glaucoma, in its many forms, is the leading cause of irreversible blindness worldwide. It is a complex family of progressive optic neuropathies where intraocular pressure (IOP) and other contributing factors lead to a characteristic pattern of optic nerve atrophy and visual field loss. Glaucomas are often classified into primary and secondary glaucomas. Primary open-angle glaucoma (POAG) is essentially a diagnosis of exclusion in which no recognizable cause of damaging IOP is identified despite meticulous clinical examination. In many cases, a cause for the pressure that produces damage can be determined, such as inflammation, trauma, or neovascularization. These are often classified as secondary glaucomas and treatment can be directed toward the specific cause. The glaucomas can also be divided on the basis of the nature of the anterior chamber angle. In angle-closure glaucoma, the pressure becomes elevated as a consequence of the resistance to aqueous out-flow due to contact or adhesions between the iris and the trabecular meshwork. In contrast, in the open-angle glaucomas, aqueous humor has clear access to the trabecular meshwork. The primary glaucomas are often further characterized according to the age of onset of the condition. Those occurring at or shortly after birth are termed *congenital*, those occurring after infancy and before age 40 years are termed *juvenile glaucomas*, and those first becoming apparent after the age of 40 are termed *adult-onset open-angle glaucoma*. The glaucomas occurring in infants represent a separate group and are discussed elsewhere in this book (see Chapter 11).

DEFINITION

The definition of glaucoma has changed dramatically since it was first used in ancient Greece; the word has come to mean different things to different people. The definition is still evolving and, as a consequence, there can be unfortunate and disturbing confusions during communication. Figure 12-1 illustrates a rough timeline of these changes.

Until the late 19th century, the definition of glaucoma was based largely on the presence of symptoms such as blindness or pain. The development of statistical theory, the availability of the tonometer, and the concept of disease as a "deviation from normal," all led to glaucoma being defined solely in terms of elevated IOP above 21 or 24 mm Hg, pressures greater than two and three standard deviations above the mean, respectively.

Studies conducted largely in the 1960s showed that only around 5% of individuals with an IOP above 21 mm Hg actually developed optic nerve damage and visual field loss. Other studies showed that around one-third of the patients who had characteristic optic nerve and visual field changes of glaucoma had IOPs in the range of normal. These two observations forced a total rethinking of the definition of glaucoma. Many authors began using the terms "low-tension glaucoma" or "normal-pressure glaucoma" or "high-tension glaucoma." As more attention became focused on the idea of glaucoma as an "optic neuropathy," the idea that glaucoma could be related solely to elevated pressure, as occurs in the angle-closure glaucomas, became less recognized. This led to the strange situation of a person with an IOP of 80 mm Hg in exquisite pain being considered to have "angle closure," but not being considered to have "angle-closure glaucoma." Recently, some authors have sub-divided glaucoma into pressure-dependent and pressure-independent types. Although it is certain that there are factors that increase or decrease the susceptibility of the ocular tissues to damage by IOP, it is not clear that these factors ever act alone and without some contribution from the effects of IOP, even when the IOP is in the normal or subnormal range.

In Figure 12-1, glaucoma is defined as the process leading to characteristic progressive ocular tissue damage, at least partially caused by IOP, regardless of the level of IOP. Findings and symptoms of early or moderate glaucoma are found in almost all people, even those who do not have glaucoma. There is nothing diagnostic, for example, about a cup-to-disc ratio of 0.5. Although this could represent a significant glaucomatous change, it may also occur in a person without glaucoma. Furthermore, there is nothing diagnostic about an IOP of 25 mm Hg. This is a common finding in people who do not have glaucoma. Thus, identification of characteristics that occur *only* (or almost only) in glaucoma is important (Fig. 12-2).

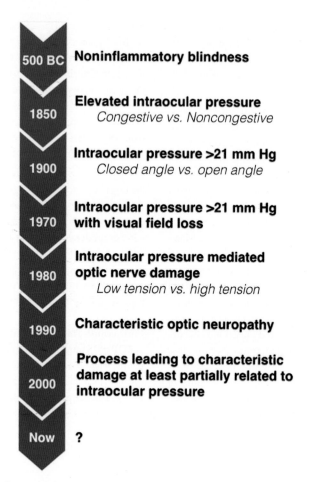

FIGURE 12-1. Definition of glaucoma. The changing definition of glaucoma over the years.

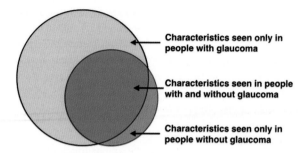

FIGURE 12-2. Glaucoma characteristics. Overlap of characteristics that occur in patients with and without glaucoma.

EPIDEMIOLOGY

Glaucoma affects individuals of all ages, all races, and in all geographic areas. It is not surprising that estimates of the prevalence of glaucoma vary widely. This variation is related to the differing definitions of glaucoma, differing methods of examination, and different expressions of the constellation of loosely related conditions called POAG.

Congenital glaucoma represents a distinct entity that is extremely rare. Most juvenile glaucoma is genetically determined, and although much more common than the congenital types of open-angle glaucoma, it is still relatively uncommon.

The majority of patients with glaucoma are older than 60 years of age and the prevalence of glaucoma increases with age.

It is difficult to generalize the amount of blindness caused by glaucoma. Again, glaucoma is a variable condition, with variable definitions. However, the incidence clearly increases markedly with age and especially in African Americans. The prevalence of glaucoma in African Americans over the age of 80 may be more than 20%.

Worldwide, the incidence of glaucoma is estimated at around 2.5 million per year. The prevalence of blindness due to POAG is probably around 3 million. In the United States, around 100,000 individuals are blind in both eyes as a result of glaucoma.

PATHOPHYSIOLOGY

The hallmark of glaucoma is ocular tissue damage, especially to the optic nerve and retinal nerve fiber layer (RNFL).

Figure 12-3 illustrates possible ways in which the tissue damage can develop. An initiating factor is IOP within the normal or the elevated range, causing mechanical deformation and leading to subsequent damage. Also illustrated are additional factors related to the structural deformation caused by IOP.

Toxic agents or autoimmune mechanisms may cause damage and eventual death of the retinal ganglion cells, leading to loss of tissue and structural damage, which itself may facilitate the IOP-related damage. Abnormal autoregulation of blood flow to the optic nerve has also been postulated to play a role in glaucomatous optic neuropathy.

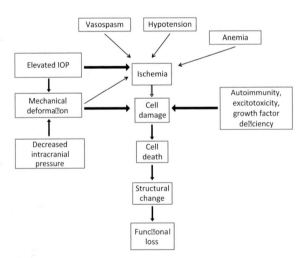

FIGURE 12-3. Pathogenesis of glaucoma. Pathogenesis of ocular tissue damage in glaucoma. IOP, intraocular pressure.

The final common pathway in all the POAGs is the death, sometimes by necrosis, but usually by apoptosis, of the retinal ganglion cells. This may lead to further damage in the retina, optic nerve, and brain. Feedback loops make this oversimplified schema far more complex. For example, "structural change" itself predisposes to cell damage. Some of the factors that may be involved in this cascade of events are shown in **Table 12-1.**

TABLE 12-1. Some Factors Involved in the Development of Tissue Damage in Glaucoma

Mechanical Injury

Stretching of lamina cribrosa, blood vessels, corneal endothelial cells, etc.

Abnormal Glial, Neural, or Connective Tissue

Metabolic Deprivation

Direct compression of neurons, connective tissue, and vasculature by intraocular pressure

Lack of neurotrophins

Secondary to mechanical blockade of axons

Genetically determined

Deficient nerve growth factors

Ischemia and hypoxia

Abnormal autoregulation of retinal and choroidal vessels

Decreased perfusion

Acute/chronic

Primary/secondary

Abnormal oxygen transfer

Autoimmune Mechanisms

Defective Protective Measures

Deficient or inhibited nitric oxide synthase

Abnormal heat-shock protein

Toxicity to Retinal Ganglion Cells and Other Tissues

Glutamate

Genetic Predisposition

Abnormal optic nerve structure

Large laminar pores

Large scleral canal

Abnormal connective tissue

Abnormal vasculature

Abnormal trabecular meshwork

Decreased permeability of extracellular matrix

Abnormal endothelial cells

Abnormal molecular biology

HISTORY

A thorough history is the single most important part of the examination of a patient with POAG, even though the disease is relatively free of symptoms in its early stages. The history is the part of the examination that develops the relationship between the patient and the physician that is essential to successful diagnosis and management of glaucoma. In

TABLE 12-2. Risk Factors for the Development of Glaucoma

Genetic Make-Up

Positive family history of glaucomatous visual loss

Identification of glaucoma-related gene

Intraocular Pressure Considerations

mm Hg	Likelihood of Eventually Developing Glaucoma
> 21	5%
> 24	10%
> 27	50%
> 39	90%

Age

Age in Years*	Prevalence of Glaucoma
< 40	Rare
40–60	1%
60–80	2%
> 80	4%

Vascular Factors

Migraine

Vasospastic disease

Raynaud disease

Hypotension

Hypertension

Myopia

Obesity

*These figures are for Europeans and Asians; the prevalence in Africans is approximately four times higher.

addition, a meticulous history will frequently uncover symptoms of the disease, even in relatively early or moderate stages. For example, patients may note difficulty seeing in the dark, mild eye ache, or a sense that vision simply is not as good as it was in the past. Furthermore, taking a history leads to eliciting the risk factors for glaucoma and, even more importantly, the risk factors for becoming blind from glaucoma (**Tables 12-2 and 12-3**).

Average-pressure glaucoma has been associated with various vascular risk factors (i.e., migraine, low blood pressure, sleep apnea). Particular attention should be placed on these issues in patients suspected of having this type of glaucoma.

The essential question in history taking is "How are you?" The physician must stress that the most important part of the question is the word "you." Glaucoma is a frightening condition that frequently decreases the patient's quality of life simply as a result of the patient knowing he or she has glaucoma. There is a long history of associating glaucoma with IOP. The physician at every appropriate opportunity must indicate to the patient that both the patient's and physician's concern relates to the patient's health, not primarily to the patient's IOP. An evaluation of health requires taking a competent, compassionate history.

TABLE 12-3. Risk Factors for Becoming Blind from Glaucoma

Disease process capable of causing blindness*

Lack of access to care
    Geographic
    Economic
    Care unavailable

Lack of self-care competence
    Intellectual limitation
    Emotional limitation
    Socioeconomic deprivation

*There is a great variation of disease severity with primary open-angle glaucoma; some patients do not get worse even in the absence of any treatment, whereas others go rapidly blind even with treatment.

CLINICAL EXAMINATION

The clinical examination of the patient suspected of having POAG differs only from the standard examination in emphasis. An essential part of the examination is a meticulous search for the presence or absence of a relative afferent pupillary defect (APD). An APD can be present before detectable field loss. In addition, the presence of APD indicates that there is definite optic nerve damage, which triggers a necessary search for the cause of that damage. Checking the patient for an APD is a part of every complete examination of the patient with glaucoma.

External and Biomicroscopic Examination

Biomicroscopic examinations of the patient with glaucoma differ from the standard biomicroscopic examination only in that the physician searches for the topical side effects of the medications that the patient may be using (Fig. 12-4) and findings that may be associated with glaucoma, such as a Krukenberg spindle.

Gonioscopy

Gonioscopy is an essential part of the evaluation of a patient with glaucoma. The examiner needs to search for the signs of pigment dispersion syndrome, exfoliation syndrome, and angle recession. Gonioscopy needs to be repeated at about yearly intervals, because anterior chamber angles that are initially deep may become increasingly narrow with age, leading eventually to chronic or, in rare cases, acute angle closure. Because miotics can cause marked shallowing of the anterior chamber angle, gonioscopy should be performed after any miotic is started or after a concentration of a miotic is changed. The Spaeth gonioscopic grading system provides a rapid, quantitative, and clinically useful method of describing and recording the anterior chamber angle (see Chapter 3).

Posterior Pole

POAG is primarily a disease of the optic disc. Consequently, knowledgeable, extensive evaluation of the optic nerve is a mandatory part of the evaluation of the patient suspected of having glaucoma and of the continuing evaluation of the patient. In the *diagnosis* of POAG, evaluation of the optic nerve is the single most important aspect of the assessment. In the *management* of glaucoma, the nature of the optic disc is the second most important aspect of the examination, a meticulous history being the first.

The optic disc is best examined with the pupil in a dilated state. After dilation the optic nerve is examined stereoscopically at the biomicroscope using a strong plus lens such as a 60- or 66-diopter lens. This is best done with the beam narrowed to a thin slit and the magnification on high (1.6 or 16×) using a Haag-Streit 900 series slit-lamp biomicroscope. The examiner gains an idea of the disc topography by this method. Also, the size of the disc is measured. To measure the vertical height of the disc, the beam is widened so that the horizontal extent of the beam is the same width as the width of the optic nerve (Fig. 12-5). The beam is then narrowed vertically until the vertical diameter of the optic disc exactly matches the vertical extent of the beam. The vertical diameter of the disc is determined by reading the reticule on the slit lamp and applying the appropriate correction factor. Although these factors vary slightly with the Volk and the Nikon lenses, a rough approximation is that for the 60-diopter lens, one multiplies the reading on the reticule by 0.9; for the 66-diopter lens, no correction factor is needed; and for the 90-diopter lens, the measurement on the reticule is multiplied by 1.3. The normal disc has a diameter between 1.5 and 1.9 mm vertically.

The next step employs the direct ophthalmoscope. The beam of the ophthalmoscope should be narrowed so that it projects a beam on the retina approximately 1.3 mm in diameter. This is the size of the middle-sized beam on some Welch-Allyn ophthalmoscopes and of the smallest beam on some other Welch-Allyn ophthalmoscopes. The examiner should determine the size of the beam for the ophthalmoscope he or she is using. This can be readily done by projecting the beam on the retina next to the optic nerve, noting the height of that beam relative to the previously determined height of the optic nerve as described earlier. Once the size of the beam has been established, the size of the optic nerve can be determined relatively accurately with the direct ophthalmoscope itself. In eyes with more than 5 diopters of hyperopia or 5 diopters of myopia, the disc size will be abnormally large or abnormally small, respectively, when viewed with the strong plus lens because of magnification or minification.

The optic nerve is best examined using a direct ophthalmoscope, with both the patient and the examiner in the seated position. The examiner's head must be in a position to avoid obstructing the patient's gaze with the other eye, because that other eye must fixate firmly to allow for careful evaluation of the eye being examined. The examiner directs primary attention to the 6- and 12-o'clock positions of the nerve: What is the rim width? Is an acquired pit or a disc hemorrhage present? Is there peripapillary atrophy? Are the vessels displaced, bent, engorged, narrowed, or "bayoneted"? The examiner also estimates the width of the neuroretinal rim at the 1-, 3-, 5-, 7-, 9-, and 11-o'clock positions. This is done in terms of a rim-to-disc ratio, that is, the relative width of the rim in comparison to the diameter of the optic nerve in that axis. Thus, the maximum rim-to-disc ratio is 0.5.

In Figure 12-6, the rim-to-disc ratio at 1-o'clock position is 0.2; at 3-o'clock position, 0.15; at 5-o'clock position, 0.0; at 7-o'clock position, 0.25; at 9-o'clock position, 0.20, and at 11-o'clock position, 0.25. Figure 12-7A illustrates a disc with a narrow rim that respects Jonas's ISNT criteria. This refers to the fact that the width of the neuroretinal rim of healthy optic discs tends to vary depending on its location. The rim of a healthy disc is usually widest inferiorly, next widest superiorly, narrower nasally, and narrowest temporally. For example, the disc illustrated in Figure 12-7B has a large cup, but respects the ISNT criteria; there is no field loss. These criteria are rough guidelines, and not definitive aspects of normalcy or pathology. The width of the rim tends also to reflect the shape of the disc, which is usually vertically oval. Figure 12-8 shows a disc with a relatively small "cup-to-disc ratio," but a rim-to-disc ratio of 0 at the inferior pole. Cup-to-disc ratios are misleading and should not be used. Figure 12-9 shows two discs of different sizes. Figure 12-9A is a small disc with a disc diameter of approximately 1.2 mm. Figure 12-9B is a large disc with a disc diameter of approximately 2.2 mm. The examiner may be misled by the relative size of the cup in these two discs and incorrectly conclude that the disc in Figure 12-9B is less healthy than that in Figure 12-9A. In actuality, it is the other way around.

The rim area is relatively constant in all healthy discs. Thus, in large discs, the rim area is spread over a much greater area (recall that area involves the square of the radius). The consequence of this is that the normal rim of the large, *healthy* disc is narrower than the normal rim of the small, *healthy* disc. The rim area in Figure 12-9B is actually greater than the rim area in Figure 12-9A.

The relative health of the optic nerve can be estimated by staging the disc according to the system illustrated in Figure 12-10.

In younger patients, or patients whose optic nerves are in the relatively early stages of glaucomatous damage, specifically stages 0 to 3 (see glaucoma graph), evaluation of the nerve fiber layer can be helpful. The examiner focuses meticulously on the retinal surface, preferably with a red-free light in the direct ophthalmoscope, and looks for lines that would follow the course of the nerve fiber layers.

A trough can indicate the presence of such a defect illustrated in Figure 12-11. In most cases, however, the topography of the optic nerve provides more valuable clues than does the nature of the nerve fiber layer.

The optic nerves of the two eyes should be symmetric. Where asymmetry is present, one of the nerves is almost always abnormal, unless the optic nerves are of different sizes, as indicated in Figure 12-9. Figure 12-12 shows the right and left eyes of a patient with unilateral optic nerve damage resulting from glaucoma.

The examiner should search out the presence of an acquired pit of the optic nerve. These localized defects immediately adjacent to the outer edge of the rim, just temporal to the inferior or superior pole of the disc, are pathognomonic for glaucomatous damage. The observer also specifically looks for the presence of a disc hemorrhage on the retina crossing the rim. Such hemorrhages may be signs that the glaucomatous process is out of control. However, these hemorrhages may have other etiologies, such as anticoagulation or posterior vitreous detachment. They are not reliable signs of poor glaucoma control. Disc hemorrhages are seen more often in patients with average-pressure glaucoma. Further information about the optic disc is found in Chapter 5.

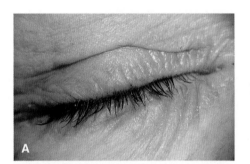

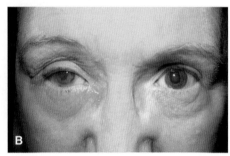

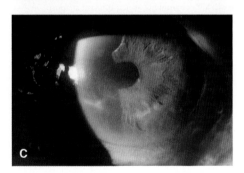

FIGURE 12-4. **Glaucoma medication sides effects.** **A.** External examination showing erythema and edema from an allergic reaction to timolol. **B.** Contact dermatitis involving the left periorbital area characterized by edema, erythema, and hyperkeratosis. This patient also exhibits conjunctival hyperemia. **C.** Corneal epithelial pseudodendrites as a result of topical latanoprost. (Photograph courtesy of Christopher Rapuano, MD, Wills Eye Hospital, Philadelphia, PA.)

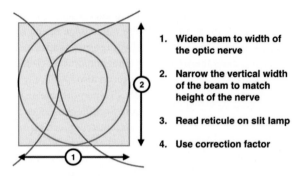

1. **Widen beam to width of the optic nerve**

2. **Narrow the vertical width of the beam to match height of the nerve**

3. **Read reticule on slit lamp**

4. **Use correction factor**

FIGURE 12-5. **Measuring the disc.** Method of measuring vertical diameter of the disc.

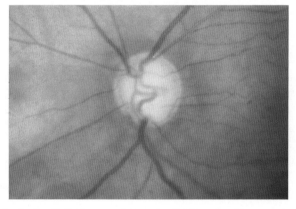

FIGURE 12-6. **Acquired optic pit.** Optic nerve photograph of a left eye showing an acquired pit at approximately 5-o'clock position.

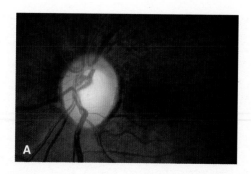

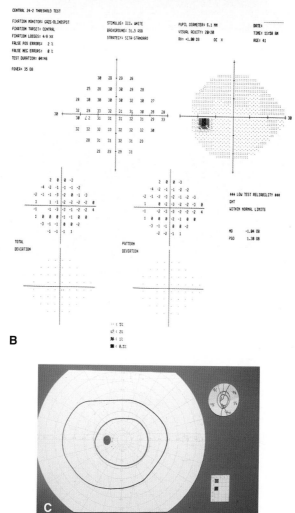

FIGURE 12-7. Jonas's ISNT rule. A. A disc with a narrow rim that respects Jonas's ISNT rule. **B.** Corresponding Goldmann visual field showing no abnormality. **C.** Corresponding Humphrey visual field showing no abnormality.

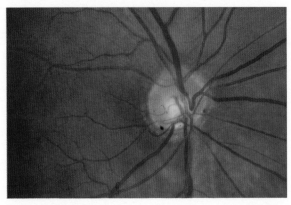

FIGURE 12-8. **Small cup-to-disc ratio.** A disc with a relatively small cup-to-disc ratio, but a rim-to-disc ratio of 0 at the inferior pole.

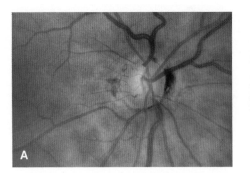 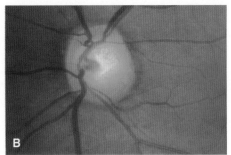

FIGURE 12-9. **Two discs of different sizes. A.** Small disc with a disc diameter of approximately 1.2 mm. **B.** Large disc with a disc diameter of approximately 2.2 mm.

DDLS Stage	Narrowest width of rim (rim/disc ratio)			DDLS Stage	Examples		
	For Small Disc <1.50 mm	For Average Size Disc 1.50-2.00 mm	For Large Disc >2.00 mm		1.25 mm optic nerve	1.75 mm optic nerve	2.25 mm optic nerve
1	0.5 or more	0.4 or more	0.3 or more	0a			
2	0.4 to 0.49	0.3 to 0.39	0.2 to 0.29	0b			
3	0.3 to 0.39	0.2 to 0.29	0.1 to 0.19	1			
4	0.2 to 0.29	0.1 to 0.19	less than 0.1	2			
5	0.1 to 0.19	less than 0.1	0 for less than 45°	3			
6	less than 0.1	0 for less than 45°	0 for 46° to 90°	4			
7	0 for less than 45°	0 for 46° to 90°	0 for 91° to 180°	5			
8	0 for 46° to 90°	0 for 91° to 180°	0 for 181° to 270°	6			
9	0 for 91° to 180°	0 for 181° to 270°	0 for more than 270°	7a			
10	0 for more than 180°	0 for more than 270°		7b			

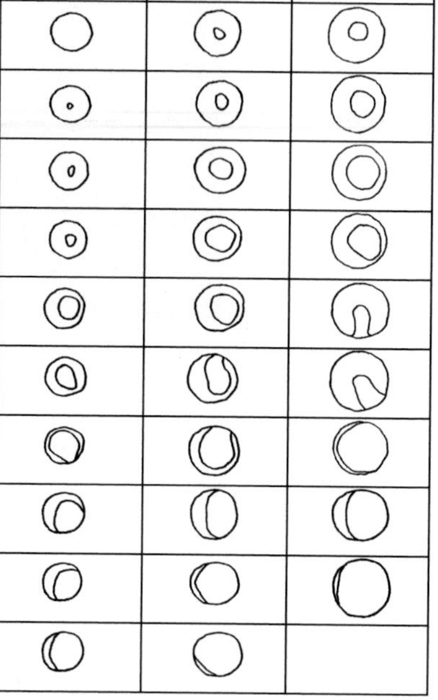

FIGURE 12-10. The DDLS. The Disc Damage Likelihood Scale (DDLS) is a way to describe quantitatively and simply the changes that occur in the optic nerve head (the disc). It is used to quantify the health of the optic disc, specifically as it relates to glaucoma.

The DDLS is based on two characteristics of the disc: (1) the width of the neuroretinal rim and (2) the size of the optic disc. The DDLS scale goes from 1 to 10, 1 being the most normal and 10 the most pathologic. The width of the neuroretinal rim is described in terms of the rim-to-disc ratio. Thus, the widest possible neuroretinal rim would be a rim-to-disc ratio of 0.5. The narrowest would be 0.0.

First, one measures the size of the optic disc and classifies the disc as small, average, large, or very large. Small is less than 1.5 mm in height, average between 1.5 and 2.0 mm in height, large between 2 and 3 mm in height, and very large greater than 3 mm. The size is easily measured with the slit lamp or, better, by using the beam of an ophthalmoscope. Next, one looks for where the neuroretinal rim is the narrowest. (Please note: "thin" is the wrong word, as thin refers to the thickness of the tissue, not to its width.) The narrowest rim would be 0.0 and the widest rim possible would be 0.5. When the width of the rim is between 0.4 and 0.5 rim-to-disc ratio, then it is stage 1; between 0.3 and 0.4, it is stage 2; between 0.2 and 0.3, it is stage 3; between 0.1 and 0.2, it is stage 4; and less than 0.1 but still present, it is stage 5—all in average-sized discs. Five is the area of indecision. A value of 5 can occasionally be normal, but usually it is pathologic and associated with visual field loss. The DDLS also depends on disc size, so the width of the rim must be corrected for disc size. In a small disc, one unit should be added to the DDLS. In a large disc, one unit should be subtracted. In a very large disc, two units should be subtracted. Thus, an average-sized disc with a rim-to-disc ratio of 0.25 would be a DDLS of 3; a small disc with a rim-to-disc ratio of 0.25 would be a DDLS of 4; a large-sized disc with the same rim-to-disc ratio of 0.25 would be a DDLS of 2; and in a very large disc with the same rim-to-disc ratio would be a DDLS of 1.

Some patients with glaucoma lose an area of the neuroretinal rim completely. When this happens, one then uses the circumferential amount of rim loss to determine the DDLS score. If the amount of rim loss is less than 45 degrees, then it is a DDLS of 6; between 90 and 180 degrees, a DDLS of 7; and between 90 and 180 degrees, a DDLS of 8. If the amount of rim loss is greater than 180 degrees, but less than 270 degrees, then it is a DDLS of 9, and if there is virtually no rim left, then it is a DDLS of 10. Again, all of these numbers refer to the average-sized disc. Consider a disc with a notch in which there is no rim for 30 degrees. In an average-sized disc, it would be a DDLS of 6, and in a small disc, a DDLS of 7. In a large disc, it would be a DDLS of 5, and in a very large disc, it would be a DDLS of 4. Discs with DDLS of 6 or more are never normal.

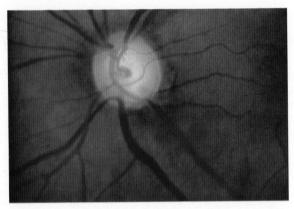

FIGURE 12-11. Inferotemporal notch. A disc with an inferotemporal notch and a nerve fiber layer defect inferotemporally.

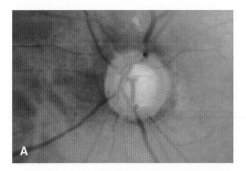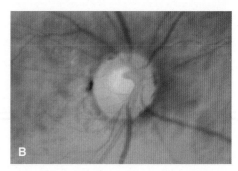

FIGURE 12-12. **Unilateral glaucoma. A** and **B.** Unilateral optic nerve damage from glaucoma. Right and left eyes of a patient with unilateral optic nerve damage caused by glaucoma. There is a loss of inferior rim tissue in the right eye.

SPECIAL TESTS

Optic nerve examination is supplemented by visual field evaluation. Visual field deficits, ideally, should correlate with anatomic changes. Monocular, automated static perimetry has become the method of choice used in diagnosis and monitoring of glaucomatous change. The different platforms available include the Humphrey visual field and the Octopus visual field. The platform, program, and settings should remain consistent with subsequent fields when assessing for progression. Progression is difficult to establish. This is especially true once there are advanced visual field changes. When this situation exists, function is most accurately evaluated with the patient's subjective symptoms. The Esterman field is a binocular program that is useful in evaluating the level of overall functional loss caused by glaucoma. Detailed discussion of visual fields can be found in Chapter 7.

There is debate in the literature about the pattern of visual field defects observed in average-pressure glaucoma. We, and others, have found visual field defects to be more dense and closer to center in average-pressure glaucoma as compared to POAG at higher pressures. Other groups have observed no difference between the two groups.

Imaging modalities of the optic nerve head (ONH) and RNFL attempt to provide objective and accurate quantitative data. It is hoped that in the future these technologies can be used to detect ganglion cell loss at the earliest stage of the glaucoma process. Although software continues to evolve, none of the available modalities has been shown to be unequivocally superior in detecting progression over time. Each technology comes with strengths, limitations, and nuances that need to be fully understood to interpret the data each provides. As with visual fields, ONH/RNFL imaging is used in conjunction with optic nerve examination. Detailed discussion of imaging technology can be found in Chapter 19.

TREATMENT

As previously stated, glaucoma is a process that results in characteristic changes to the optic disc. In POAG, this process is usually slow. The course of average-pressure glaucoma seems to be more variable and, possibly, less linear. It has been shown that 40% of the ganglion cell axons that compose the optic nerve can be lost before functional deficits are detected on visual field tests. Optimally, one would like to intervene in the process of glaucoma when accelerated ganglion cell loss is confirmed but before functional loss is noted. Unfortunately, none of the current interventions available come without at least some risk of accelerated vision loss or other side effects. Appropriate management of POAG requires thoughtful balance of (1) the risks of pain or functional loss in the face of no intervention, (2) the potential benefit of an intervention (in terms of retardation or stabilization of deterioration of visual function or actual improvement), and (3) the potential risks introduced by the intervention itself (**Tables 12-4** and **12-5**).

The "process" of glaucoma is not visible. It becomes visible only through the effects of that process over time. The goal of managing a patient with POAG is to maintain or enhance the patient's health. Both the physician and the patient wish to ensure that the patient does not develop functional loss before his or her death. Estimating the need to start treatment or the need to change the vigor of treatment requires that the physician have a good idea of the likelihood that the patient's glaucoma will ultimately cause functional problems. To make this determination appropriately, the physician must consider four issues: (1) the stage of the glaucoma, (2) the rate of change of the glaucoma, (3) the duration that the glaucoma will continue to exist, and (4) socioeconomic matters. The use of the "Glaucoma Graph" can be of great help in

TABLE 12-4. Risks and Benefits of Treatment

Risks Attendant to No Intervention	Risks Attendant to Intervention	Benefits of Intervention
Pain	Local side effects	Improvement of ability to do
Visual loss	Pain	visually related activities
Minimal	Redness	Stabilization of the ability to
Moderate	Cataract	do visually related activities
Total	Infection	Retardation of the rate of
Visual loss	Bleeding	deterioration of ability to do
Minimal	Allergy	visually related activities
Moderate	Abnormal flashes	
Total	Increased pigmentation	
	Other	
	Systemic side effects	
	Fatigue	
	Malaise	
	Cardiovascular changes	
	Neurologic changes	
	Psychological changes	
	Pulmonary changes, etc.	
	Expense	
	Inconvenience	
	Embarrassment	
	Decreased quality of life	

TABLE 12-5. Risk of Losing Function If No Intervention

Low with:

Healthy optic nerve

Negative family history of visual loss due to glaucoma

Good self-care skills

Good access to good care

Estimated years remaining less than 10 years

Intraocular pressure below 15 mm Hg

No exfoliation or pigment dispersion syndrome changes

Normal cardiovascular status

Moderate with a Situation Between "Low" and "High"

High with:

Optic nerve already damaged by glaucoma

Positive family history of visual loss due to glaucoma or presence of recognized "gene" for glaucoma

Poor self-care skills

Poor access to good care

Estimated years remaining over 15 years

Intraocular pressure over 30 mm Hg

Exfoliation syndrome

Poor cardiovascular status

this regard (Fig. 12-13). Stage of the glaucoma is determined by utilizing the Disc Damage Likelihood Scale (DDLS) (Fig. 12-10). Rate of change is determined by serial evaluations of the history and optic nerve. The duration the glaucoma will continue to cause damage is, in most cases, determined by a reasonable estimate of the patient's remaining years of life.

IOP reduction decreases the rate of disease progression in patients with glaucoma. To date, lowering IOP is the only treatment proved to be beneficial for patient with glaucoma. In the United States, the usual treatment algorithm for glaucoma progresses from topical medications, laser trabeculoplasty, and culminates with incisional surgery. Because of its relative risk, surgery is typically reserved for patients who do not respond to other measures (Tables 12-6 and 12-7).

There is little to support this treatment algorithm. Treatment options should be tailored to the individual, taking into consideration patient factors such as age and access to medications and disease factors such as stage and rate of progression. It is important to recall that all glaucoma interventions carry risk. Although generally safe, topical medications carry the risk of local and occasionally life-threatening

TABLE 12-6. Expected Benefit of Treatment Related to Amount of Lowering of Intraocular Pressure*

Expected benefit great if intraocular pressure lowering greater than 30%
Expected benefit possible to probable if intraocular pressure lowering is 15%–30%
No benefit expected if intraocular pressure lowering is less than 15%

*In some cases, stabilization of intraocular pressure appears to be beneficial in itself.

systemic adverse events. Furthermore, medications require daily adherence to a daily schedule. As the number of medications prescribed to a patient increases, the likelihood of the patient maintaining such a schedule decreases. Therefore the "risk" of medication nonadherence should be considered as well. In our practice, patients with POAG, pigmentary glaucoma and exfoliation glaucoma are offered laser trabeculoplasty as first-line therapy.

The current gold standard glaucoma surgery continues to be trabeculectomy (guarded filtration procedure). Despite significant improvements to the technique, this surgery still

TABLE 12-7. Relative Effect of Various Treatments on Intraocular Pressure and on Development of Side Effects

Usual Decrease in Intraocular Pressure:	
In response to medications	~15% (range 0%–50%)
In response to argon laser trabeculoplasty	~20% (range 0%–50%)
In response to filtering surgery	~40% (range 0%–80%)
Likelihood of Side Effects As a Result of Treatment	
From medications	~30%
From argon laser trabeculoplasty	Almost no lasting side effects
From selective laser trabeculoplasty	Rare, but some permanent and disabling
From incisional surgery	~60%*

*The lower the final intraocular pressure, the greater the likelihood of side effects from the surgery; the rate varies with the type of surgery, severity of condition, and skill and judgment of the surgeon.

carries a significant risk of complications that can lead to decrease in vision, loss of vision, or loss of the eye. Other procedures include tube shunts (glaucoma drainage devices) and an emerging class of surgeries classified as microinvasive or minimally invasive glaucoma surgeries (MIGS). The former of these is well established with advantages and disadvantages of its own. MIGS procedures have been developed in an effort to achieve the IOP lowering observed with trabeculectomy while avoiding the complications associated with this surgery. To date, none of the MIGS procedures have yet been proved to satisfy these qualifications and risk of complications seems to be inexorably linked to efficacy. Further studies may provide evidence to support adoption of one or more of these techniques. The continued pursuit of new surgical options highlights the need for improvement upon what is currently available for the care of medically refractive patients.

The amount that the IOP should be lowered to prevent deterioration, stabilize the condition, or result in improvement varies from individual to individual; but guidelines have been developed. A target pressure is an IOP level believed likely to be low enough to prevent further damage. One method of arriving at a target pressure is shown in Figure 12-14. It is important to remember, however, that the target IOP is only a relative, tentative guide to treatment. The only valid method of establishing the state of control in a patient with POAG is by determining stability or instability of the optic nerve or visual field, or both. Thus, if the optic nerve and visual field are stable despite an IOP higher than the calculated target pressure, it is not wise to attempt to lower the pressure more vigorously to achieve the target IOP. Conversely, if the target pressure is achieved, but the optic nerve or visual field continues to deteriorate, then the target pressure is too high, there is another cause for the continuing deterioration other than glaucoma, or the neurons are so badly damaged that deterioration will progress no matter what level of IOP is achieved.

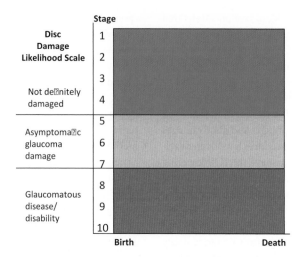

FIGURE 12-13. Glaucoma graph and explanation. The glaucoma graph is a way of determining and understanding the clinical course of glaucoma in an individual patient.

Green Zone: When a person has a Disc Damage Likelihood Scale (DDLS) of 2, 3, or 4, one cannot be sure that optic nerve damage is not present, even though one knows that visual field loss is not present. It is possible that at an earlier date the patient had a smaller DDLS, in which case the present larger DDLS would represent a deterioration. If this were the case, the patient still would not have visual field loss and the need for treatment would be determined by the four factors that always determine if treatment is necessary: the amount of damage that is present, the rate of change, the duration that the change will continue, and socioeconomic considerations. Valid serial measurements allow establishing a trend, such as a rate of deterioration of field or disc. If the rate of change is sufficiently rapid that the person would get into the red zone before death, then treatment is clearly necessary. On the other hand, if the rate of change is so slow that the person will probably not get into the red zone before death, then treatment is not likely justified.

Yellow Zone: When a patient is in the yellow zone (with a DDLS of 5 to 7), the optic nerve is definitely damaged, but the person is asymptomatic. Even though asymptomatic, it is certain that the eye is not normal. Nobody starts with DDLS scores in those ranges. The person's optic nerve must have become worse. In such a situation it is likely that the patient will need treatment, although this is not always the case. For example, a person could have developed damage in the past which then became stabilized. Or, a person's anticipated number of years to live could be so short that even without treatment he/she would not move from the yellow to the red zone. Such individuals would not need treatment.

Red Zone: When a person is already in the red zone, that is, the person has a decreased quality of life or impaired ability to perform the activities of daily living (with a DDLS of 8, 9, or 10), there is already a disability. Consequently, the goal is preventing any worsening of the disability, because any increase in damage makes the patient symptomatically worse. Therefore, the remaining years of life is no longer a consideration in patients who already have disability. In such a situation, the only reason for not treating the patient is if the disability is totally stable without treatment.

IOP*– [IOP*/100 × IOP*] − D − E = Target IOP

Where: IOP* = Intraocular pressure known to be associated with progressive disc or field damage or maximum IOP

D = 0 if Disc Damage Likelihood Scale is less than 5

D = 1 if Disc Damage Likelihood Scale = 6–8

D = 2 if Disc Damage Likelihood Scale is greater than 8

E = 0 if estimated years remaining is less than 10 years

E = 1 if estimated years remaining = 11–20 years

E = 2 if estimated years remaining is greater than 20 years

FIGURE 12-14. A method of estimating target intraocular pressure.

A CONCEPTUAL APPROACH TO THE TREATMENT OF GLAUCOMA

The feature common to all the types of glaucoma is IOP high enough to damage the optic nerve. It is important to stress that "high enough" pressure is not a synonym for elevated pressure. It should also not be construed to mean a specific number. In this section, we stress the difficulty, or the likely impossibility, of determining what tonometrically determined IOP is damaging and what is not damaging to the optic nerve.

What IOP is high enough to damage the optic nerve? This is a critically important question when considering treatment for glaucoma. At this moment, it can only be partially answered. IOP above the retinal arterial pressure acutely causes nerve damage. However, arterial pressure varies from person to person, and it is not possible to know with certainty what specific IOP will damage a particular person. IOP below retinal arterial pressure can also damage the optic nerve, but only after a relatively period of days, weeks, months, or perhaps years. Again, solid figures are not established for how long a particular pressure needs to be at a particular level before it damages the optic nerve.

On the basis of ophthalmodynamometry studies evaluating retinal vessel collapse pressures, it is reasonable to set a threshold for damage at somewhere around 30 mm Hg. Although there will be some individuals whose optic nerves can withstand such pressures for a prolonged duration, there are likely few. The other practical consideration is that IOP at this level will predispose retinal vein occlusions. Because retinal vein occlusion causes immediate and potentially permanent vision loss, this rough, admittedly arbitrary, threshold has significant clinical significance.

Determining the lower threshold in which no damage occurs is even more challenging. It is certain that this lower threshold varies from person to person. What is also certain is that standard statistical theory is of no help in establishing a safe lower pressure. A significant proportion of glaucoma patients experience disease progression despite a constant IOP in the average range. Unfortunately, many physicians have adopted the incorrect belief that there is a particular level of IOP that is safe for all patients.

We believe it is wise to assume that there is no lower threshold that can be generalized for all persons, and it is impossible to predict accurately what level of IOP is safe. Currently, the only way to determine if a specific IOP is too high with certainty is to demonstrate optic nerve deterioration at that pressure. On the other hand, one can determine that IOP is low enough if damage is halted. Therefore, while IOP is an important barometer for monitoring glaucoma, a careful and meticulous evaluation of the optic nerve structure and function is of primary importance when considering treatment of glaucoma.

REVERSIBILITY OF GLAUCOMA

Previously, we made the case for not assuming or trying to calculate a particular safe level of IOP for a specific patient. Here, we refer to the reversibility of structure and function that characterizes most individuals with glaucoma. It is now indisputable that when IOP is lowered there can be an improvement in the appearance of the optic nerve and in the visual field.

In 1869, von Jaeger showed in his drawings that lowering IOP can reverse structural damage. Many studies since then have confirmed that this is not just an occasional occurrence, but is quite frequent. Whether change in visual field has been a real consequence of lowered pressure, however, has been far more controversial. Nevertheless, it now also seems indisputable that improvement in visual field is a consequence of adequate lowering of IOP in an individual with glaucoma. Given this fact, we raise two questions: (1) Does the presence of such improvements serve as a sign that IOP has been lowered adequately? (2) Is the absence of such an improvement a sign that a "safe" IOP has not been reached? We believe the answers to these questions are, "yes." However," believe" and "know" are different words with different meanings. Furthermore, not all ophthalmologists have access to instruments that are necessary to detect such improvements in the optic disc or visual field. We await further studies and clinical experimentation with this idea of using improvement as a method to establish a level of IOP that is safe.

Secondary Open-Angle Glaucoma

Jonathan S. Myers and Scott Fudemberg ■

PIGMENT DISPERSION SYNDROME

Pigment dispersion syndrome (PDS) is a condition in which an abnormal amount of pigment is dislodged from the pigmented epithelium on the posterior surface of the iris and then deposited on various structures throughout the anterior segment. Obstruction of the trabecular meshwork by pigment, and subsequent damage to the meshwork, can lead to elevated intraocular pressure (IOP) and secondary open-angle glaucoma.

Epidemiology

- PDS occurs most frequently in young (aged 20 to 45 years), myopic, Caucasian men.
- Approximately one-third of PDS patients go on to develop pigmentary glaucoma.

Pathophysiology

Currently, it is believed that the iris of predisposed individuals is abnormal and also posteriorly bowed so that the iris pigment epithelium contacts underlying packets of lens zonular fibers, leading to liberation of the pigment into the aqueous.

Pigment becomes trapped in and damages the trabecular meshwork, leading to reduced aqueous outflow, increase in IOP, and, ultimately, optic nerve damage if uncontrolled.

History

- Myopia and a family history of glaucoma
- Jarring exercise, strenuous physical activity, or, rarely, dilation may lead to dramatically increased pigment dispersion, a so-called pigment storm, leading to sudden elevations of IOP. Patients may then experience blurred vision and headaches.

Clinical Examination

- Slit lamp (**Figs. 13-1** to **13-7**): Characteristic findings include Krukenberg spindle (pigment carried from the posterior iris surface by aqueous convection currents passes through the pupil and deposits on the central corneal endothelium in a vertical pattern), pigment deposition on the anterior surface of the iris (usually concentric rings in furrows on the iris surface), mid-peripheral iris transillumination defects (best seen on retroillumination with a small beam through the pupil), and pigment deposition on the zonular fiber attachments near the equator of the lens (also called a Scheie stripe).

- Gonioscopy: Patients typically have posterior bowing of the peripheral iris, leading to lens–iris contact. The angle is very widely open, with moderate to heavy pigmentation, which is relatively homogeneously spread over the entire circumference of the angle. A Sampaolesi line is often present and represents pigment deposition on Schwalbe line.

- Posterior pole: Characteristic glaucomatous optic atrophy is seen with prolonged elevation of IOP or intermittent pressure spikes. Myopic patients, and possibly especially those with PDS, are prone to peripheral retinal tears, necessitating close examination.

Treatment

- The goal of therapy is to control IOP in patients with significantly elevated pressure or glaucomatous nerve changes, usually through aqueous suppressants.

- Miotics reduce pigment shedding and reduce IOP, but are often poorly tolerated in this young population and may increase the risk of retinal detachment while making monitoring of the retina periphery more difficult.

- Laser peripheral iridotomy also may reduce pigment shedding, because it allows the posteriorly bowed iris to move anteriorly as any built-up fluid pressure in the anterior chamber is then normalized with the posterior chamber (relief of the so-called reverse pupillary block). This may help prevent glaucoma in individuals at higher risk but who have not yet developed uncontrolled pressure (although clear evidence supporting iridotomy in pigmentary glaucoma is lacking).

- Laser trabeculoplasty is effective, although there are reports of increased postoperative elevations in IOP. Lower energies are indicated to reduce the risk of pressure spikes, given the heavily pigmented trabecular meshwork.

- Efficacy of glaucoma filtration surgery in these patients is similar to that in primary open-angle glaucoma.

BIBLIOGRAPHY

Campbell DG. Pigmentary dispersion and glaucoma: a new theory. *Arch Ophthalmol.* 1997;97:1667.

Gandolfi SA, Vecchi M. Effect of a YAG laser iridotomy on intraocular pressure in pigment dispersion syndrome. *Ophthalmology.* 1996;103:1693–1695.

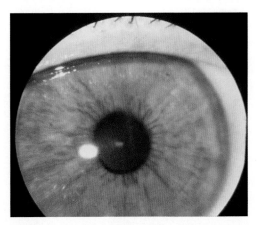

FIGURE 13-1. Krukenberg spindle. A vertical endothelial deposition of pigment characteristic of pigment dispersion syndrome (PDS). It may slowly resolve when pigment shedding stops but may persist for many years or forever. Pattern of deposition is thought to be related to convection currents of aqueous within the eye.

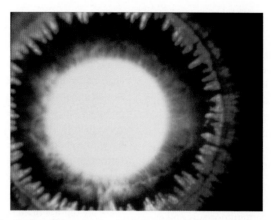

FIGURE 13-2. **Transillumination defects in pigment dispersion syndrome (PDS).** Marked peripheral and mid-peripheral transillumination defects in PDS. Many patients may present with only several mild radial spoke-like defects.

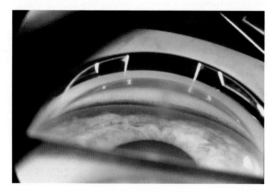

FIGURE 13-3. **Pigment dispersion syndrome, dense pigmentation, and Krukenberg spindle.** Krukenberg spindle (foreground), heavily pigmented deep angle (background). Characteristic homogeneous dense pigmentation of trabecular meshwork.

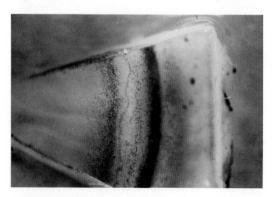

FIGURE 13-4. **Pigment dispersion syndrome, pigment deposition.** Pathology specimen showing pigment deposition on trabecular meshwork and anterior to meshwork.

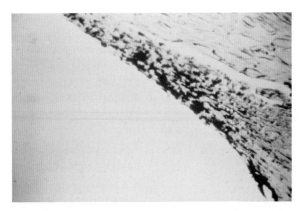

FIGURE 13-5. Pigment dispersion syndrome, pigment deposition. Pathology specimen showing pigment deposition within beams of trabecular meshwork.

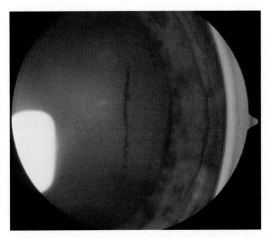

FIGURE 13-6. Pigment dispersion syndrome, Zentmeyer line. Deposition of pigment near equator of lens, at insertion of lens zonular fibers. Variously referred to as Zentmeyer line or Scheie stripe.

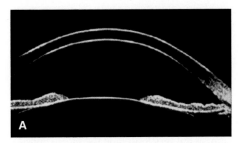
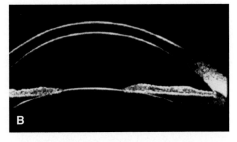

FIGURE 13-7. Pigment dispersion syndrome (PDS), bowing of peripheral iris. A. Ultrasound biomicroscopy (UBM) of patient with PDS, showing backward-bowing peripheral iris in contact with lens surface. **B.** UBM of the same patient, following iridotomy, showing anterior relaxation of iris with reduced contact with lens.

PSEUDOEXFOLIATION SYNDROME

Pseudoexfoliation syndrome (PXFS) is a systemic condition that can lead to secondary open-angle glaucoma. The characteristic flaky white pseudoexfoliation material, seen throughout the anterior segment, can obstruct the trabecular meshwork and has also been isolated in tissues throughout the body.

Epidemiology

- PXFS ranges in prevalence from near 0% in Eskimos to near 30% in people in Scandinavian countries. Presentation may be highly asymmetric, but its incidence and likelihood of binocular findings increase with age and time.

- Although patients with PXFS are at an increased risk for the development of glaucoma (estimated in the Blue Mountains Eye Study at fivefold greater), the majority of these patients do not develop glaucoma.

Pathophysiology

- The exact nature of the pseudoexfoliation material is not well understood, but the material has been isolated from the iris, lens, ciliary body, trabecular meshwork, corneal endothelium, and endothelial cells in blood vessels throughout the eye and orbit, as well as the skin, myocardium, lung, liver, gallbladder, kidney, and cerebral meninges. The material leads to blockage of and damage to the trabecular meshwork and thereby a secondary open-angle glaucoma. It also leads to iris peripapillary ischemia and posterior synechiae. This results in pigment release, increasing the burden on the trabecular meshwork, and increased pupillary block, predisposing to angle closure.

- Patients with pseudoexfoliation syndrome are at risk of weakened lens zonular support and complications of cataract surgery.

- Recent research has not fully uncovered the causes of PXFS, but links to the LOXL1 gene and solar exposure may be factors.

History

- Although patients rarely have symptomatic elevations of IOP, most patients have no contributory history.

- Some patients report a family history, but no clear hereditary pattern is known.

- A history of complicated cataract surgery is potentially suggestive.

Clinical Examination

- Slit lamp (**Figs. 13-8** to **13-12**): The hallmark of PXFS is the flaky white material seen most often at the edge of the pupil and on the surface of the anterior lens capsule, where it forms a ring spread from the position and diameter of the dilated pupil to the constricted pupil.

- This material may also be seen deposited on the iris, angle structures, corneal endothelium, lens implant, and vitreous face in aphakic patients.

  - Peripapillary transillumination defects and atrophy of the pigmented ruff are often seen. Peripapillary pigment deposition is also frequent.

  - Affected eyes are often more miotic and dilate poorly secondary to synechiae and iris ischemia.

  - Pigment liberation with dilation may cause significant pressure spikes. Cataract formation is more frequent.

- Gonioscopy: The anterior chamber angle is often more narrow in PXFS, especially inferiorly relative to superiorly, which may relate to zonular laxity and lens position. Acute angle-closure glaucoma is a risk when the lens zonules are very loose, and therefore continued monitoring of the angle is necessary.

▪ There is irregular pigmentation of the meshwork, with large, dark pigment particles. In contrast to the pigmented trabecular meshwork of pigment dispersion patients, in PXFS the pigmentation appears more black than brown. A Sampaolesi line may be present.

● Posterior pole: Characteristic glaucomatous optic atrophy is seen with prolonged elevation of IOP or intermittent pressure spikes.

Treatment

● PXFS-related glaucoma often leads to higher pressures with greater diurnal fluctuation.

● Topical medications are appropriate, but have been reported to be less effective.

● Laser trabeculoplasty is effective, although there are reports of increased postoperative elevations in IOP. Lower energies are indicated to reduce the risk of pressure spikes, given the heavily pigmented trabecular meshwork.

● The results of filtration surgery are similar to those seen in primary open-angle glaucoma.

● Cataract surgery should be performed with extra caution, given the known fragility of the capsule and zonular fibers in these patients.

BIBLIOGRAPHY

Mitchell P, Wang JJ, Hourihan F. The relationship between glaucoma and pseudoexfoliation: the Blue Mountains Eye Study. *Arch Ophthalmol*. 1999;117: 1319–1324.

Ritch R, Schlotzer-Schrehardt U. Exfoliation syndrome. *Surv Ophthalmol*. 2001;45:265–315.

Thorleifsson G, Magnusson KP, Sulem P, et al. Common sequence variants in the LOXL1 gene confer susceptibility to exfoliation glaucoma. *Science*. 2007; 317(5843):1397–1400.

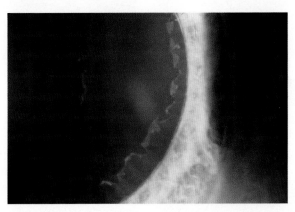

FIGURE 13-8. Exfoliation syndrome. Exfoliation material on anterior lens capsule with clear zone in the region between undilated pupil zone and more peripheral lens. Presumably, the movement of the iris clears exfoliative material from this area.

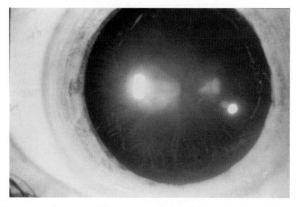

FIGURE 13-9. Exfoliation syndrome, exfoliation material. Exfoliation material on lens surface. Note typical scrolled edges.

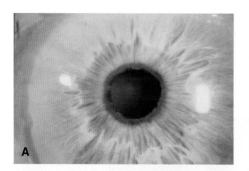

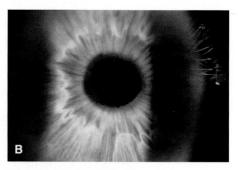

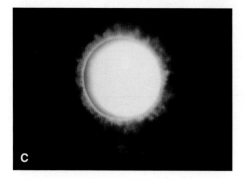

FIGURE 13-10. Comparison of exfoliation syndrome (XFS) and normal eyes. Slit-lamp photos of affected (**A**) and clinically unaffected (**B**) eyes. In **A**, there is atrophy of the pigmented ruffs, seen in XFS, whereas it is preserved in **B**. (**C**). Peripapillary transillumination corresponding to iris pigment epithelial atrophy in **A**.

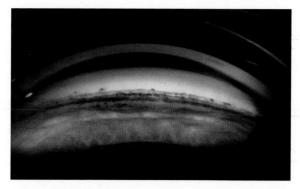

FIGURE 13-11. Exfoliation syndrome (XFS), angle structures. Heavy, dark, irregular pigmentation of angle structures in XFS.

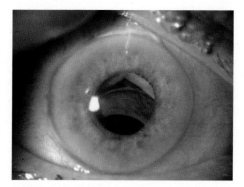

FIGURE 13-12. Exfoliation syndrome (XFS), dislocated lens. Spontaneously dislocated lens in a patient with XFS highlights fragility of zonular support. (Courtesy of Brandon Ayers, MD Wills Eye Hospital.)

STEROID-RESPONSIVE GLAUCOMA

Secondary open-angle glaucoma may result from nearly any route of steroid administration. Elevations in IOP may be severe and prolonged.

Epidemiology

• The incidence of steroid-induced glaucoma in the general population is unknown. Significant elevations in IOP in response to topical steroids have been reported in 50% to over 90% of glaucoma patients and 5% to 10% of patients with normal pressure.

• The incidence of the steroid response is related to the type, dose, duration of treatment, and route of steroid administration.

  ▪ Elevated IOP has been observed with topical, intraocular, periocular, inhaled, oral, intravenous, and dermatologic administrations of steroids, as well as with endogenous elevations of steroids in Cushing's syndrome.

  ▪ Steroid-induced pressure elevation is not uncommon following intravitreal injection of steroids or insertion of some depot steroid devices in the posterior segment.

  ▪ Following intravitreal injection, approximately 50% experience an elevation of IOP, but a low percentage require surgical intervention to lower IOP.

Pathophysiology

• Increased glycosaminoglycans in the trabecular meshwork in response to steroids impede aqueous outflow and lead to elevated IOPs. Steroids may reduce the membrane permeability of the trabecular meshwork, as well as reduce local phagocytic activity by cells and the breakdown of extracellular and intracellular structural proteins, further contributing to reduced meshwork permeability.

• The myocilin/TIGR (trabecular meshwork–inducible glucocorticoid response) gene has been shown to be upregulated in trabecular meshwork endothelial cells in response to steroid application.

History

• Steroid use of any type is a crucial aspect of the history. Prior use of steroids in the distant past with subsequent normalization of IOP may present as an apparent normal-tension glaucoma (**Figs. 13-13** to **13-15**).

• Typically, oral steroid use must be for a prolonged period of time (at least 2 weeks) to stimulate an IOP elevation.

• A history of asthma, skin disorders, allergies, autoimmune disorders, or other conditions that often require steroid treatment may therefore suggest possible past or current steroid use.

• Occasionally, patients note changes in vision related to advanced visual field loss.

• **Table 13-1** gives a clinical example.

Clinical Examination

• Slit lamp: Usually unremarkable. Even in cases with extreme elevations of IOP, the chronicity usually prevents the microcystic corneal edema that occurs with acute IOP elevation.

• Gonioscopy: Usually unremarkable.

• Posterior pole: Typical glaucomatous optic nerve changes are noted if elevation of IOP is sufficiently high and prolonged.

• Special tests: Discontinuation of the steroids, if possible, may lead to a steady reduction of IOP. The time course of IOP reduction after steroid withdrawal is variable and may be prolonged in cases of prolonged steroid use. In cases in which there is concern regarding halting an ocular steroid (e.g., a corneal graft at high risk of rejection), contralateral steroid challenge may demonstrate IOP elevation and confirm the diagnosis.

TABLE 13-1. Clinical Example: Steroid-Induced Glaucoma Following Subconjunctival Depot Steroid Injection

Postoperative Day	IOP (mm Hg)	Course and Medications
Surgery #1: Vitrectomy/Membranectomy with Subconjunctival Depot Steroid		
1	25	Prednisolone, hyoscine, erythromycin
6	45	Add timolol, iopidine, acetazolamide
16	20	Stop acetazolamide
30	29	Add dorzolamide, taper prednisolone
48	19	Take off prednisolone
72	27	Continue timolol, apraclonidine, dorzolamide
118	44	Add latanoprost; consult glaucoma
154	31	Arrange steroid depot excision
Surgery #2: Excise Depot Steroid		
1	32	Add timolol, dorzolamide
4	28	Continue same
23	24	Continue same
38	14	Stop dorzolamide

Note: Patient later discontinued timolol; IOP has been 10–14 mm Hg since discontinuation of drug.
IOP, intraocular pressure.

Treatment

- Discontinuation of the steroids, if possible, or excision of depot steroids may yield complete resolution.

- If topical steroids are used, weaker or less pressure–inducing steroids may help (e.g., loteprednol, rimexolone, fluorometholone).

- Patients with significant uveitis present a special challenge because they may require steroids to control the uveitis. In addition, the uveitis may itself lead to various forms of glaucoma, or may mask glaucoma with aqueous hyposecretion.

- Topical antiglaucoma medications of all types are often helpful for steroid-induced elevations of IOP.

- In general, laser trabeculoplasty is less effective for these patients than for those with other types of glaucomas, but has been reported to be effective in selected cases.

- Filtering surgery has results similar to those in primary open-angle glaucoma.

BIBLIOGRAPHY

Johnson DH, Bradley JM, Acott TS. The effect of dexamethasone on glycosaminoglycans of human trabecular meshwork in perfusion organ culture. *Invest Ophthalmol Vis Sci.* 1990;31:2568–2571.

Johnson D, Gottanka J, Flugel C, et al. Ultrastructural changes in the trabecular meshwork of human eyes treated with corticosteroids. *Arch Ophthalmol.* 1997;115:375–383.

Jones R, Rhee DJ. Corticosteroid-induced ocular hypertension and glaucoma: a brief review and update of the literature. *Curr Opin Ophthalmol.* 2006;17:163–167.

Mitchell P, Cumming RG, Mackey DA. Inhaled corticosteroids, family history, and risk of glaucoma. *Ophthalmology.* 1999;106:2301–2306.

Oh DJ, Martin JL, Williams AJ, et al. Analysis of expression of matrix metalloproteinases and tissue inhibitors of metalloproteinases in human ciliary body following latanoprost. *Invest Ophthalmol Vis Sci.* 2006;47:953–963.

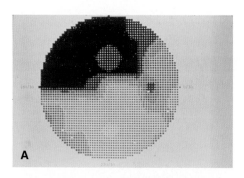

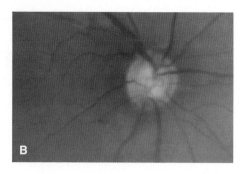

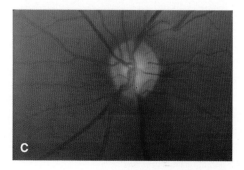

**FIGURE 13-13. Steroid-responsive glaucoma.
A.** Visual field defect seen in a 28-year-old internal medicine resident self-medicating atopic blepharocon-junctivitis with topical steroids. **B** and **C.** Intraocular pressures were greater than 40 mm Hg, with advanced optic nerve cupping and associated visual field loss. The patient later underwent a trabeculectomy.

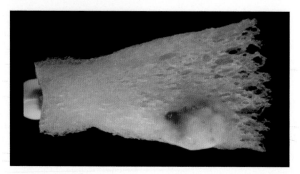

FIGURE 13-14. Steroid-responsive glaucoma. Excised steroid depot 5 months following vitrectomy for Eales disease on a Weck cell sponge.

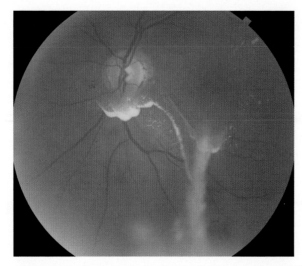

FIGURE 13-15. Steroid-responsive glaucoma. Fundus photograph taken immediately following an intravitreal injection of triamcinolone. White-colored crystals seen beginning to disperse in the vitreous of this patient with diabetic macular edema.

Uveitic Glaucomas

Nicole Benitah, Ronald Buggage, and George N. Papaliodis ■

INTRODUCTION

The development of increased intraocular pressure and glaucoma in patients with uveitis is a multifactorial process that can be viewed as a complication of the intraocular inflammation. Both directly and by the induction of structural changes, inflammation in the eye can alter the aqueous humor dynamics, resulting in high, normal, or low intraocular pressures. The glaucomatous optic nerve damage and visual field defects that occur in patients with uveitis are primarily an effect of the uncontrolled intraocular pressure. The primary treatment objective for patients with uveitis-induced ocular hypertension and glaucoma is the control of the inflammatory disease and the prevention of permanent structural alterations to aqueous outflow by the use of appropriate anti-inflammatory therapy. Management of the intraocular pressure, either medically or surgically, is a secondary objective.

This chapter defines and discusses the pathophysiologic mechanisms, diagnosis, and treatment strategies for patients with uveitis and elevated intraocular pressure or secondary glaucoma. The chapter concludes with a description of specific uveitic entities in which increased intraocular pressure and glaucoma most commonly occur.

In common usage, the term *uveitis* is used to encompass all causes of intraocular inflammation. Uveitis can cause acute, transient, or chronic elevations in the intraocular pressure. The terms *inflammatory glaucoma* and *uveitic glaucoma* are commonly used to refer to any patient with uveitis and increased intraocular pressure. In patients with uveitis and no demonstrable "glaucomatous" optic nerve damage or "glaucomatous" visual field defects, it is more correct, however, to use terms such as *uveitis-induced ocular hypertension, ocular hypertension secondary to uveitis,* or *secondary ocular hypertension* to refer to those with uveitis and only elevated intraocular pressure. With resolution or appropriate management of the intraocular inflammation, the increased intraocular pressure need not progress to secondary glaucoma.

The terms *inflammatory glaucoma, uveitic glaucoma,* or *glaucoma secondary to uveitis* should be reserved for those patients with uveitis, increased intraocular pressure, and "glaucomatous" optic nerve or "glaucomatous" visual field defects. In most cases of uveitic glaucoma, the glaucomatous optic nerve injury is primarily a sequela of the elevated intraocular pressure;

therefore, the diagnosis of uveitic glaucoma should be questioned in a patient with no known history of increased intraocular pressure. In addition, the diagnosis of glaucoma secondary to uveitis should be questioned in any patient with visual field defects atypical for glaucoma and a normal-appearing optic nerve head. This is because many types of uveitis, particularly those affecting the posterior segment, are characterized by chorioretinal and optic nerve lesions that can produce visual field defects that do not represent glaucoma. This distinction is important, because the visual field defects in patients with active inflammatory disease may resolve or improve with appropriate therapy, whereas true glaucomatous visual field defects in patients with uveitis are irreversible.

EPIDEMIOLOGY

Uveitis may account for 5% to 10% of legal blindness in the United States and Europe, and up to 25% of blindness in the developing world.[1] The prevalence of uveitis in the United States from all causes has been estimated between 114.5 and 204 cases per 100,000 persons, with an annual incidence between 17 and 50 cases per 100,000 person-years.[2,3] Uveitis is found in patients of all ages; although earlier reports indicated a peak incidence between ages 25 and 44, more recent data indicate increasing incidence rates with increasing age.[2,3] Children constitute 5% to 10% of patients with uveitis, but children with uveitis are at relatively high risk of vision loss.[4] Common causes of visual loss in patients with uveitis include secondary glaucoma, cystoid macular edema, cataract, hypotony, retinal detachment, subretinal neovascularization or fibrosis, and optic nerve atrophy.

About 25% of all patients with uveitis will develop increased intraocular pressure at some time during the course of their inflammatory disease.[5] In general, uveitis-induced ocular hypertension and uveitic glaucoma are more

commonly complications of anterior uveitis and panuveitis because the inflammation in the anterior segment can interfere directly with the aqueous outflow route (**Table 14-1**). Uveitic glaucoma is also more common in cases of granulomatous than in nongranulomatous uveitis. When all causes of uveitis are considered, the prevalence of glaucoma secondary to uveitis in adults is estimated between 5.2% and 19%.[6] The overall prevalence of glaucoma in children with uveitis is similar to that in adults, ranging from 5% to 13.5%; however, the reported visual prognosis for children with uveitic glaucoma is worse.[6,7]

ETIOLOGY

The intraocular pressure depends on the balance of aqueous secretion and aqueous outflow. In most cases of uveitis, no single mechanism can account for the development of elevated intraocular pressure; rather, it is the result of a combination of several pathologic factors. The final common pathway of all mechanisms contributing to increased intraocular pressure in uveitis, however, is the impairment of aqueous outflow through the trabecular meshwork. Intraocular inflammation can impair aqueous outflow by causing derangements in aqueous secretion, producing changes in aqueous content, infiltrating ocular tissues, and inducing irreversible alterations in the anterior segment anatomy such as peripheral anterior synechiae and posterior synechiae that can lead to angle closure. These changes can produce a glaucoma that is not only severe but also resistant to all medical therapies. Paradoxically, the treatment of the uveitis with corticosteroids can also contribute to the development of elevated intraocular pressure.

The pathophysiologic mechanisms resulting in the development of elevated intraocular pressure in patients with uveitis can be simply classified as either open angle or closed angle. This classification is clinically useful because

TABLE 14-1. Uveitic Conditions Commonly Associated with Secondary Glaucoma

Anterior Uveitis

Juvenile rheumatoid arthritis

Fuchs heterochromic uveitis

Glaucomatocyclitic crisis (Posner-Schlossman syndrome)

HLA-B27–associated uveitis (ankylosing spondylitis, Reiter syndrome, psoriatic arthritis)

Herpetic uveitis

Lens-induced uveitis (phacoantigenic uveitis, phacolytic glaucoma, lens particle, phacomorphic glaucoma)

Panuveitis

Sarcoidosis

Vogt-Koyanagi-Harada syndrome

Behçet syndrome

Sympathetic ophthalmia

Syphilitic uveitis

Intermediate Uveitis

Intermediate uveitis of the pars planitis subtype

Posterior Uveitis

Acute retinal necrosis

Toxoplasmosis

the initial treatment approach differs between these two groups.

OPEN-ANGLE MECHANISMS

Abnormal Aqueous Secretion

Inflammation of the ciliary body usually results in decreased aqueous production. Decreased aqueous secretion in eyes with normal outflow facility results in the decreased intraocular pressure or hypotony that is frequently encountered in eyes with acute uveitis. If, however, there is concomitant or greater impairment of the aqueous outflow in eyes with decreased aqueous production as may happen due to decreased aqueous perfusion of the trabecular meshwork, the intraocular pressure may be normal or possibly increased.[8] There is a disagreement as to whether aqueous hypersecretion can result from the breakdown of the blood–aqueous barrier

in uveitic eyes. If this was possible, increased aqueous production could contribute to the development of high intraocular pressure in uveitic eyes. Relative to ciliary body function, the most likely explanation for the elevated intraocular pressure in eyes with intraocular inflammation, however, is that the aqueous production remains normal while the aqueous outflow is reduced.

Aqueous Humor Proteins

Alteration in the aqueous humor content was one of the first hypotheses offered to explain the onset of elevated intraocular pressure associated with uveitis. The influx of proteins into the eye resulting from the breakdown of the blood–aqueous barrier is the earliest change in uveitic eyes that can affect the balance of aqueous flow and increase the intraocular pressure.[9] In normal eyes, the protein content of the aqueous humor is approximately 100 times less than that in normal serum.[10] However, when the blood–aqueous barrier is disrupted, the aqueous protein concentration can resemble that of undiluted serum. An increased aqueous protein concentration can impair aqueous outflow by decreasing the flow rate of aqueous into the anterior chamber angle, mechanically obstructing the trabecular meshwork, and causing dysfunction of the endothelial cells lining the trabecular meshwork beams. In addition, the proteins promote the development of posterior or peripheral anterior synechiae. If the integrity of the blood–aqueous barrier is restored, the effect of the aqueous protein concentration on the aqueous outflow and intraocular ocular pressure can be reversed. However, if the permeability of the blood–aqueous barrier is permanently damaged, leakage of serum proteins into the anterior chamber may persist even after the intraocular inflammation has resolved.

Inflammatory Cells

An influx of inflammatory cells that secrete inflammatory mediators such as prostaglandins and cytokines occurs shortly after the protein influx in eyes with uveitis. Inflammatory cells in the anterior segment are believed to have a more direct effect on the intraocular pressure than aqueous proteins. Inflammatory cells can increase the intraocular pressure by infiltrating the trabecular meshwork and Schlemm canal, creating a mechanical obstruction to aqueous outflow. The risk for increased intraocular pressure is higher in granulomatous uveitis because of the greater infiltration of macrophages and lymphocytes compared with nongranulomatous uveitis entities in which the cellular infiltrate may contain higher proportions of polymorphonuclear cells.[5] Chronic, severe, or recurrent episodes of uveitis can cause permanent damage to the trabecular meshwork from injury to the trabecular endothelial cells, scarring in the trabecular meshwork and Schlemm canal, or from the formation of a hyaline membrane overlying the trabeculum.[6] Inflammatory cells and cellular debris in the anterior chamber angle can also contribute to the formation of peripheral anterior and posterior synechiae.

Prostaglandins

Prostaglandins are known to produce many of the signs of ocular inflammation, including vasodilatation, miosis, and increased vascular permeability, and have complex interactions on the intraocular pressure.[11,12] Whether or not prostaglandins are directly responsible for increased intraocular pressure in uveitic eyes is unclear. Through their action on the blood–aqueous barrier, they may indirectly contribute to increased intraocular pressure by enhancing the influx of aqueous protein, cytokines, and inflammatory cells. Alternatively, they can also decrease the intraocular pressure by the enhancement of uveoscleral outflow.

Trabeculitis

Trabeculitis is diagnosed when the intraocular inflammatory response is localized to the trabecular meshwork. Clinically, trabeculitis is characterized by the presence of inflammatory precipitates on the trabecular meshwork in the absence of other signs of active intraocular inflammation such as keratic precipitates, aqueous cells, or flare. The aqueous outflow in trabeculitis is decreased by mechanical obstruction of the trabecular meshwork resulting from the accumulation of inflammatory cells, swelling of the trabecular beams, and decreased phagocytosis of the trabecular endothelial cells. Because aqueous production in the ciliary body function is usually unaffected, the intraocular pressure in eyes with trabeculitis can be significantly elevated from the reduced aqueous outflow.[6]

Steroid-Induced Ocular Hypertension

Corticosteroids are considered first-line drug therapy for patients with uveitis. Whether given topically, systemically, or by periocular or sub-Tenon injection, corticosteroids are known to accelerate the formation of cataracts and cause increased intraocular pressure via increased outflow resistance.[13] This may happen in three ways: by inducing physical and mechanical changes in trabecular meshwork microstructure, by increasing the deposition of substances in the trabecular meshwork, and by decreasing the breakdown of substances in the trabecular meshwork.[13] Inhibition of prostaglandin synthesis is another mechanism by which corticosteroids may impair outflow facility.

The terms *steroid-induced ocular hypertension* and *steroid responder* are used to refer to patients who develop elevated intraocular pressures related to corticosteroid therapy. After 4 to 6 weeks of topical steroid treatment, 35% of the population will have an increase in intraocular pressure of at least 5 mm Hg, and 5% will have greater than a 16 mm Hg rise.[14] The risk of a steroid response is related to the duration and the dose of corticosteroid therapy. Patients with glaucoma, glaucoma suspects, first-degree relatives of people with glaucoma, the elderly, patients with connective tissue disease, type 1 diabetics, high myopes, and children younger than 10 years are at greatest risk for a steroid response.[6,13] Although steroid-induced ocular hypertension may occur at any time after the induction of corticosteroid therapy, it is most frequently detected within 2 to 8 weeks of the treatment being started. Compared with the other routes of administration, local steroids are most frequently associated with a steroid response. Periocular and intravitreal steroid injections can cause an acute pressure rise in susceptible patients that may be difficult to control. In most cases, the intraocular pressure returns to normal after discontinuation of the corticosteroid; however, in some cases, particularly following a steroid depot injection, the intraocular pressure can remain elevated for 18 months or longer. In these cases, surgical removal of the depot steroid or filtration surgery may be required if the intraocular pressure cannot be controlled medically (Fig. 14-1). For this reason, depot steroids should be avoided when possible in known steroid responders. A more recent steroid-delivery method for the treatment of posterior uveitis, the fluocinolone acetonide implant (Retisert), is associated with a 71% risk of an increase in intraocular pressure over 3 years; a combined surgery implanting the steroid device and a glaucoma drainage device may be beneficial in select patients.[15,16]

When a patient with uveitis who is being treated with corticosteroids develops an increased intraocular pressure, it is often difficult to know if the pressure rise is a result of the restored aqueous secretion, the impaired aqueous outflow caused by the intraocular inflammation, a steroid response, or a combination of all three. Although a fall in the intraocular pressure as the steroid is tapered may be evidence of steroid-induced ocular hypertension, the decline in pressure could also be secondary to improved outflow through the trabecular meshwork or a recurrence of inflammation with aqueous hyposecretion. If a steroid response that cannot be easily controlled medically is suspected in a patient who maintains active intraocular inflammation requiring systemic corticosteroids, this may be an indication for the initiation of a steroid-sparing agent. If steroid-induced ocular hypertension is suspected in a patient with controlled or quiescent uveitis, a reduction in the concentration, dose, or frequency of the corticosteroid used should be attempted.

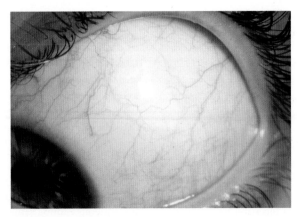

FIGURE 14-1. Periocular steroid injection in a steroid responder. Periocular steroid injections, useful in treating both anterior and posterior uveitis, can sometimes induce a severe elevation in the intraocular pressure in patients with ocular hypertension and known steroid responders. The anteriorly placed steroid depot in this 16-year-old patient with presumed sarcoidosis was removed when medical therapy failed to control his elevated intraocular pressure. Subsequently, his pressures normalized.

CLOSED-ANGLE MECHANISMS

Morphologic changes in the anterior chamber structures as a result of uveitis are often irreversible and lead to significant elevations in the intraocular pressure by altering or preventing the flow of aqueous from the posterior chamber to the trabecular meshwork. The structural changes that typically lead to secondary angle closure include peripheral anterior synechiae, posterior synechiae, and pupillary membranes that can cause pupillary block and, less commonly, forward rotation of the ciliary body.

Peripheral Anterior Synechiae

Peripheral anterior synechiae are adhesions between the iris and the trabecular meshwork or cornea that can completely block or impair access of the aqueous to the trabecular meshwork. Best detected by gonioscopy, peripheral anterior synechiae are a common complication of anterior uveitis and occur more commonly in granulomatous than nongranulomatous causes of uveitis. Peripheral anterior synechiae result from the organization of inflammatory material that pulls the iris surface into the angle. They develop more frequently in eyes with preexisting narrow angles or those narrowed by iris bombé. The iris attachments are usually broad, covering large segments of the angle, but can also be patchy or peaked, affecting only small portions of the trabecular meshwork or cornea (Fig. 14-2). In cases of peripheral anterior synechiae related to uveitis, even though large portions of the angle may remain open, the patient may still have increased intraocular pressure because the remaining angle is functionally compromised because of prior inflammatory damage that may not be detectable by gonioscopy.[5]

In cases of recurrent or chronic uveitis, continued peripheral anterior synechiae formation can result in complete angle closure. Neovascularization

of the iris and the angle should be sought in all cases of uveitis presenting with angle closure or extensive peripheral anterior synechiae. Contraction of the fibrovascular tissue in the angle or anterior iris surface may rapidly induce a complete and severe angle closure. Neovascular glaucoma secondary to uveitis is typically resistant to medical and surgical therapy and has a poor prognosis (Fig. 14-3).

Posterior Synechiae

Inflammatory cells, protein, and fibrin in the aqueous humor can stimulate posterior synechiae formation. Posterior synechiae are adhesions between the posterior iris surface and the anterior lens capsule, the vitreous face in aphakic patients, or the intraocular lens in pseudophakic individuals. The likelihood of developing posterior synechiae is related to the type, duration, and severity of the uveitis. The greater the extent of the posterior synechiae, the less the pupil is able to dilate and the greater the risk for further synechiae formation in subsequent uveitic recurrences.

The term *pupillary block* is used to denote impaired aqueous flow between the posterior and anterior chamber through the pupillary aperture as a result of posterior synechiae. Seclusio pupillae, posterior synechiae that extend for 360 degrees around the pupil, and pupillary membranes can cause complete pupillary block. In this condition, there is no flow of aqueous from the posterior to the anterior chamber. The buildup of aqueous in the posterior chamber may produce a severe elevation of the intraocular pressure that causes forward bowing of the iris into the anterior chamber, or iris bombé (Fig. 14-4). Iris bombé in an eye with ongoing inflammation may result in the rapid development of angle closure caused by the formation of peripheral anterior synechiae owing to appositional iridocorneal contact, even in an eye that may have previously had an open angle.[17] In some cases of uveitis with pupillary block, if the iridolenticular adhesions are sufficiently broad, only the peripheral iris may bulge forward, and the iris bombé may be difficult to diagnose without the use of gonioscopy.

Forward Rotation of the Ciliary Body

Acute intraocular inflammation can cause ciliary body swelling and supraciliary or suprachoroidal effusions that may result in the forward rotation of the ciliary body, causing angle closure not associated with pupillary block. Elevated intraocular pressure because of this type of angle closure occurs most often in patients with iridocyclitis, annular choroidal detachments, and posterior scleritis and can be seen in the acute stage of Vogt-Koyanagi-Harada syndrome.[5]

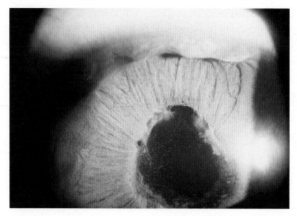

FIGURE 14-2. HLA-B27–associated anterior uveitis. Both posterior synechiae and a broad area of peripheral anterior synechiae obliterating the anterior chamber angle and extending onto the cornea (superior) are seen in this patient with HLA-B27–associated anterior uveitis following a severe exacerbation of intraocular inflammation.

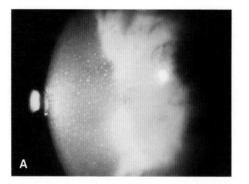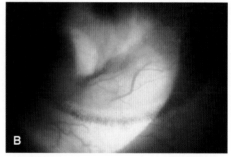

FIGURE 14-3. Neovascular glaucoma. This patient with granulomatous panuveitis developed intractable neovascular glaucoma, one of the most severe complications of uveitis. Note the diffuse, mutton fat keratic precipitates and iris bombé (**A**) and the neovascularization in the broad peripheral anterior synechiae (**B**).

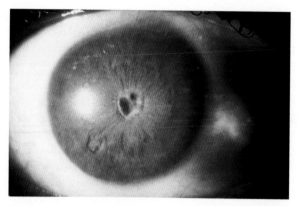

FIGURE 14-4. Posterior synechiae causing pupillary block and iris bombé. This patient with Vogt-Koyanagi-Harada syndrome presented with anterior segment inflammation and increased intraocular pressure as a result of posterior synechiae causing pupillary block with iris bombé. The uveitis was managed with topical and systemic corticosteroids, and the elevated intraocular pressure normalized following a laser iridotomy.

DIAGNOSIS

The accurate diagnosis and management of glaucoma in patients with uveitis relies on a thorough ophthalmic examination and the appropriate use of ancillary tests. Slit-lamp examination is required to establish the classification of the uveitis, the degree of inflammatory activity, and the type of inflammatory reaction. Uveitis can be classified anatomically as anterior, intermediate, posterior, or panuveitis according to the primary site of the inflammation in the eye.

The likelihood of uveitic glaucoma is greater in cases of anterior uveitis and panuveitis in which the structures involved in the aqueous outflow are more likely to be damaged by intraocular inflammation. The severity of the intraocular inflammation can be determined by assessing the aqueous cells and flare in the anterior chamber and the vitreous cells and haze. In addition, the structural changes in the ocular architecture induced by the inflammatory disease, such as peripheral anterior and posterior synechiae, should be noted.

The inflammatory response in eyes with uveitis can be either granulomatous or nongranulomatous. Signs of granulomatous uveitis in the anterior segment include mutton fat keratic precipitates and iris nodules (Figs. 14-3 and 14-5). Granulomatous uveitis is associated with a higher incidence of uveitic glaucoma than nongranulomatous uveitis.

Gonioscopy is the most critical part of ophthalmic examination in patients with uveitis and increased intraocular pressure and should be performed using a lens that indents the central cornea and pushes the aqueous into the angle. Gonioscopic examination reveals the presence of inflammatory material, peripheral anterior synechiae, and neovascularization in the angle, allowing differentiation between open-angle and closed-angle glaucoma.

On fundus examination, particular attention should be directed to the optic nerves, which should be assessed for excavation, hemorrhage, edema, or hyperemia. The retinal nerve fiber layer should also be evaluated. The diagnosis of uveitic glaucoma should not be made without documented glaucomatous disc damage and or visual field loss. Although retinal or chorioretinal lesions in the posterior pole do not contribute to the development of uveitic glaucoma, the presence and location of lesions that may manifest as a visual field defect and result in an incorrect diagnosis of uveitic glaucoma should be noted (Fig. 14-6).

Applanation tonometry is required during every clinical assessment, and reliable personnel should routinely perform visual field testing. Other ancillary tests that may be useful for the diagnosis and follow-up of patients with uveitis and increased intraocular pressure include laser flare photometry and ocular ultrasonography. Laser flare photometry is able to detect slight changes in the aqueous humor flare or protein content that cannot be assessed by the slit-lamp examination. The changes detected by the photometer have been shown to be useful in determining the activity of the uveitis.[5] B-scan ultrasonography and ultrasound biomicroscopy are useful in the assessment of uveitic glaucoma by demonstrating the morphology of the ciliary body and iridocorneal angle, which is helpful in determining the cause of both elevated and abnormally low intraocular pressures in patients with uveitis.[5]

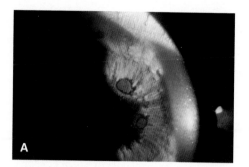
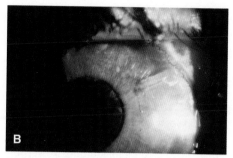

FIGURE 14-5. Sarcoidosis and active granulomatous panuveitis. A. This patient with sarcoidosis presented with an active granulomatous panuveitis, including Busacca nodules (seen here in the iris stroma) and secondary glaucoma resulting from posterior synechiae with pupillary block. Despite management with topical and systemic corticosteroids and topical antiglaucoma medications, his intraocular pressures were uncontrolled. Examination of the optic nerve head and visual field testing were consistent with glaucoma. **B.** Two months following tube shunt placement for uveitic glaucoma, the intraocular pressures were controlled and the iris nodules were resolved.

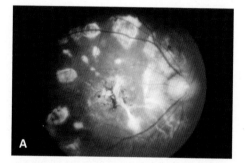
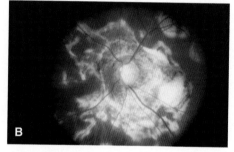

FIGURE 14-6. Multifocal choroiditis. This patient with multifocal choroiditis demonstrates the need for careful examination of the optic nerve for evidence of glaucoma in patients with uveitis. Because of the extensive posterior pole lesions, visual field testing did not reliably demonstrate the development of glaucoma in the left eye, evidenced by the progressive cupping off the optic disc. **A.** Right eye. **B.** Left eye.

MANAGEMENT

The first goal in the treatment of patients with uveitis-induced ocular hypertension or uveitic glaucoma is the control of the intraocular inflammation and prevention of permanent structural changes in the eyes. In some patients, resolution of the intraocular inflammation with appropriate therapy alone may normalize the intraocular pressure. In addition, irreversible consequences of uveitis such as peripheral anterior and posterior synechiae can be prevented with early anti-inflammatory therapy combined with mydriatics and cycloplegics.

The first-line treatment in most cases of uveitis requires the use of corticosteroids topically, locally via periocular or sub-Tenon injection, or systemically. Topical corticosteroids are useful for anterior segment inflammation; but alone, they are inadequate therapy for a phakic patient with active posterior segment inflammation. The frequency of administration of the topical corticosteroids depends on the severity of the inflammation in the anterior segment. Prednisolone acetate 1% (Pred Forte) is the most commonly used topical corticosteroid formulation for the control of anterior segment inflammation. Likewise, it is also the topical steroid formulation that is likely to cause steroid-induced intraocular hypertension and posterior subcapsular cataracts. A newer topical steroid, difluprednate (Durezol), has been shown to have equal efficacy to prednisolone acetate 1% with less frequent dosing; data on its propensity to cause elevated intraocular pressure have been reported.[18] Birnbaum et al. published a case series of patients with anterior uveitis treated with difluprednate and demonstrated that 39% had an increase in intraocular pressure of ≥ 10 mm Hg; 28% had an increase in intraocular pressure of ≥ 15 mm Hg; and 13% had an increase in intraocular pressure of ≥ 20 mm Hg.[19] Less-potent topical steroid formulations such as rimexolone, fluorometholone, medrysone,

and loteprednol etabonate (Lotemax) are less likely to cause a steroid response, but they are also less effective in controlling the intraocular inflammation. In our experience, topical nonsteroidal anti-inflammatory agents play no significant role in the treatment of uveitis or prevention of its complications.

Periocular steroid injections of triamcinolone (Kenalog, 40 mg per mL) into sub-Tenon space or transseptally through the lower lid, or intravitreal injections of preservative-free formulations of triamcinolone, can be effective for the control of both anterior and posterior segment intraocular inflammation. The main drawback of periocular and intraocular steroids is their greater potential to cause elevated intraocular pressure and cataract in susceptible patients. It is therefore inadvisable to administer periocular injections of depot steroid in patients with uveitis and intraocular hypertension because of their long-lasting effect, which cannot be readily discontinued.

Oral corticosteroids are the mainstay of uveitis therapy, with starting doses as high as 1 mg/kg/day, depending on the severity of the disease. Systemic steroids should be tapered once the intraocular inflammation is controlled. If sustained control of the intraocular inflammation using corticosteroids alone is not possible because of their side effects or because of persistent disease activity, a second-line immunosuppressant or a steroid-sparing medication may be needed. Steroid-sparing agents commonly used for the treatment of uveitis include cyclosporine, methotrexate, azathioprine, mycophenolate mofetil, and more recently tumor necrosis factor-alpha inhibitors and other biologic agents.[20-22] Alkylating agents such as cyclophosphamide and chlorambucil are generally reserved for severe cases of uveitis.[20]

Mydriatic and cycloplegic agents are used in the treatment of patients with anterior segment intraocular inflammation to relieve the pain and discomfort associated with ciliary muscle and iris sphincter spasm. Because these agents also dilate the pupil, they are also useful in preventing and breaking synechiae, which can alter aqueous flow and contribute to elevated intraocular pressure. Commonly prescribed agents for this purpose are atropine, scopolamine, homatropine, phenylephrine, cyclopentolate, and tropicamide. Some clinicians prefer relatively short-acting agents to reduce the risk of posterior synechiae forming in a dilated position.

Medical Therapy

Once the intraocular inflammation has been adequately addressed, specific therapy should also be administered to control the intraocular pressure. In general, the medical therapy for uveitis-induced ocular hypertension and uveitic glaucoma relies primarily on aqueous suppressants for pressure control. Antiglaucoma medications used in the treatment of uveitic glaucoma include beta-blockers, carbonic anhydrase inhibitors, adrenergic agents, and hyperosmotic agents for emergent control of acute pressure elevations. As a group, miotic agents and prostaglandin-like agents are generally avoided in patients with uveitis because they may exacerbate the intraocular inflammation. Topical adrenergic antagonists are the drugs of choice for the treatment of increased intraocular pressure in patients with uveitic glaucoma because they decrease aqueous humor production without affecting the pupil size. Beta-blockers commonly used in patients with uveitis include timolol, betaxolol, carteolol, and levobunolol. Betaxolol, which has fewer pulmonary side effects, may be safer to use in patients with sarcoid uveitis and known pulmonary disease. Metipranolol has been reported to cause a granulomatous iridocyclitis in some patients and should probably be avoided in patients with uveitis.[23]

Carbonic anhydrase inhibitors that reduce intraocular pressure by inhibiting aqueous humor production can be given topically, orally, or intravenously. The oral carbonic anhydrase inhibitor acetazolamide (Diamox) has been reported to reduce cystoid macular edema, which is a common cause of visual loss in patients with uveitis.[24] Topical carbonic anhydrase inhibitors are unlikely to have a similar effect on macular edema because sufficient concentrations probably do not reach the retina.

Adrenergic agents used in the treatment of uveitic glaucoma include apraclonidine, particularly to control acute intraocular pressure elevations that can occur after a neodymium (Nd):YAG capsulotomy and brimonidine; both are alpha-2 agonists that lower intraocular pressure by decreasing aqueous humor production and increasing uveoscleral outflow. Granulomatous anterior uveitis has also been reported as a late adverse effect of treatment with brimonidine (11 to 15 months after starting treatment).[17] Although they are now used infrequently, epinephrine and dipivefrin, which both lower intraocular pressure primarily by increasing aqueous outflow, also cause mydriasis, which could be helpful in the prevention of synechiae in uveitic eyes.

Prostaglandin analogs are thought to reduce intraocular pressure by increasing uveoscleral outflow.[5] Although effective at lowering intraocular pressure, the benefit of this class of agents in the treatment of uveitis is questioned because latanoprost (Xalatan) has been reported to induce intraocular inflammation and cystoid macular edema.[25,26] However, randomized controlled trials have not established a causal relationship.[17] More recently, there have been comparison studies in patients with uveitic glaucoma treated with latanoprost versus combination dorzolamide/timolol and there was no statistical difference between the two groups in regard to relapse of inflammatory disease.[27]

Hyperosmotic agents rapidly lower intraocular pressure, primarily by a reduction in the vitreous volume, and are helpful in the management of uveitic patients with acute angle closure. Glycerin and isosorbide can be administered orally, whereas mannitol is given intravenously.

Cholinergic agents such as pilocarpine, echothiophate iodide, eserine, and carbachol are generally avoided in patients with uveitis. This is because the induced miosis caused by these agents may potentiate formation of posterior synechiae, aggravate ciliary body muscle spasm, and contribute to a prolongation of the ocular inflammatory response by enhancing the breakdown of the blood–aqueous barrier.

MANAGEMENT OF ANGLE-CLOSURE GLAUCOMA

Iris bombé and angle closure caused by pupillary block are frequently the cause of severe intraocular pressure elevations and secondary glaucoma in patients with uveitis. When pupillary block is responsible for the obstruction of aqueous outflow, a communication between the posterior and anterior chambers can be reestablished using an argon or Nd:YAG laser iridotomy or a surgical iridotomy. Laser iridotomy may worsen or reactivate anterior chamber inflammation. To lessen the likelihood of this complication, the patient should be treated aggressively with topical corticosteroids before and after the procedure. Compared with the argon laser, the Nd:YAG laser requires the delivery of less energy and induces less postoperative inflammation. Because laser iridotomies are prone to closure, particularly in eyes with active inflammation, several iridotomies should be performed to ensure adequate aqueous flow (Fig. 14-7). Repeat procedures are needed in approximately 40% of uveitic eyes.[6] To reduce the risk of endothelial damage, laser iridotomy should not be performed in eyes with severe active uveitis or corneal edema, or in the areas of peripheral anterior synechiae.

Surgical iridectomy is indicated when laser iridotomies are unsuccessful or the use of laser is contraindicated. Surgical iridectomy is reported to be successful in uveitic eyes with peripheral anterior synechiae that involves less than 75% of the angle.[6] Although generally more effective than laser iridotomy, the procedure can lead to severe surgically induced postoperative inflammation that may be blunted by the use of aggressive preoperative and postoperative anti-inflammatory therapy; intravenous corticosteroids at the time of the procedure may also be beneficial. Compared with a laser iridotomy, a large-sector surgical iridectomy may delay cataract progression.

In uveitic eyes in which the angle closure is caused by forward rotation of the ciliary body without evidence of pupillary block, laser iridotomy and surgical iridectomy are of no use. The angle closure and elevated intraocular pressure in this rare group of patients are best treated with immunosuppressive therapy and aqueous suppressants. A surgical filtration procedure may be required in these cases if the intraocular pressure cannot be controlled medically and the angle closure cannot be reversed because of the formation of peripheral anterior synechiae.

Goniosynechialysis has been reported to be successful in lowering the intraocular pressure and establishing a normal anterior chamber angle in cases of acute angle closure resulting from extensive and recent formation of peripheral anterior synechiae. Trabeculodialysis, the disinsertion of the trabeculum from the scleral spur using a goniotomy knife, allows the aqueous direct access into Schlemm canal and has been used in children and young adults with uncontrolled uveitic glaucoma.[6]

Argon laser trabeculoplasty is not recommended for the treatment of uveitis-induced ocular hypertension or the treatment of uveitic glaucoma because the thermal energy and additional laser-induced inflammation may further damage the previously injured trabecular meshwork.

In secondary uveitic glaucoma, the damaging mechanism is nearly always intraocular hypertension. Because there is usually no primary disc pathology and because patients with uveitis are relatively young, there is a tendency to tolerate hypertension for longer periods and to tolerate higher levels of intraocular pressure before using surgical intervention. However, when the intraocular pressure remains uncontrolled in patients receiving maximal medical therapy or there is evidence of optic nerve injury or visual field defects, surgical intervention to control the intraocular pressure is required.

Surgical procedures performed in patients with uveitic glaucoma include trabeculectomy with and without the use of antimetabolites and tube shunt procedures such as the Ahmed, Baerveldt, and Molteno implants[5,6,28] (**Fig. 14-8**). The best surgical procedure for patients with uveitic glaucoma has not been established.

All surgical procedures performed on patients with uveitis carry the risk of a postoperative flare of intraocular inflammation, which typically occurs in the first postoperative week. Postoperative inflammation or reactivation of uveitis has been reported to occur in 5.2% to 31.1% cases of uveitic glaucoma treated surgically.[29] The risk of a postoperative flare is decreased in eyes that are quiescent before the surgical procedure. For elective surgeries, we require that the eyes remain quiet for at least 3 months before the operative procedure. To help decrease the risk of a postoperative flare, approximately 1 week before the planned surgery day, the patient's topical or systemic immunosuppressive regimen, or both, is increased and tapered postoperatively according to inflammatory response. Intraoperatively, periocular, intraocular, and/or intravenous steroids are routinely given. For emergent glaucoma procedures in patients with active disease, an exacerbation of the existing inflammation should be expected; therefore, aggressive topical therapy and the use of high-dose oral (0.5 to 1.5 mg/kg/day)

or intravenous corticosteroids may be required in the perioperative period. For many patients, we prefer a single intraoperative dose of 250 to 1,000 mg of intravenous methylprednisolone, as a single pulse dose not requiring a gradual taper.

Reported success rates for trabeculectomy in patients with uveitis glaucoma range from 62% to 81%.[17,30] However, depending to some extent on the follow-up interval, the true significance of such findings is not entirely clear. In trabeculectomy cases performed in patients with uveitis, the postoperative inflammatory response is believed to accelerate the wound-healing process and cause failure of the filtering procedure.[31] The outcome of trabeculectomies in patients with uveitis may be improved by the use of aggressive perioperative anti-inflammatory therapy and antimetabolites such as mitomycin C, which is favored over 5-fluorouracil.[6] The higher success rates of filtering surgery with the use of wound-modulating agents, however, is associated with an elevated risk for hypotony, bleb leaks, and endophthalmitis, which has been reported in up to 9.4% of eyes following trabeculectomy.[31] Cataract progression is also very common after filtration surgery for uveitic glaucoma.

Implant drainage procedures have also been used for the treatment of uveitic glaucoma, most commonly in patients who have failed previous filtering procedures.[6,28] They have been reported to be more successful than a repeat trabeculectomy in patients with uveitis.[30] Glaucoma drainage devices are also used as a primary treatment for uveitic glaucoma with increasing frequency, and further study is needed to definitively compare this approach with trabeculectomy.[17] Postoperative complications such as choroidal effusion, choroidal hemorrhage, and shallow anterior chambers may be greater in eyes with uveitic glaucoma as compared with eyes with primary open-angle glaucoma (**Fig. 14-9**).

Nonpenetrating glaucoma surgery may also have a role in the surgical management of uveitic glaucoma, although it is not an option in eyes with extensive anterior synechiae obstructing the trabecular meshwork. Viscocanalostomy has been shown to be effective in patients with open-angle glaucoma with a lower rate of complications than trabeculectomy. A small series has reported successful intraocular pressure control using nonpenetrating surgery in eyes with uveitic glaucoma. However, additional study is needed to validate the safety and efficacy of nonpenetrating surgery in uveitic glaucoma.[17] Deep sclerectomy is a nonpenetrating surgical procedure for the treatment of open-angle glaucoma (including uveitic glaucoma). A recent British publication demonstrated long-term efficacy and safety in this patient population.[32]

Ciliary body destructive procedures should be considered as a last resort for the treatment of uveitic glaucoma in which intraocular pressure is not amenable to any other medical or surgical glaucoma treatment. Cyclocryotherapy and contact and noncontact laser cycloablation procedures are generally similar in their ability to successfully lower the intraocular pressures. The primary disadvantage of cycloablative treatments is the induction of a severe intraocular inflammatory response and the development of phthisis bulbi in about 10% of treated eyes.[33]

REFERENCES

1. London NJS, Rathinam SR, Cunningham ET. The epidemiology of uveitis in developing countries. *Int Ophthalmol Clin.* 2010;50(2):1–17.
2. Gritz DC, Wong IG. Incidence and prevalence of uveitis in northern California: The northern California epidemiology of uveitis study. *Ophthalmology.* 2004;111:491–500.
3. Darrell RW, Wagener HP, Kurland LT. Epidemiology of uveitis: Incidence and prevalence in a small urban community. *Arch Ophthalmol.* 1962;68:502–514.
4. Cunningham ET Jr. Uveitis in children. *Ocul Immunol Inflamm.* 2000;8:251–261.
5. Tran VT, Mermoud A, Herbort CP. Appraisal and management of ocular hypotony and glaucoma associated with uveitis. *Int Ophthalmol Clin.* 2000;40:175–203.
6. Moorthy RS, Mermoud A, Baerveldt G, et al. Glaucoma associated with uveitis. *Surv Ophthalmol.* 1997;41:361–394.
7. Kanski JJ, Shun-Shin GA. Systemic uveitis syndromes in childhood: an analysis of 340 cases. *Ophthalmology.* 1984;91:1247–1252.
8. Johnson DH. Human trabecular meshwork cell survival is dependent on perfusion rate. *Invest Ophthalmol Vis Sci.* 1996;37(6):1204–1208.
9. Elliot R. *A Treatise on Glaucoma.* London, UK: Oxford Medical Publications; 1918.
10. Peretz WL, Tomasi TB. Aqueous humor proteins in uveitis. Immunoelectrophoretic and gel diffusion studies on normal and pathological human aqueous humor. *Arch Ophthalmol.* 1961;65:20–23.
11. Beitch BR, Easkins KE. The effects of prostaglandins on the intraocular pressure of the rabbit. *Br J Pharmacol.* 1969;37:158–167.
12. Bhattacherjee P. The role of arachidonate metabolites in ocular inflammation. *Prog Clin Biol Res.* 1989;312:211–227.
13. Jones R III, Rhee DJ. Corticosteroid-induced ocular hypertension and glaucoma: a brief review and update of the literature. *Curr Opin Ophthalmol.* 2006;17:163–167.
14. Weinreb RN, Mitchell MD, Polansky JR. Prostaglandin production by human trabecular cells: in vitro inhibition by dexamethasone. *Invest Ophthalmol Vis Sci.* 1983;24:1541–1545.
15. Goldstein DA, Godfrey DG, Hall A, et al. Intraocular pressure in patients with uveitis treated with fluocinolone acetonide implants. *Arch Ophthalmol.* 2007;125:1478–1485.
16. Malone P, Herndon LW, Muir KW, et al. Combined fluocinolone acetonide intravitreal insertion and glaucoma drainage device placement for chronic uveitis and glaucoma. *Am J Ophthalmol.* 2010;149:800–806.
17. Kuchtey RW, Lowder CY, Smith SD. Glaucoma in patients with ocular inflammatory disease. *Ophthalmol Clin North Am.* 2005;18:421–430.
18. Foster CS, Davanzo R, Flynn TE, et al. Durezol (difluprednate ophthalmic emulsion 0.05%) compared with Pred Forte 1% ophthalmic suspension in the treatment of endogenous anterior uveitis. *J Ocul Pharmacol Ther.* 2010;26(5):475–483.
19. Jabs DA, Rosenbaum JT, Foster CS, et al. Guidelines for the use of immunosuppressive drugs in patients with ocular inflammatory disorders: recommendations of an expert panel. *Am J Ophthalmol.* 2000;130:492–513.
20. Larkin G, Lightman S. Mycophenolate mofetil. A useful immunosuppressive in inflammatory eye disease. *Ophthalmology.* 1999;106:370–374.
21. Heiligenhaus A, Thurau S, Hennig M, et al. Anti-inflammatory treatment of uveitis with biological:

new treatment options that reflect pathogenetic knowledge of the disease. *Graefes Arch Clin Exp Ophthalmol.* 2010;248:1531–1551.

22. Akingbehin T, Villada JR. Metipranolol-associated granulomatous anterior uveitis. *Br J Ophthalmol.* 1991;75:519–523.

23. Whitcup SM, Csaky KG, Podgor MJ, et al. A randomized, masked, cross-over trial of acetazolamide for cystoid macular edema in patients with uveitis. *Ophthalmology.* 1996;103:1054–1062.

24. Warwar RE, Bullock JD, Ballal D. Cystoid macular edema and anterior uveitis associated with latanoprost use. Experience and incidence in a retrospective review of 94 patients. *Ophthalmology.* 1998;105: 263–268.

25. Da Mata A, Burk SE, Netland PA, et al. Management of uveitic glaucoma with Ahmed glaucoma valve implantation. *Ophthalmology.* 1999;106: 2168–2172.

26. Markomichelakis NN, Kostakou A, Halkiadakis I, Chalkidou S, Papakonstantinou D, Georgopoulos G. Efficacy and safety of latanoprost in eyes with uveitic glaucoma. *Graefes Arch Clin Exp Ophthalmol.* 2009;247(6):775–780.

27. Prata JA Jr, Neves RA, Minckler DS, et al. Trabeculectomy with mitomycin C in glaucoma associated with uveitis. *Ophthalmic Surg.* 1994;25:616–620.

28. Hill RA, Nguyen QH, Baerveldt G, et al. Trabeculectomy and Molteno implantation for glaucomas associated with uveitis. *Ophthalmology.* 1993;100:903–908.

29. Skuta GL, Parrish RK II. Wound healing in glaucoma filtering surgery. *Surv Ophthalmol.* 1987;32:149–170.

30. Wolner B, Liebmann JM, Sassani JW, et al. Late bleb-related endophthalmitis after trabeculectomy with adjunctive 5-fluorouracil. *Ophthalmology.* 1991;98:1053–1060.

31. Schuman JS, Bellows AR, Shingleton BJ, et al. Contact transscleral Nd:YAG laser cyclophotocoagulation. Midterm results. *Ophthalmology.* 1992;99:1089–1094.

32. Mercieca K, Steeples L, Anand N. Deep sclerectomy for uveitic glaucoma: long-term outcomes. *Medscape. Eye (Lond).* 2017;31(7):1008–1019.

33. Birnbaum AD, Jiang Y, Tessler HH, Goldstein DA. Elevation of intraocular pressure in patients with uveitis treated with topical difluprednate. *Arch Ophthalmol.* 2011;129(5):667–668.

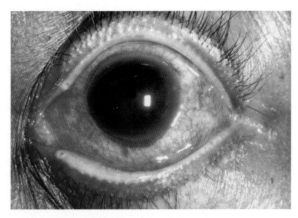

FIGURE 14-7. Recurrent iris bombé. This patient presented with acute eye pain and increased intraocular pressure from recurrent iris bombé when the previous laser iridotomy site closed during a uveitic flare associated with the tapering of her systemic immunosuppression.

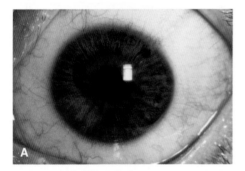 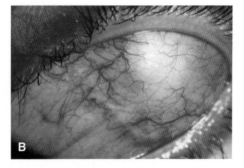

FIGURE 14-8. Bilateral Baerveldt implants in patient with juvenile rheumatoid arthritis. This 16-year-old female patient developed bilateral anterior uveitis at the age of 3 years that has been well managed with a combination of topical and systemic anti-inflammatory therapy. Because of uncontrolled intraocular pressure, she underwent bilateral Baerveldt implants as a primary glaucoma procedure with excellent results. **A.** Right eye showing the implant tube in the anterior chamber. **B.** Right eye looking down and nasally, revealing the conjunctival bleb over the implant.

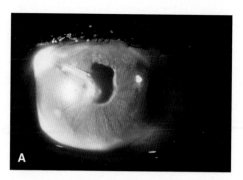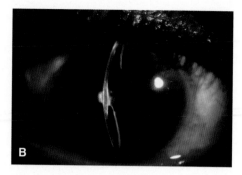

FIGURE 14-9. Complications of glaucoma surgery in a patient with uveitis. Hypotony with choroidal effusion and a shallow anterior chamber (**A,** diffuse illumination; **B,** slit beam) is a common complication of implant drainage procedures in patients with uveitis.

SPECIFIC ENTITIES

FUCHS HETEROCHROMIC IRIDOCYCLITIS

Fuchs heterochromic iridocyclitis is typically a unilateral, chronic, low-grade, nongranulomatous anterior uveitis that is associated with secondary posterior subcapsular cataract and glaucoma in 13% to 59% of cases.[1] The heterochromia that characterizes the condition is a result of intraocular inflammation leading to iris atrophy in the affected eye.

Epidemiology

- Fuchs heterochromic iridocyclitis is thought to be a relatively uncommon cause of anterior uveitis, accounting for 1.2% to 3.2% of all uveitis cases, although recently reported to comprise 12% of patients evaluated at a tertiary referral center.[2,3]

- The condition is unilateral in 90% of cases and appears to affect men and women equally.

- The disease is most commonly diagnosed in the third to fourth decades of life.

- Estimates of the overall incidence of glaucoma in Fuchs patients range from 13% to 60% and may be higher in patients with bilateral disease and in African-American patients.[4,6]

Etiology

- A growing body of evidence correlates Fuchs uveitis with the presence of intraocular antibodies to Rubella virus.[5]

- The increased intraocular pressure in Fuchs heterochromic iridocyclitis is thought to be the result of decreased aqueous outflow caused by inflammatory cells or a hyaline membrane obstructing the trabecular meshwork.

History

- Patients with this condition are typically asymptomatic, although some patients may have mild ocular discomfort and blurred vision.

- They are not known to have associated systemic disease. They frequently come to medical attention because of decreased vision associated with cataract progression.

Differential Diagnosis

- The differential diagnosis for Fuchs heterochromic iridocyclitis includes herpetic uveitis, the Posner Schlossman syndrome, sarcoidosis, syphilis, and, in those cases with posterior pole lesions, toxoplasmosis.

Diagnostic Evaluation

Ophthalmic Examination

- External examination typically reveals a white, quiet eye. The anterior segment generally shows a unilateral, low-grade, nongranulomatous anterior uveitis. The cornea shows stellate keratic precipitates scattered over the entire endothelium, which are an important clue to the diagnosis (**Fig. 14-10A**).

- In patients with dark irides, the stromal atrophy that results from the intraocular inflammation may cause the iris in the affected eye to appear lighter in color (**Fig. 14-10B**) or may cause only a flattening of iris details and a moth-eaten appearance.[4] In patients with light irides, however, the stromal atrophy will cause the affected eye to appear darker in color because of the exposure of the iris pigment epithelium.

- Another important diagnostic finding in patients with Fuchs heterochromic iridocyclitis is the identification of iris neovascularization or neovascularization of the angle by gonioscopy. Despite the chronicity of the intraocular inflammation in these patients, peripheral anterior synechiae and posterior synechiae almost never form. However, posterior subcapsular cataract is very common.

Laboratory Studies

- There are no laboratory studies that allow for the diagnosis of Fuchs heterochromic iridocyclitis. Lymphocytes and plasma cells have been identified in aqueous humor from affected patients; the antibody index to rubella virus may be elevated if checked, but this is generally unnecessary.[5]

- The diagnosis is made clinically based on the distribution of the keratic precipitates, the low-grade anterior uveitis typically unresponsive to steroids, iris heterochromia, absence of synechiae, and the lack of ocular symptoms.

Course

- The anterior uveitis in Fuchs heterochromic iridocyclitis is insidious and slowly progressive. The neovascularization of the iris and angle may cause mild intraocular hemorrhage spontaneously or with minor trauma, but does not cause peripheral anterior synechiae or neovascular glaucoma.

- Cataract and glaucoma are the most common complications.

    - Cataract formation has been reported in more than 80% of patients with the condition.[4] Cataract extraction, when required, is generally uncomplicated and is less likely to be complicated by the postoperative inflammation that is characteristic of other types of uveitis.[6] Posterior lens implantation is considered to be safe.

    - The glaucoma associated with Fuchs heterochromic iridocyclitis closely resembles the course of primary open-angle glaucoma.

Management

- Despite the presence of a chronic anterior uveitis, aggressive topical therapy with corticosteroids and the use of systemic immunosuppressive therapy are not recommended for the treatment of Fuchs heterochromic iridocyclitis because of the poor response to treatment. In fact, the use of topical steroids may be contraindicated because they may accelerate the development of cataract and glaucoma. Medical therapy is recommended for the control of the glaucoma; however, as many as 66% of patients may require surgical management.[7]

- The best surgical procedure for patients with Fuchs heterochromic iridocyclitis is unknown. Argon laser trabeculoplasty is not effective because of the formation of a hyaline membrane over the trabecular meshwork and should not be used.

REFERENCES

1. O'Connor GR. Doyne lecture. Heterochromic iridocyclitis. *Trans Ophthalmol Soc U K.* 1985;104:219–231.
2. Bloch-Michel E. Physiopathology of Fuchs's heterochromic cyclitis. *Trans Ophthalmol Soc U K.* 1981;101: 384–386.
3. Birnbaum AD, Little DM, Tessler HH, et al. Etiologies of chronic anterior uveitis at a tertiary referral center over 35 years. *Ocul Immunol Inflamm.* 2011;19(1):19–25.
4. Bonfioli AA, Curi AL, Orefice F. Fuchs' heterochromic cyclitis. *Semin Ophthalmol.* 2005;20(3):143–146.
5. Ruokonen PC, Metzner S, Ücer A, et al. Intraocular antibody synthesis against rubella virus and other microorganisms in Fuchs' heterochromic cyclitis. *Graefes Arch Clin Exp Ophthalmol.* 2010;248:565–571.
6. Tejwani S, Murthy S, Sangwan V. Cataract extraction outcomes in patients with Fuchs' heterochromic cyclitis. *J Cataract Refract Surg.* 2006;32:1678–1682.
7. Liesegang TJ. Clinical features and prognosis in Fuchs' uveitis syndrome. *Arch Ophthalmol.* 1982;100: 1622–1626.

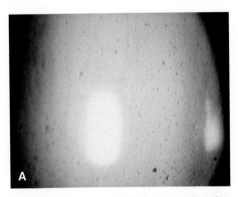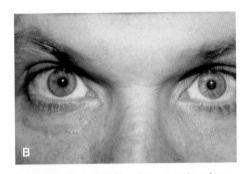

FIGURE 14-10. **Fuchs heterochromic iridocyclitis. A.** Fuchs heterochromic iridocyclitis is a unilateral, non-granulomatous anterior uveitis commonly characterized by the triad of heterochromia, cataract, and glaucoma in the affected eye. Patients with this condition characteristically show stellate keratic precipitates distributed over the entire corneal endothelium. **B.** The iris heterochromia and cataract in the left eye are a result of the chronic unilateral inflammation in the left eye.

GLAUCOMATOCYCLITIC CRISIS (POSNER-SCHLOSSMAN SYNDROME)

Glaucomatocyclitic crisis is a syndrome of recurrent episodes of mild, idiopathic, unilateral, nongranulomatous anterior uveitis accompanied by marked elevation in the intraocular pressure. Although this syndrome was probably first described in 1929, it carries the eponym of Posner and Schlossman who reported the syndrome in 1948.[1]

Epidemiology

- Glaucomatocyclitic crisis typically occurs in patients between the ages of 20 and 50 years.
- Although bilateral cases are reported, it is a unilateral disease in the overwhelming majority of cases.

Etiology

- The cause of glaucomatocyclitic crisis is unclear, but studies have implicated cytomegalovirus or herpes simplex virus (HSV) in at least some cases.[2,3] The increased intraocular pressure is believed to result from an acute decrease in the aqueous outflow during the attack.
- Prostaglandins have been demonstrated to play a role in the disease pathogenesis, with elevated levels in the aqueous humor correlating with the increase in intraocular pressure during an acute attack.[4] Prostaglandins break down the blood–aqueous barrier, resulting in an influx of proteins and inflammatory cells that can impair aqueous outflow and increase the intraocular pressure.
- Some patients with glaucomatocyclitic crisis have abnormal aqueous humor dynamics between episodes and may have an underlying primary open-angle glaucoma.

History

- Patients have a history of recurring symptoms of mild ocular pain or discomfort and blurred vision without ocular injection.
- Some patients may also describe halos that may indicate the presence of corneal edema.

Differential Diagnosis

Diseases to be considered in the differential diagnosis of glaucomatocyclitic crisis include Fuchs heterochromic iridocyclitis, herpes simplex or zoster uveitis, sarcoidosis, HLA-B27–associated anterior uveitis, and idiopathic anterior uveitis.

Diagnostic Evaluation

Ophthalmic Examination

- External ocular examination is frequently normal.
- Anterior segment examination typically reveals few keratic precipitates distributed over the inferior corneal endothelium. In some cases, particularly if the intraocular pressure is sufficiently elevated, the cornea may show microcystic edema.
- Keratic precipitates may occasionally be seen on gonioscopy, suggesting the presence of a trabeculitis.
- The anterior chamber characteristically shows only mild aqueous cells and flare.
- If pressure is significantly elevated, the pupil may be slightly dilated; however, peripheral anterior synechiae and posterior synechiae do not occur.
- Infrequently, heterochromia may be noted as a result of stromal atrophy caused by the recurrent unilateral inflammatory attacks.
- The intraocular pressure is generally much greater than would be expected for the degree of intraocular inflammation, typically measuring greater than 30 mm Hg, often in the 40 to 60 mm Hg range.
- The fundus examination is typically normal.

Laboratory Studies

• Glaucomatocyclitic crisis is a clinical diagnosis, and there are no laboratory studies that are specific for the diagnosis.

Course

• Posner-Schlossman syndrome is a self-limited ocular hypertension that resolves spontaneously regardless of treatment.

• The recurrent inflammatory attacks tend to occur at intervals of a few months to years and may last from several hours to a few weeks before spontaneously resolving.

• The development of optic nerve damage and visual field defects in glaucomatocyclitic crisis may occur as a result of the repeated bouts of extremely elevated intraocular pressure superimposed on an underlying primary open-angle glaucoma.[5]

Management

• Posner-Schlossman syndrome is treated initially with topical corticosteroids to control the anterior uveitis.

• If the intraocular pressure does not respond to topical anti-inflammatory therapy, antiglaucoma medications may be required to lower the intraocular pressure. Mydriatic and cycloplegic agents are not commonly needed because ciliary muscle spasm is uncommon and synechiae rarely form. Oral indomethacin, 75 to 150 mg daily—a prostaglandin antagonist—has been reported to lower the intraocular pressure in patients with glaucomatocyclitic crises faster than standard antiglaucoma medications.[4] Topical nonsteroidal anti-inflammatory medications might likewise be an effective treatment option for patients with ocular hypertension, but evidence is lacking to support this.

• Miotics and argon laser trabeculoplasty are generally not effective. Between attacks, prophylactic anti-inflammatory therapy is not required.

• Surgical filtration procedures are rarely required and, if performed, do not prevent the recurrent inflammatory attacks.

REFERENCES

1. Moorthy RS, Mermoud A, Baerveldt G, et al. Glaucoma associated with uveitis. *Surv Ophthalmol.* 1997;41:361–394.
2. Chee SP, Bacsal K, Jap A, et al. Clinical features of cytomegalovirus anterior uveitis in immunocompetent patients. *Am J Ophthalmol.* 2008;145(5):834–840.
3. Yamamoto S, Pavan-Langston D, Tada R, et al. Possible role of herpes simplex virus in the origin of Posner-Schlossman syndrome. *Am J Ophthalmol.* 1995;119(6):796–798.
4. Masuda K, Izawa Y, Mishima SS. Prostaglandins and glaucomato-cyclitis crisis. *Jpn J Ophthalmol.* 1975;19:368.
5. Kass MA, Becker B, Kolker AE. Glaucomatocyclitic crisis and primary open-angle glaucoma. *Am J Ophthalmol.* 1973;75:668–673.

HERPETIC KERATOUVEITIS

In the eye, infection with the HSV can manifest as several distinct, recurrent, unilateral ocular diseases such as blepharoconjunctivitis, epithelial keratitis, stromal keratitis, and uveitis. Although ocular involvement may occur with primary herpes zoster infection (chickenpox), it more commonly accompanies herpes zoster ophthalmicus, a reactivation of herpes zoster in older adults affecting the distribution of the ophthalmic branch of cranial nerve V. Uveitis associated with both HSV and herpes zoster infections typically follows previous episodes of keratitis and accounts for about 5% of all uveitis cases seen in adults.[1] Elevated intraocular pressure that can progress to a secondary glaucoma is a prominent feature of recurrent herpetic uveitis.

Epidemiology

• Approximately 0.15% of the US population has a history of external HSV infection.[2]

• Stromal keratitis and uveitis, which together account for the greatest visual morbidity from all forms of recurrent herpes simplex ocular disease, develop in fewer than 10% of patients with primary ocular herpes simplex infection.[1]

• The incidence of herpes zoster has been increasing, and ocular involvement occurs in two-thirds of all cases of herpes zoster ophthalmicus.[3] Uveitis and ocular hypertension in patients with zoster may be associated with either epithelial or stromal keratitis. The incidence of increased intraocular pressure in patients with herpetic uveitis varies from 28% to 40%.[4]

• The incidence of secondary glaucoma in patients with herpes simplex uveitis and herpes zoster uveitis is about 10% and 16%, respectively.[4,5]

Etiology

• It remains unclear whether the uveitis associated with herpes simplex keratitis is a secondary inflammatory response to the corneal disease or whether it is induced by invasion of the virus into the anterior uvea. The elevated intraocular pressure in herpes simplex and herpes zoster uveitis is the result of normal aqueous secretion in eyes, with impaired outflow resulting from trabeculitis, direct inflammation of the trabecular meshwork. In herpes zoster uveitis, ischemia resulting from an occlusive vasculitis may also contribute to the increased intraocular pressure.[6] HSV has been cultured from the anterior chamber of patients with herpetic uveitis, and its presence is positively correlated with ocular hypertension.

• Prolonged steroid use may also contribute to ocular pressure in patients with herpetic uveitis.

History

• Patients with herpetic uveitis typically present with a complaint of unilateral ocular redness, pain, photophobia, and, often, decreased vision.

• A prior history of recurrent keratitis is commonly given.

• Patients with uveitis related to herpes zoster are generally older and report a history of herpes zoster ophthalmicus. Ocular disease related to HSV is rarely bilateral, whereas herpes zoster ophthalmicus only occurs unilaterally.

Differential Diagnosis

• The differential diagnosis for herpetic uveitis includes Fuchs heterochromic iridocyclitis, glaucomatocyclitic crisis, and sarcoidosis.

• The presence of corneal hypoesthesia may be helpful in the diagnosis of herpetic uveitis.

DIAGNOSTIC EVALUATION

Ophthalmic Examination

• External ocular examination may reveal evidence of previous cutaneous lesions with herpes zoster and conjunctival injection and ciliary flush in either type of herpetic disease.

• Corneal sensation is often decreased in the affected eye.

• The cornea in patients with herpes keratouveitis may show a range of findings related to the prior epithelial or stromal disease, including epithelial dendrites, ghost dendrites, active disciform or necrotizing stromal keratitis, neovascularization, or scarring.

• Diffuse, nongranulomatous, stellate keratic precipitates or granulomatous precipitates can be found in both forms of herpetic uveitis. In severe cases of herpetic uveitis, posterior synechiae and angle closure may be found.

• Iris atrophy is a characteristic finding in uveitis resulting from both herpes simplex and zoster and may be patchy or segmental (Fig. 14-11).

- In patients with herpes zoster, the iris atrophy may be the result of an occlusive vasculitis in the iris stroma.

Laboratory Studies

- The diagnosis of herpetic uveitis is clinical and does not routinely rely on laboratory testing.

- Viral serologies for HSV and varicella zoster virus, if negative, exclude the diagnosis.

- The detection of viral DNA in the aqueous by polymerase chain reaction is supportive but not diagnostic of herpetic uveitis.

Course

- Similar to the other ocular manifestations of herpes eye disease, the uveitis is recurrent and may or may not be associated with recurrent keratitis.

- Elevated intraocular pressure is typically present during the course of the intraocular inflammation and may normalize or remain elevated after the uveitis has subsided.

- Approximately 12% of patients will have persistently elevated intraocular pressure that will require antiglaucoma therapy or filtering surgery.[4]

Management

- Uveitis associated with HSV and herpes zoster should be treated with topical corticosteroids.

- Cycloplegic agents may also be necessary if there is ocular pain resulting from ciliary spasm. An antiviral agent should be used with the topical steroids to lessen the likelihood of a reactivation of the epithelial keratitis.

- Oral acyclovir or valacyclovir in patients with herpes zoster ophthalmicus has been found to ameliorate the incidence and severity of dendritic keratitis, stromal keratitis, and uveitis.[7]

- Patients with increased intraocular pressure should be treated as needed with antiglaucoma therapy, although control of inflammation often leads to resolution of ocular hypotension.

- Filtration surgery may occasionally be required. Argon laser trabeculoplasty is not considered effective in the management of herpetic uveitis.

REFERENCES

1. Barron BA, Gee L, Hauck WW, et al; Herpetic Eye Disease Study. A controlled trial of oral acyclovir for herpes simplex stromal keratitis. *Ophthalmology.* 1994;101:1871–1882.
2. Parrish CM. Herpes simplex virus eye disease. In: *Focal Points: Clinical Modules for Ophthalmologists.* Vol. 15. San Francisco, CA: American Academy of Ophthalmology; 1997:2.
3. Leung J, Harpaz R, Molinari NA, et al. Herpes zoster incidence among insured persons in the United States, 1993–2006: evaluation of impact of varicella vaccination. *Clin Infect Dis.* 2011;52(3):332–340.
4. Falcon MG, Williams HP. Herpes simplex keratouveitis and glaucoma. *Trans Ophthalmol Soc UK.* 1978;98:101–104.
5. Panek WC, Holland GN, Lee DA, et al. Glaucoma in patients with uveitis. *Br J Ophthalmol.* 1990;74:223–227.
6. Johns KJ, O'Day DM, Webb RA, et al. Anterior segment ischemia in chronic herpes simplex keratouveitis. *Curr Eye Res.* 1991;10(suppl):117–124.
7. Sanjay S, Huang P, Lavanya R. Herpes zoster ophthalmicus. *Curr Treat Options Neurol.* 2011;13(1):79–91.

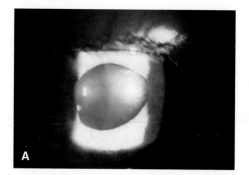
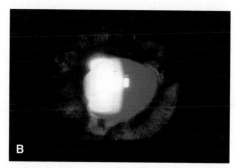

FIGURE 14-11. Herpetic uveitis because of herpes simplex. In patients presenting with unilateral anterior uveitis and elevated intraocular pressure, assessment of corneal sensation and transillumination of the pupil are helpful in making a clinical diagnosis of herpetic uveitis. Diffuse illumination of the iris (**A**) does not reveal the patchy atrophy of the iris stoma seen on transillumination (**B**). After the patient started oral acyclovir, he was able to discontinue topical antiglaucoma therapy.

SYPHILITIC INTERSTITIAL KERATITIS

Ocular syphilis may occur congenitally or may be acquired by sexual transmission. Congenital syphilis mainly affects the anterior segment of the eye, causing interstitial keratitis and anterior uveitis, whereas acquired syphilis more frequently causes both anterior and posterior uveitis. With the advent of effective diagnostic tests and antibiotic therapy, syphilitic interstitial keratitis and secondary glaucoma have become rare.

Epidemiology

- Ocular involvement in both congenital and acquired syphilis can be associated with increased intraocular pressure and secondary glaucoma that may occur during the active inflammatory stage or many years after the intraocular inflammation has become quiescent.

- Secondary glaucoma has been reported in 15% to 20% of adults with a history of interstitial keratitis caused by congenital syphilis.[1]

- Secondary glaucoma is less common in patients with acquired syphilis.

Etiology

- The pathologic mechanism of the increased intraocular pressure during the active stage of the disease is likely obstruction to the aqueous outflow by inflammatory cells and aqueous proteins.

- Synechiae formation, ocular maldevelopment, and lens subluxation may contribute to the development of narrow-angle or angle-closure glaucoma.

- Endothelialization of the angle demonstrated by histopathology is believed to be the underlying mechanism of the late-onset glaucoma in patients with congenital syphilis.

History

- Patients with ocular disease resulting from congenital syphilis typically present in the first or second decade of life with acute symptoms of ocular pain, photophobia, tearing, and decreased vision.

- The condition is bilateral in 90% of cases.

- Nonocular signs of congenital syphilis that may be present include dental deformities such as notched incisors and mulberry molars; skeletal abnormalities including a saddle nose, palatal perforation, saber shins, and frontal bossing; deafness; rhagades; and mental retardation.[2]

- Patients with acquired ocular syphilis are more likely to present with unilateral symptoms.

Differential Diagnosis

- The differential diagnosis for the active stage of ocular syphilis characterized by interstitial keratitis and anterior uveitis includes diseases such as herpes simplex and zoster infections, *Mycobacterium tuberculosis* and *leprae,* Lyme disease, rubeola (measles), Epstein–Barr virus (infectious mononucleosis), leishmaniasis and onchocerciasis, sarcoidosis, and Cogan syndrome.

Diagnostic Evaluation

Ophthalmic Examination

- Ocular examination of patients with congenital syphilis may show a variety of findings, including acute and chronic anterior uveitis, cataracts, chorioretinitis, retinal vasculitis, optic neuritis, and scleritis. Of these, interstitial keratitis is the most characteristic manifestation.

- The cornea in patients with active interstitial keratitis typically shows sectoral edema, opacification, and deep stromal vascularization that may be so pronounced as to give the cornea a pink salmon patch appearance.[3]

- Anterior uveitis commonly accompanies syphilitic interstitial keratitis and is often associated with elevated intraocular pressure.

- Ocular findings in patients with acquired syphilis frequently include anterior uveitis, chorioretinitis, and optic neuritis.

- Interstitial keratitis rarely develops in patients with acquired syphilis; and when it occurs, it is typically unilateral.

- Nodular iris lesions often accompany the anterior uveitis in patients with acquired syphilis.[4]

Laboratory Studies

- Ocular syphilis is diagnosed on the basis of a positive serology. The nontreponemal tests such as the Venereal Disease Research Laboratory or the rapid plasma reagin alone are insufficient and a treponemal test, such as the fluorescent treponemal antibody absorption test or the microhemagglutination test, *Treponema pallidum*, must be obtained.

- Any patient with syphilitic uveitis should have a spinal fluid examination to rule out asymptomatic neurosyphilis.

Course

- The interstitial keratitis and anterior uveitis typically persist for several weeks to months before spontaneously resolving, leaving ghost vessels in the deep corneal stroma.

- Glaucoma is a late complication of patients with congenital syphilis that typically develops in eyes without evidence of ongoing intraocular inflammation decades after the interstitial keratitis has subsided.

- Both open-angle and narrow-angle glaucoma have been described in these patients with equal frequency.

Management

- During the active stage of the disease, management of the increased intraocular pressure relies on topical corticosteroids, cycloplegic

agents, and antiglaucoma medications as needed.

- Systemic syphilis should be treated with an appropriate antibiotic course; when affecting the eyes, it should be treated as would be neurosyphilis.

- Laser iridotomy or surgical iridectomy should be performed in patients with narrow-angle or closed-angle glaucoma.

- Patients with late-onset open-angle glaucoma are less responsive to antiglaucoma medications and may require a filtering procedure.

- Argon laser trabeculoplasty is of little benefit because of the angle endothelialization.

REFERENCES

1. Lichter PR, Shaffer RN. Interstitial keratitis and glaucoma. *Am J Ophthalmol.* 1969;68:241–248.
2. Woods CR. Congenital syphilis—persisting pestilence. *Pediatr Infect Dis J.* 2009;28(6):536–537.
3. Lee ME, Lindquist TD. Syphilitic interstitial keratitis. *JAMA.* 1989;262(20):2921.
4. Aldave AJ, King JA, Cunningham ET Jr. Ocular syphilis. *Curr Opin Ophthalmol.* 2001;12(6):433–441.

JUVENILE IDIOPATHIC ARTHRITIS

Juvenile idiopathic arthritis (JIA), formerly known in the United States as juvenile rheumatoid arthritis, is a common cause of pediatric uveitis often complicated by increased intraocular pressure and glaucoma. Three subtypes of JIA with different risks for the development of uveitis can be diagnosed on the basis of the extent of articular and systemic involvement within the first 3 months of presentation. Systemic-onset JIA, or Still disease, is commonly seen in boys younger than 4 years of age and is an acute systemic disease consisting of a cutaneous rash, fever, polyarthritis, hepatosplenomegaly, leukocytosis, and polyserositis. Young girls more commonly present with the oligoarticular (fewer than five joints, also known as pauciarticular) and polyarticular (five or more joints) forms of JIA that lack the systemic features.

Epidemiology

- The incidence of uveitis in JIA varies from 2% to 30%, depending on the subtype.[1,2]
- Uveitis is typically not associated with Still disease or systemic-onset JIA.
- Anterior uveitis is more common in patients with the oligoarticular form (19% to 29%) than in those with the polyarticular form (2% to 5%) of JIA.[3,4]
- Children with the oligoarticular or monoarticular onset of joint involvement account for more than 90% of the JIA patients with uveitis.
- Secondary glaucoma is seen in approximately 14% to 22% of patients with chronic anterior uveitis associated with JIA.[1]

Etiology

- The development of increased intraocular pressure and glaucoma in patients with JIA is most often caused by progressive angle closure as a result of synechiae.
- Open-angle glaucoma also occurs and may be the result of chronic inflammatory damage to the trabecular meshwork or steroid-induced glaucoma resulting from prolonged topical steroid treatment.

History

- Although arthritis develops first in the majority of cases, JIA-associated uveitis may be the presenting sign.
- Because the anterior uveitis associated with JIA is mild, asymptomatic, and rarely causes ocular redness, the disease may go unnoticed for a long period of time until visual loss, cataract, or an irregular pupil is noted.
- The uveitis in patients with JIA is bilateral in almost all cases.

Differential Diagnosis

- The differential diagnosis for chronic anterior uveitis in children includes sarcoidosis, pars planitis, HLA-B27–associated diseases, and idiopathic anterior uveitis.

Diagnostic Evaluation

Ophthalmic Examination

- Band keratopathy is found in up to 50% of children with anterior uveitis, and its presence is thought to be associated with the chronicity of the disease.[1]
- The anterior uveitis in patients with JIA is nongranulomatous in the vast majority of cases.
- Keratic precipitates are generally distributed over the inferior half of the cornea.
- Miotic pupils resulting from posterior synechiae or pupillary membranes, iris bombé, and peripheral anterior synechiae are frequent findings in affected patients that can contribute to the development of glaucoma.
- Anterior and posterior subcapsular cataracts are present in up to one-third of affected patients. Posterior segment examination in patients with JIA may show papillitis and cystoid macular edema, which can contribute to visual loss.

Laboratory Studies

- Up to 80% of patients with anterior uveitis and JIA are antinuclear antibody positive and rheumatoid factor negative.

Course

- The uveitis associated with JIA is a chronic disease that is difficult to control despite treatment.
- In patients with JIA, there is no direct correlation between the activity of the ocular disease and the joint disease.

- The incidence of secondary complications, such as band keratopathy, cataract, and glaucoma, increases with the duration of the disease.

- The prognosis for children with uveitic glaucoma, previously considered poor, is improving with more effective surgical management.

Management

- The initial treatment approach for the management of intraocular inflammation in patients with JIA includes topical corticosteroids and cycloplegic agents to prevent the formation of synechiae.

- Often, periocular steroid injections and even systemic steroids are necessary to control anterior uveitis. Oral nonsteroidal agents are also used in JIA patients. Methotrexate alone or in combination with other immunosuppressive agents such as prednisone or cyclosporine has been used to treat the ocular and joint manifestations of JIA. Newer biologic agents such as infliximab (Remicade), adalimumab (Humira), and abatacept (Orencia), shown to be of benefit for the joint disease in JIA, are currently being evaluated for their efficacy in the treatment of uveitis in these patients.

- Elevated intraocular pressure in JIA is treated initially with antiglaucoma medications. Medical management is initially effective in only about 50% of patients with JIA, with only 30% of patients being controlled medically over the long term.[4]

- Laser iridotomy or surgical iridectomy may be necessary to relieve the pupillary block in patients with posterior synechiae.

- Surgical management is required for patients who are unresponsive to medical therapy. To increase the likelihood of a good outcome, if possible, surgical intervention should be deferred until the intraocular inflammation has been adequately controlled for a period of at least 3 months.

- Operative procedures most commonly used in children with JIA include trabeculectomy and tube shunts (see Fig. 14-8).

- Improved success has been reported with the use of antimetabolites in patients undergoing trabeculectomy.[1]

- Trabeculodialysis in a small case series has been shown to be safe and effective for controlling the pressure in patients with JIA for up to 2 years.[5]

REFERENCES

1. Moorthy RS, Mermoud A, Baerveldt G, et al. Glaucoma associated with uveitis. *Surv Ophthalmol.* 1997;41:361–394.
2. Ravelli A, Felici E, Magni-Manzoni S, et al. Patients with antinuclear antibody-positive juvenile idiopathic arthritis constitute a homogeneous subgroup irrespective of the course of joint disease. *Arthritis Rheum.* 2005;52:826–832.
3. Calabro JJ, Parrino GR, Atchoo PD, et al. Chronic iridocyclitis in juvenile rheumatoid arthritis. *Arthritis Rheum.* 1970;13:406–413.
4. O'Brien JM, Albert DM. Therapeutic approaches for ophthalmic problems in juvenile rheumatoid arthritis. *Rheum Dis Clin North Am.* 1989;15:413–437.
5. Kanski JJ, McAllister JA. Trabeculodialysis for inflammatory glaucoma in children and young adults. *Ophthalmology.* 1985;92:927–930.

LENS-INDUCED UVEITIS AND GLAUCOMA

The liberation of lens proteins through an intact or disrupted lens capsule into the anterior chamber or vitreous cavity can trigger a severe intraocular inflammatory reaction that may impair aqueous outflow and cause an acute elevation in the intraocular pressure or glaucoma. Leakage of lens proteins is typically the result of accidental or surgical trauma to the lens capsule or may be associated with cataract progression. Clinical entities characterized by lens-induced uveitis and glaucoma include phacoantigenic uveitis, phacolytic glaucoma, lens particle glaucoma, and phacomorphic glaucoma. Uveitis and glaucoma may also be a complication of intraocular lens placement.[1]

Epidemiology

• Although the condition is well described, the exact incidence of glaucoma caused by various forms of lens-induced uveitis is not known.

• In one study of patients with phacoanaphy-lactic uveitis (phacoantigenic uveitis), 17% of patients were diagnosed with glaucoma.[2]

History

• Phacoantigenic uveitis, also referred to as phacoanaphylactic uveitis or phacoanaphy-lactic endophthalmitis, is a granulomatous uveitis initiated by the release of lens proteins through a ruptured lens capsule.

• The onset of the inflammation is days to weeks after the traumatic or surgical injury to the lens. Patients present with a red, painful eye.

• Rarely, phacoantigenic uveitis is associated with sympathetic ophthalmia and the development of an inflammatory reaction in the fellow eye.[3]

• Phacolytic glaucoma typically seen in older patients arises when lens proteins leak from a mature or hypermature cataract through an intact but permeable lens capsule. Patients with phacolytic glaucoma commonly present with the abrupt onset of ocular pain and redness in a poorly seeing eye with a known cataract.

• Lens particle glaucoma, also known as pha-cotoxic uveitis, occurs following any ocular injury that results in the liberation of lens cortical material into the anterior chamber. In most cases, the onset of increased intraocular pressure is detected days or weeks after the inciting injury.

• In cases of phacomorphic glaucoma, the lens capsule is not typically violated and the eye generally does not show significant intraocular inflammation. Patients typically present with a redness and pain from angle closure in an eye with decreased vision caused by a cataract.

• The uveitis–glaucoma–hyphema syndrome was a frequent cause of postoperative intraocular inflammation and glaucoma in patients following implantation with the first generation of rigid, anterior chamber intraocular lenses. The syndrome was attributed to poor intraocular lens size selection or manufacturing defects in the lens material, causing mechanical irritation to anterior chamber structures.

• Chronic or severe postoperative inflammation can also result in pseudophakic inflammatory glaucoma in patients with posterior chamber intraocular lens implants.

Etiology

• Obstruction of aqueous outflow at the level of the trabecular meshwork is the common mechanism in the lens-induced glaucomas.

  ▪ In phacoantigenic uveitis, there is a granulomatous inflammatory response to the elaborated lens proteins that can induce the formation of synechiae and blockage of the trabecular meshwork.

  ▪ In phacolytic glaucoma, the released lens proteins and macrophages engorged with lens proteins obstruct the trabecular meshwork, whereas in lens particle glaucoma, it is the actual fragments of lens cortical material that are believed to injure the trabecular meshwork.

• Unlike the other lens-induced glaucomas, in which the anterior chamber angle is typically open, in phacomorphic glaucoma the intumescent lens can cause pupillary block or dislocate the iris forward, resulting in a shallowed anterior chamber or acute angle closure. In pseudophakic eyes, intraocular inflammation may be the result of a preexisting uveitis, a delayed-onset postsurgical endophthalmitis, or irritation of the uveal tissue by the intraocular lens. Glaucoma may arise because of damage to the trabecular meshwork or formation of synechiae on the lens implant, causing pupillary block, and peripheral anterior synechiae formation, resulting in angle closure.

Differential Diagnosis

- The main differential diagnoses for phacoantigenic and lens particle glaucoma are post-traumatic and postsurgical endophthalmitis.

- Other causes of acute angle closure should be considered in patients with phacomorphic glaucoma.

Diagnostic Evaluation

Ophthalmic Examination

- External examination of patients with acute lens-induced uveitis and glaucoma commonly reveals conjunctival injection and ciliary flush. There may also be external evidence of a prior ocular injury.

- If the pressure is significantly elevated, the cornea is often edematous.

- The anterior chamber typically contains anterior chamber cells and flare, with granulomatous or nongranulomatous keratic precipitates. White, flocculent material and fragments of lens cortex may be seen circulating within the aqueous and in the anterior chamber angle, which may be open, narrowed, or closed. Peripheral anterior and posterior synechiae are not uncommon.

- In cases of phacoantigenic uveitis and lens particle glaucoma, evidence of injury to the native lens or retained lens material can usually be found. In cases of phacolytic and phacomorphic glaucoma, examination reveals a hypermature or intumescent cataract, respectively, and in cases of pseudophakic inflammatory glaucoma, an intraocular lens is present.

- Posterior segment examination may show vitreous cells and haze, lens material in the vitreous cavity, and other findings related to the ocular injury.

Laboratory Studies

- The diagnosis of lens-induced uveitis and glaucoma is clinical and does not rely on laboratory testing.

- Histopathologic examination of the lens in patients with phacoantigenic uveitis reveals a zonal granulomatous inflammation centered at the site of lens injury.

Course

- The clinical course of the lens-induced glaucomas tends to be relatively brief because they are effectively managed with surgical intervention.

Management

- Cataract extraction or removal of the retained lens material or lens implant is the definitive therapy for lens-induced uveitis and glaucoma.

- Before surgical intervention, the intraocular inflammation is treated with topical corticosteroids and the increased intraocular pressure is controlled with antiglaucoma medications.

  ▪ In some patients with uveitic glaucoma related to an intraocular lens, medical management may be adequate, and the inflammation may resolve over time, avoiding the need for surgery.

- In patients with phacomorphic glaucoma, after the intraocular pressure is lowered medically, laser iridotomy can be used to temporize the condition if cataract extraction needs to be delayed or cannot be performed.

REFERENCES

1. Ellant JP, Obstbaum SA. Lens-induced glaucoma. *Doc Ophthalmol.* 1992;81(3):317–338.
2. Thach AB, Marak GE Jr, McLean IW, et al. Phacoanaphylactic endophthalmitis: a clinicopathologic review. *Int Ophthalmol.* 1991;15:271–279.
3. Allen JC. Sympathetic uveitis and phacoanaphylaxis. *Am J Ophthalmol.* 1967;63:280–283.

SARCOIDOSIS

Sarcoidosis is a systemic disease characterized by noncaseating, granulomatous, inflammatory infiltrates affecting the lungs, skin, liver, spleen, central nervous system, and eyes. Ocular disease occurs in 10% to 38% of patients with systemic sarcoidosis.[3] Sarcoidosis, which can present as anterior, intermediate, posterior, or panuveitis, is the prototype for a chronic, granulomatous uveitis.

Epidemiology

- Sarcoidosis is 8 to 10 times more frequent among African Americans than whites, having an estimated prevalence of 82 per 100,000 in this population.[1]

- Although sarcoidosis can develop at any age, the disease is typically diagnosed in adults between 20 and 50 years of age. Sarcoidosis accounts for 5% of all uveitis cases in adults but about 1% of uveitis cases in children.[2]

- Sarcoidosis involves the anterior segment in up to 70% of cases with ocular involvement, whereas the posterior segment is affected in less than 33% of cases.[3]

- Secondary glaucoma occurs in approximately 11% to 25% of all patients with sarcoidosis and is more commonly a complication of the anterior segment disease.[4]

- African-American patients with sarcoidosis have a higher incidence of uveitic glaucoma and blindness.

Etiology

- Ocular hypertension and glaucoma in patients with sarcoidosis results from obstruction of the trabecular meshwork by the chronic granulomatous inflammation and angle closure caused by the formation of peripheral anterior and posterior synechiae with iris bombé.

- Anterior segment neovascularization and the prolonged use of steroids can also contribute to the impairment of aqueous outflow.

History

- Most adult patients with sarcoidosis present with pulmonary involvement that may manifest as cough, shortness of breath, wheezing, or dyspnea on exertion.

- Another common presentation of sarcoidosis is with generalized symptoms such as fever, fatigue, and weight loss.

- Many patients are asymptomatic at the time of diagnosis.

- Patients with ocular involvement typically present with complaints of ocular pain, redness, photophobia, floaters, and blurred or decreased vision.

Differential Diagnosis

- The differential diagnosis of sarcoidosis includes the other causes of granulomatous panuveitis such as the Vogt-Koyanagi-Harada syndrome, sympathetic ophthalmia, and tuberculosis.

- Syphilis, Lyme disease, primary intraocular lymphoma, and pars planitis should also be considered.

Diagnostic Evaluation

Ophthalmic Examination

- The ocular disease of sarcoidosis is typically bilateral, although it may be unilateral or very asymmetric.

• Most frequently a cause of granulomatous uveitis, sarcoidosis may also cause a nongranulomatous uveitis.

• Ophthalmic findings in the anterior segment include orbital and cutaneous granulomas, enlarged lacrimal glands, and palpebral and bulbar conjunctival nodules.

■ The cornea most commonly shows large, mutton fat keratic precipitates, with nummular corneal infiltrates and inferior areas of endothelial opacification being noted less frequently.

■ Posterior and peripheral anterior synechiae, when extensive, result in elevated intraocular pressure or secondary uveitic glaucoma caused by angle closure or iris bombé.

■ Koeppe and Busacca-type iris nodules are often seen in the more severe cases of anterior segment disease (see Fig. 14-5).

• Posterior segment involvement in sarcoidosis occurs less frequently than anterior segment disease.

■ The vitreous frequently shows a vitritis with vitreous snowballs and inferior inflammatory debris.

■ Examination of the posterior pole may reveal a variety of findings, including peripheral retinal vasculitis, peripheral exudates similar to snowbanks, hemorrhages, retinal exudates, and perivascular nodular granulomatous lesions, Dalen-Fuchs nodules, and retinal, subretinal, or disc neovascularization. Granulomas in the retina, choroid, and optic nerve may also be seen.

• Visual loss in sarcoidosis is most often a result of cystoid macular edema, optic neuritis caused by granulomatous infiltration of the optic nerve, and secondary glaucoma.

Laboratory Studies

• The diagnosis of sarcoidosis is confirmed with a tissue biopsy showing noncaseating or nonnecrotizing granulomas or granulomatous inflammation in a patient in whom all other causes of granulomatous disease, such as tuberculosis and fungal infections, have been excluded.

• An initial diagnostic evaluation for sarcoidosis should include a chest X-ray and serum angiotensin-converting enzyme (ACE) level. Serum lysozyme levels may also be elevated in patients with sarcoidosis; this test may have a better combination of sensitivity, specificity, positive predictive value, and negative predictive value than ACE level.[5]

• Additional studies that may be useful in confirming the diagnosis include anergy testing, pulmonary function testing, gallium scan, computed tomographic scan of the thorax, bronchoalveolar lavage, and transbronchial biopsy.

• Because ACE levels may be high in normal children, serum ACE level is a less useful diagnostic test for sarcoidosis in children. Elevated ACE levels have been reported in the aqueous humor and cerebrospinal fluids of patients with ocular and central nervous system sarcoid uveitis and neurosarcoidosis, respectively.

Course

• The clinical course of ocular sarcoidosis can be acute and self-limited or chronic, recurrent, and relentless.

• The chronic form of sarcoid uveitis has the worse prognosis because of the onset of complications such as glaucoma, cataract, and macular edema.

Management

• The mainstay of therapy for both systemic and ocular sarcoidosis is corticosteroids.

• Anterior segment disease may be managed with topical or periocular corticosteroid injections. Systemic therapy is typically required for bilateral posterior segment uveitis. Other immunosuppressive agents such as methotrexate and infliximab have demonstrated therapeutic benefit in the management of sarcoidosis and should be considered early for patients with chronic sarcoidosis requiring prolonged steroid therapy.[6,7] Cyclosporine and etanercept do not appear to have benefit in the treatment of sarcoidosis.[8–10]

● The glaucoma should be treated medically with aqueous suppressants for as long as possible.

● Argon laser trabeculoplasty is frequently ineffective.

● Laser iridotomy and surgical iridectomy are the treatments of choice for patients with pupillary block.

● If the intraocular pressure remains uncontrolled, surgical intervention with either a filtering procedure or a tube shunt is required.

● Surgical success is improved if the intraocular inflammatory disease can be controlled before the surgical procedure.

REFERENCES

1. Nussenblatt RB, Whitcup SM, Palestine AG. Sarcoidosis. In: *Uveitis: Fundamentals and Clinical Practice.* St Louis, MO: Mosby; 1996:289–298.

2. Hoover DL, Khan JA, Giangiacomo J. Pediatric ocular sarcoidosis. *Surv Ophthalmol.* 1986;30:215–228.

3. Jabs DA, Johns CJ. Ocular involvement in chronic sarcoidosis. *Am J Ophthalmol.* 1986;102:297–301.

4. Obenauf CD, Shaw HE, Sydnor CF, et al. Sarcoidosis and its ophthalmic manifestations. *Am J Ophthalmol.* 1978;86:648–655.

5. Herbort CP, Rao NA, Mochizuki M; Members of Scientific Committee of First International Workshop on Ocular Sarcoidosis. International criteria for the diagnosis of ocular sarcoidosis: results of the first International Workshop on Ocular Sarcoidosis (IWOS). *Ocul Immunol Inflamm.* 2009;17(3):160–169.

6. Chan ES, Cronstein BN. Molecular action of methotrexate in inflammatory diseases. *Arthritis Res.* 2002;4(4):266–273.

7. Baughman RP, Drent M, Kavuru M, et al. Infliximab therapy in patients with chronic sarcoidosis and pulmonary involvement. *Am J Respir Crit Care Med.* 2006;174(7):795–802.

8. Wyser CP, van Schalkwyk EM, Alheit B, et al. Treatment of progressive pulmonary sarcoidosis with cyclosporine A: a randomized controlled trial. *Am J Respir Crit Care Med.* 1997;156(5):1371–1376.

9. Martinet Y, Pinkston P, Saltini C, et al. Evaluation of the in vitro and in vivo effects of cyclosporine on the lung T-lymphocyte alveolitis of active pulmonary sarcoidosis. *Am Rev Respir Dis.* 1988;138(5):1242–1248.

10. Utz JP, Limper AH, Kalra S, et al. Etanercept for the treatment of stage II and III progressive pulmonary sarcoidosis. *Chest.* 2003;124(1):177–185.

Lens-Associated Open-Angle Glaucomas

Michele C. Lim and Ashley G. Lesley ■

INTRODUCTION

Lens-associated open-angle glaucomas are composed of three separate diagnoses with similar clinical presentations. Lens protein glaucoma, lens particle glaucoma, and lens-associated uveitis (LAU) may each present with intraocular inflammation, an abnormal lens, and elevated intraocular pressure (IOP), although hypotony may commonly occur in the latter. Distinguishing among the three entities requires careful examination and an understanding of the mechanisms that define each diagnosis (**Table 15-1**).

TABLE 15-1. Clinical Presentation of Lens-Associated Open-Angle Glaucomas

	Lens Particle Glaucoma	Lens Protein Glaucoma	LAU
Mechanism	Lens material obstructs TM	HMW lens proteins obstruct TM	Loss of immune tolerance
IOP	Elevated	Elevated	Low or elevated
Gonioscopy	Open angle	Open angle	Open angle
Lens status	Disruption to lens capsule with release of lens particles	Mature or hypermature cataract	Disruption to lens capsule; exposure of large lens fragments
Management	Antiglaucoma medication, steroids, surgical removal of lens material	Antiglaucoma medication, topical steroids, cataract removal	Antiglaucoma topical medication, topical steroids, removal of lens fragments

HMW, heavy-molecular-weight; IOP, intraocular pressure; LAU, lens-associated uveitis; TM, trabecular meshwork.

LENS PROTEIN OR PHACOLYTIC GLAUCOMA

Lens protein glaucoma occurs in the presence of a mature or a hypermature cataract (Fig. 15-1). Soluble lens proteins seep into the anterior chamber and obstruct the trabecular meshwork, causing an elevation in IOP.

Pathophysiology

- In lens protein glaucoma, heavy-molecular-weight (HMW) proteins (greater than 150×10^6 Da) obstruct trabecular meshwork outflow, causing a rise in IOP. Previously, it was thought that the rise in pressure resulted exclusively from macrophage outflow obstruction, based on the fact that they were identified in the aqueous humor and in the trabecular meshwork of patients with lens protein glaucoma[1,2] (Fig. 15-2). However, Epstein et al.[3,4] suggested that HMW proteins obstruct the trabecular meshwork based on the following experimental evidence:

1. Epstein sampled aqueous fluid of patients with phacolytic glaucoma and showed an abundance of HMW proteins, which increase in concentration as the cataract matures.

2. In vitro perfusion of cadaver eyes with HMW soluble proteins caused a 60% decrease in outflow facility after 1 hour.

3. The HMW proteins were present in high-enough concentrations in the aqueous humor of patients with lens protein glaucoma to cause obstruction of outflow.

4. Several of the eyes with phacolytic glaucoma had a paucity of macrophages.

- Lens proteins can induce the migration of peripheral blood monocytes[5] and macrophages probably function as scavengers to remove soluble lens proteins and fragments from the anterior chamber and trabecular meshwork.

History

- Patients report gradually diminishing vision from the mature or hypermature cataract and pain from inflammation and elevated IOP.

Clinical Examination

- Lens protein glaucoma occurs in the presence of a mature or hypermature cataract. These patients have an acutely elevated IOP, ocular redness, and pain. There is intense flare, which correlates with soluble proteins released from the mature cataract (Fig. 15-3). A cellular response composed mostly of macrophages is present, and the cells appear larger and more translucent than lymphocytes (Fig. 15-4). Hypopyon is uncommon.

- White patches may be observed on the lens and are thought to correspond to aggregates of macrophages phagocytosing lens proteins at leakage sites on the capsule.

- Gonioscopy reveals open angles. A retinal perivasculitis has been observed in some cases.[6]

Special Tests

- Samples taken from the aqueous humor and concentrated via Millipore filtration may reveal macrophages and an amorphous substance corresponding to lens protein.

- The diagnosis is usually made on clinical observation alone.

Treatment

- Management of lens protein glaucoma should start with medical therapy to temporize the elevated IOP. Beta-blockers, prostaglandin analogs, alpha-adrenergic drugs, and carbonic anhydrase inhibitors are the mainstays of medical therapy. Topical steroids to reduce the inflammation and cycloplegics to stabilize the blood–aqueous barrier and to reduce pain may also be used.

● Medical therapy may help partially lower the pressure, but definitive treatment can only be obtained by removal of the cataract. In developing countries, small-incision extracapsular cataract surgery has been shown in a case series to be a safe and effective method of surgical therapy with minimal morbidity.[7]

REFERENCES

1. Hogan M, Zimmerman L. *Ophthalmic Pathology: An Atlas and Textbook*. 2nd ed. Philadelphia, PA: WB Saunders; 1962:797.

2. Irvine S, Irvine A. Lens-induced uveitis and glaucoma. *Am J Ophthalmol*. 1952;35:489.

3. Epstein D, Jedziniak J, Grant W. Identification of heavy-molecular-weight soluble protein in aqueous humor in human phacolytic glaucoma. *Invest Ophthalmol Vis Sci*. 1978;17(5):398–402.

4. Epstein D, Jedziniak J, Grant W. Obstruction of aqueous outflow by lens particles and by heavy-molecular-weight soluble lens proteins. *Invest Ophthalmol Vis Sci*. 1978;17(3):272–277.

5. Rosenbaum J. Chemotactic activity of lens proteins and the pathogenesis of phacolytic glaucoma. *Arch Ophthalmol*. 1987;105:1582.

6. Uemura A, Sameshima M, Nakao K. Complications of hypermature cataract: Spontaneous absorption of lens material and phacolytic glaucoma-associated retinal perivasculitis. *Jpn J Ophthalmol*. 1988;32(1):35–40.

7. Venkatesh R, Tan CS, Kumar T, et al. Safety and efficacy of manual small incision cataract surgery for phacolytic glaucoma. *Br J Ophthalmol*. 2007;91:279–281.

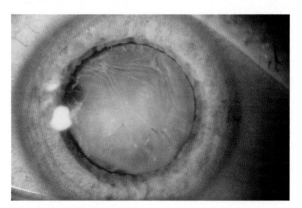

FIGURE 15-1. Mature cataract. Mature cataract with folds in the anterior capsule. (Courtesy of Donald L. Budenz, MD, MPH University, North Carolina, Chapel Hill.)

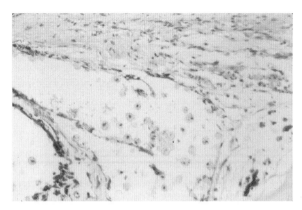

FIGURE 15-2. **Lens protein glaucoma.** Macrophages in the trabecular meshwork in lens protein glaucoma. (Courtesy of Donald L. Budenz, MD, MPH University, North Carolina, Chapel Hill.)

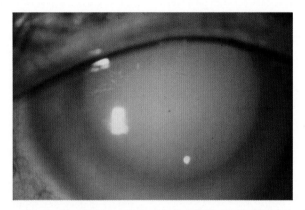

FIGURE 15-3. **Lens protein glaucoma.** Intense anterior chamber inflammation with mature cataract in lens protein glaucoma. (Courtesy of Donald L. Budenz, MD, MPH University, North Carolina, Chapel Hill.)

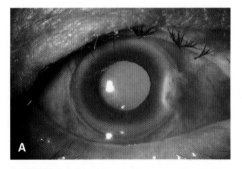
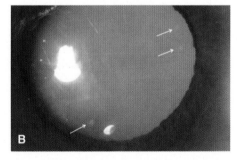

FIGURE 15-4. **Lens protein glaucoma.** Hypermature cataract (**A** and **B**) with clumps of inflammatory cells on the lens face (*white arrows*). (Courtesy James D. Brandt, Department of Ophthalmology and Vision Science, University of California, Davis, Sacramento, CA.)

LENS PARTICLE GLAUCOMA

Lens particle glaucoma occurs when the lens capsule is disrupted and lens cortex and proteins are released into the anterior chamber. This may occur after extracapsular cataract surgery, lens trauma with capsular disruption, and neodymium (Nd):YAG posterior capsulotomy in which liberated lens particles obstruct the trabecular meshwork, reducing aqueous outflow. Lens particle glaucoma after subluxation of a posterior chamber intraocular lens in a patient with pseudoexfoliation syndrome has also been reported[1] (**Figs. 15-5** and **15-6**). **Figure 15-7** shows an extreme case of lens particle glaucoma in which a hypermature cataract with phacodonesis progressed to dislocation into the anterior chamber with disruption of the capsular bag and led to high IOP.

Pathophysiology

- The elevated IOP in lens particle glaucoma can be caused by the following:

  1. Lens particles obstructing the trabecular meshwork

  2. Inflammatory cells

  3. Peripheral anterior synechiae and angle closure related to the inflammation

  4. Pupillary block from posterior synechiae

- Epstein et al.[2] perfused whole enucleated human eyes with particulate lens material as well as with HMW soluble lens proteins. Aqueous outflow facility decreased in a stepwise manner as the concentration of lens particles increased. Not all patients undergoing cataract surgery with lens particles in the anterior chamber develop elevated pressures. This suggests that a dynamic state exists between lens particle obstruction of the trabecular meshwork and lens particle clearance by phagocytic cells. Phagocytic cells in the trabecular meshwork can ingest lens particles and clear the outflow pathways. Macrophages have been observed to contain lens proteins and lens particles. Perhaps, in patients who develop lens particle glaucoma, the mechanism of meshwork clearance becomes overloaded or that phagocytic cells or the meshwork itself is abnormal.

- Elevated IOP can occur after Nd:YAG capsulotomy. Smith[3] has shown that the aqueous outflow facility after Nd:YAG capsulotomy decreases. One hour after the laser procedure, the aqueous outflow facility decreased by an average of 43% and the IOP increased by an average of 38%. At 24 hours and 1 week after the laser procedure, outflow facility drifted back to normal values. After Nd:YAG capsulotomy, lens debris consisting of lens capsule fragments and fragments of cortex can be seen on slit-lamp examination. It was suggested that this is one of the mechanisms for the decrease in outflow facility.

History

- Patients have decreased vision resulting from corneal edema and pain if the IOP is extremely high.

- In some cases, a recent history of trauma, cataract surgery, or laser procedure to the eye exists, although pressure rise can also occur years after cataract surgery.[4] One case report describes lens particle glaucoma diagnosed after vitrectomy because of inadvertent rupture of the posterior capsule.[5]

Clinical Examination

- The rise in IOP seen with lens particle glaucoma may correlate with the amount of lens particles circulating in the anterior chamber. There can be a delay of days to weeks between the release of the material and the onset of elevated IOP. Small white fragments of the lens cortex can be seen circulating in the anterior chamber and can deposit on the corneal endothelium.

- Elevated IOP can cause corneal edema, and inflammation can be marked, as evidenced by flare and cell.

- A hypopyon may be present, and one case series has also described spontaneous hyphema in the absence of trauma or neovascularization in these patients.[6]

- Early in the process, the angle is open on gonioscopy, although peripheral anterior synechiae may develop.

Special Tests

- The diagnosis is made by the observation of free lens particles floating around in the anterior chamber and an elevated IOP. If the appearance is atypical or if there is a paucity of lens particles, an aqueous sample can be taken to identify lens material histologically (Fig. 15-7).

Treatment

- Glaucoma medications mentioned previously for treatment of lens protein glaucoma should be used in conjunction with the degree of pressure elevation. A cycloplegic agent may be used to prevent posterior synechiae. Topical corticosteroids should be used, but the inflammation should not be completely suppressed or lens absorption will be delayed.

- If medical therapy is not effective, the lens particles should be removed surgically by aspiration. If surgery is delayed, the persistent inflammation may cause peripheral anterior synechiae, pupillary block, and inflammatory membranes that may extend posteriorly, placing tension on the retina. At this stage, membranes and debris must be cut out with vitrectomy instruments.

- Usually, surgical aspiration of the material is enough to bring about control of IOP and inflammation.

REFERENCES

1. Lim MC, Doe EA, Vroman DT, et al. Late onset lens particle glaucoma as a consequence of spontaneous dislocation of an intraocular lens in pseudoexfoliation syndrome. *Am J Ophthalmol.* 2001;132(2):261–263.
2. Epstein D, Jedziniak J, Grant W. Obstruction of aqueous outflow by lens particles and by heavy-molecular-weight soluble lens proteins. *Invest Ophthalmol Vis Sci.* 1978;17(3):272–277.
3. Smith C. Effect of neodynium: YAG posterior capsulotomy on outflow facility. *Glaucoma.* 1984;6:171.
4. Barnhorst D, Meyers S, Myers T. Lens-induced glaucoma 65 years after congenital cataract surgery. *Am J Ophthalmol.* 1994;188:807–808.
5. Yihua, S, Mao Z, Liu Y, et al. Late-onset lens particle glaucoma as a consequence of posterior capsule rupture after pars plana vitrectomy. *Eye Sci.* 2012;27(1):47–49.
6. Rathinam SR, Cunningham ET. Spontaneous hyphema and acute ocular hypertension associated with severe lens-induced uveitis. *Eye.* 2010;24(12):1822–1824.

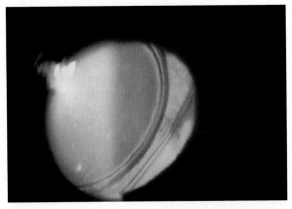

FIGURE 15-5. **Pseudoexfoliation.** Subluxed posterior chamber intraocular lens (PCIOL) in a patient with pseudoexfoliation. This patient developed lens particle glaucoma as a result of released lens cortex after the PCIOL dislocation.

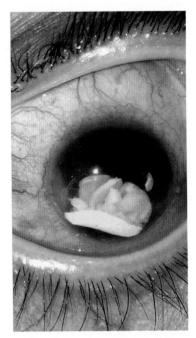

FIGURE 15-6. **Lens particle glaucoma.** Necrotic lens and capsular bag in the anterior chamber causing high intraocular pressures. (Courtesy of Stan H. Feil, MD, Visalia Eye Center, Visalia, CA.)

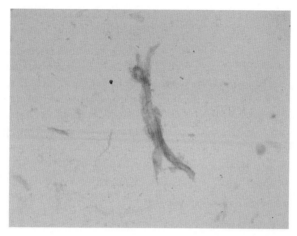

FIGURE 15-7. Lens fiber. Lens fiber recovered from aqueous aspirate of the eye shown in Figure 15-5.

LENS-ASSOCIATED UVEITIS (PHACOANAPHYLAXIS)

LAU, also known as phacoanaphylactic uveitis or endophthalmitis, can be confused with the previous two entities, although it is usually associated with hypotony. This is a rare granulomatous inflammation that develops in situations in which the immune system is exposed to lens proteins:

- After cataract extraction

- After traumatic rupture of the lens capsule

- After cataract extraction in one eye followed by cataract extraction or leaking mature cataract in the other eye

Pathophysiology

- LAU was once thought to represent an immune rejection of previously sequestered lens proteins. However, lens proteins are found in the aqueous of normal eyes. It is now thought that an alteration in immune tolerance to lens proteins occurs because not all eyes with disrupted lens capsules develop LAU, while rejection of foreign tissue grafts approaches 100%.[1] Cousins and Kraus-Mackiw[2] speculate that LAU is a spectrum of diseases that may be explained by autoimmune, infectious, and toxic mechanisms.

- The autoimmune theory has never been proven in human eyes, but experimental lens-induced granulomatous endophthalmitis in rats closely resembles LAU. The animals are sensitized to lens homogenates and, upon surgical injury to the lens, develop uveitis with histology similar to LAU. T cells have been shown to be a requirement for the induction of experimental LAU.[2] Cell-mediated immune response, macrophages, mast cells, and other elements may all make contributions. Mast-cell degranulation is regularly observed in experimental disease, and immune complexes seem to be the main mediator of the inflammatory response.[3]

- The infectious mechanism postulates that an inflammatory response is mounted against indolent bacteria such as *Propionibacterium acnes* that are found in lens material or that bacteria instigate a loss of immune tolerance in the eye. Finally, the theory of lens toxicity may be described as lens material that directly triggers an inflammatory reaction without previous immunity. All three entities are possibilities in the explanation of LAU, but none has been proved thus far.

- Unfortunately, LAU is often diagnosed after enucleation when histology can be examined. The histology of LAU may be described as a zonal granulomatous inflammation with three populations of cell types found in layers around the lens material (Fig. 15-8):

  1. *Zone 1*—Neutrophils closely surround and infiltrate the lens.

  2. *Zone 2*—A secondary zone of monocytes, macrophages, epithelioid cells, and giant cells surround the neutrophils.

  3. *Zone 3*—A nonspecific mononuclear cell infiltrate forms the outer zone of inflammation.

The inflammatory response can eventually result in fibroplasia. One case report describes an exuberant spindle-cell reaction to lens material resulting in a large intraocular inflammatory mass 47 years after the initial trauma.[1]

History

- Patients have pain, decreased vision, and red eye.

Clinical Examination

- The presentation can be variable and may present as a low-grade anterior segment inflammation, especially after cataract surgery.

Once remaining lens material is resorbed, the inflammation resolves.

• Panuveitis with a hypopyon represents a more severe presentation that is difficult to distinguish from endophthalmitis (Fig. 15-9). There is usually a history of retained lens fragments in the vitreous. The granulomatous inflammatory reaction can occur within days or months after disruption of the lens.

• LAU is usually associated with hypotony rather than with elevated IOP, although high pressures may occur.[4] Keratic precipitates are present, and synechiae can lead to pupillary block or angle-closure glaucoma.

Special Tests

• Aspirates of aqueous or vitreous with negative bacterial cultures may help differentiate LAU from bacterial endophthalmitis, but cytology is rarely helpful.

• Ultrasound may help locate large lens fragments in the vitreous chamber in the setting of cataract surgery or trauma.

Treatment

• If left untreated, a relentless uveitis can lead to phthisis. Topical, sub-Tenon, and oral steroids may be used as a temporizing measure, and conservative therapy only may be appropriate if the lens material resorbs without destructive inflammation.

• Definitive treatment involves removal of lens fragments, optimally by pars plana vitrectomy.

• Historically, the prognosis of severe cases of LAU has been very poor; but currently, with better surgical techniques and equipment, the possibility of retaining good vision is improving.[5]

REFERENCES

1. Guffey Johnson J, Margo CE. Intraocular inflammatory mass associated with lens-induce uveitis. *Surv Ophthalmol.* 2017;62(4):541–545.
2. Cousins SW, Kraus-Mackiw E. *Ocular Infection & Immunity.* 1st ed. St. Louis, MO: Mosby; 1996:1552.
3. Marak G. Phacoanaphylactic endophthalmitis. *Surv Ophthalmol.* 1992;36:325–339.
4. Rathinam S, Cunningham ET. Spontaneous hyphema and acute ocular hypertension associated with severe lens-induced uveitis. *Eye.* 2010:1–3.
5. Oruc S, Kaplan H. Outcome of vitrectomy for retained lens fragments after phacoemulsification. *Ocul Immunol Inflamm.* 2001;9(1):41–47.

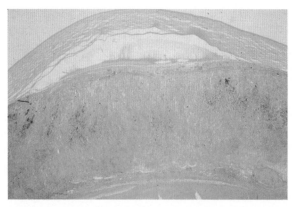

FIGURE 15-8. **Lens-associated uveitis (LAU).** Zonal granulomatous formation in a patient with LAU. (Courtesy of Donald L. Budenz, MD, MPH University, North Carolina, Chapel Hill.)

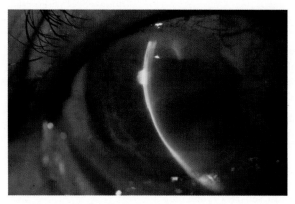

FIGURE 15-9. **Lens-associated uveitis (LAU).** Severe anterior chamber inflammation, hypopyon, and corneal edema in a patient with LAU. (Courtesy of Donald L. Budenz, MD, MPH University, North Carolina, Chapel Hill.)

PHACOMORPHIC GLAUCOMA

Phacomorphic glaucoma results from angle closure secondary to a mature or hypermature lens. It may be distinguished from the previous entities by the clinical appearance of an intumescent lens, shallow anterior chamber, and angle closure.

Pathophysiology

• Phacomorphic glaucoma is a direct sequela of a mature or hypermature lens that has become intumescent, causing crowding of the anterior segment structures.[1] In the early stage, pupillary block may cause high IOP. Later, the growing size of the lens presses forward on the iris in the periphery, blocking off outflow through the trabecular meshwork. The trabecular meshwork can also be mechanically blocked in ectopia lentis, a condition caused by a defective zonular apparatus and subluxation/dislocation of the lens. These include Weill-Marchesani syndrome, hyperlysinemia, sulfite-oxidase deficiency, and trauma. Dislocation can result in pupillary block and subsequent angle-closure glaucoma.[2]

• Phacomorphic glaucoma is a common condition in developing countries in which cataract surgery is delayed.

• The visual prognosis is poor, with one study reporting that only 57% of 49 patients with phacomorphic glaucoma attained visual acuity of 6/12 or better, although another study reported that over 80% of patients had some long-term visual improvement and IOP normalization after cataract extraction. Another study reported acuity of 6/12 or better in 72% of patients with symptoms less than 2 weeks in duration. However, optic disc damage was found in 80% of cases with symptoms lasting more than 2 weeks.[3] Better visual outcome

appears to be related to a shorter duration of elevated IOP.[4,5]

History

• Patients have chronic or acute decrease in vision, ocular pain, headache, and photophobia.[6]

Clinical Examination

• The crux of the problem is the mature or hypermature cataract causing a shallow anterior chamber (Fig. 15-10). The pupil may be mid-dilated with or without iris bombé, and gonioscopy reveals angle closure. The greatest risk factor for development is shallow anterior chamber.[3]

• The IOP is high from obstruction of aqueous outflow, and as a result, the cornea may be edematous (Fig. 15-11).

Special Tests

Anterior segment optical coherence tomography shows a small angle opening distance (AOD750, a measure of angle narrowing), anterior chamber depth, anterior chamber area, and anterior chamber width. There may be a relatively high lens vault value.[7]

Ultrasound biomicroscopy will also show a shallow anterior chamber and angle closure but can also be useful in diagnosis of intraocular lens implant induced glaucoma by delineating the position of the optic and haptic. (Fig. 15-12)[8]

Treatment

• Medical therapy to suppress aqueous formation is the first line of treatment. Miotics may increase contact between the lens and iris and should not be used.[1] Laser iridotomy should be performed to alleviate any component of pupillary block. Iridotomy may open up the angle, lower the IOP, and allow the eye to quiet before cataract removal. It may also give the clinician an opportunity to examine the angle for peripheral anterior synechiae.[6]

- The degree of scarring in the angle may signal the need for glaucoma surgery either at the time of cataract removal or in the future. One study found a 20% rate of glaucoma progression over 2 years, indicating that these patients need to be followed long term.[5] The definitive treatment for phacomorphic glaucoma is removal of the intumescent lens. One case series reported manual small-incision cataract surgery as a safe and effective treatment in developing countries where this entity is more common, but phacoemulsification has also proved an effective technique.[9,10]

- Capsulorhexis in the setting of a dense lens may be facilitated by the use of trypan blue staining of the anterior capsule.

REFERENCES

1. Liebmann JM, Ritch R. *Glaucoma Associated with Lens Intumescence and Dislocation.* Vol. 2. 2nd ed. St. Louis, MO: Mosby-Year Book; 1996:1033–1053.
2. Papaconstantinou D, Georgalas I, Kourtis N, et al. Lens-induced glaucoma in the elderly. *Clin Interv Aging.* 2009;4:331–336.
3. Sharanabasamma M, Vaibhav K. Management and visual outcome in patients of lens-induced glaucomas at a tertiary eye care hospital in South India. *J Curr Glaucoma Pract.* 2016;10(2):68–75.
4. Prajna N, Ramakrishnan R, Krishnadas R, et al. Lens induced glaucomas—visual results and risk factors for final visual acuity. *Indian J Ophthalmol.* 1996;44(3): 149–155.
5. Lee J, Lai J, Yick D, et al. Retrospective case series on the long-term visual and intraocular pressure outcomes of phacomorphic glaucoma. *Eye.* 2010;24(11):1675–1680.
6. Tomey K. Neodynium: YAG laser iridotomy in the initial management of phacomorphic glaucoma. *Ophthalmology.* 1992;99:660–665.
7. Mansouri M, Ramezani F, Moghimi S, et al. Anterior segment optical coherence tomography parameters in phacomorphic angle closure and mature cataracts. *Invest Ophthalmol Vis Sci.* 2014;55(11):7403–7409.
8. Dada T, Gadia R, Ajay S, et al. Ultrasound biomicroscopy in glaucoma. *Surv Ophthal.* 2011;56:433–450.
9. Lee S, Lee C, Kim W. Long-term therapeutic efficacy of phacoemulsification with intraocular lens implantation in patients with phacomorphic glaucoma. *J Cataract Refract Surg.* 2010;36(5):783–789.
10. Ramakrishanan R, Maheshwari D, Kader M, et al. Visual prognosis, intraocular pressure control and complications in phacomorphic glaucoma following manual small incision cataract surgery. *Indian J Ophthalmol.* 2010;58(4):303–306.

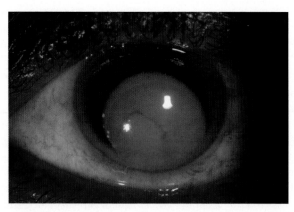

FIGURE 15-10. Phacomorphic glaucoma. A hyperdense crystalline lens causing a shallow anterior chamber. The lens is dislocated inferiorly. (Courtesy of Richard K. Lee, MD, PhD, Bascom Palmer Eye Institute, Miami, FL.)

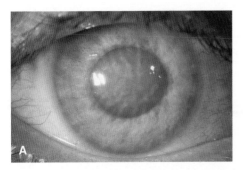
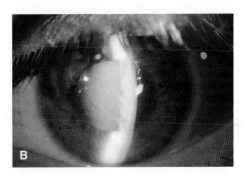

FIGURE 15-11. Phacomorphic glaucoma. A. Slit-lamp photograph of an eye with phacomorphic glaucoma. Descemet folds from an edematous cornea and darkly brunescent cataract are seen. **B.** Slit-beam photograph of the same eye shows the corneal swelling and narrow anterior chamber. (Courtesy of Douglas J. Rhee, MD, Wills Eye Hospital, Philadelphia, PA.)

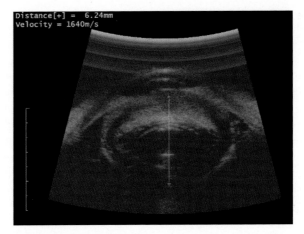

FIGURE 15-12. Phacomorphic glaucoma. Ultrasound biomicroscopy of an intumescent, phacomorphic lens resulting in angle closure and high intraocular pressures. (Courtesy of Cynthia L. Grosskreutz, MD PhD, at Massachusetts Eye and Ear and VP/Global Head of Ophthalmology at Novartis.)

Traumatic Glaucoma

Angela V. Turalba and Mary Jude Cox ■

INTRODUCTION

Following ocular trauma, patients often develop difficulties with intraocular pressure control. Intraocular pressure may be elevated or the eye may be hypotonous. Patients may have difficulty acutely or many years following the injury. In either case, a thorough history and examination will often determine the cause and severity of the intraocular damage and the appropriate course of treatment and follow-up. Open and closed globe injuries can result in damage to any of the ocular structures. This chapter focuses on traumatic hyphemas, angle recession, and cyclodialysis clefts.

TRAUMATIC HYPHEMA

The term *hyphema* refers to the blood in the anterior chamber. The amount of blood may be microscopic, termed *microhyphema*, visible only at the slit lamp as nonlayering red blood cells in the aqueous. Red blood cells may also layer or form clots in the anterior chamber (**Figs. 16-1** to **16-3**). As the blood clears from the anterior chamber, it will settle in the angle and is only visible on gonioscopy. A *total hyphema* refers to layered blood filling the entire anterior chamber (**Fig. 16-4**). A total hyphema that has clotted and appears black in color is referred to as an *eight-ball hyphema* (**Fig. 16-5**). A traumatic hyphema can result from either blunt or penetrating injury to the globe. The majority of hyphemas resolve gradually without sequelae; however, complications such as rebleeding, increased intraocular pressure, and corneal blood staining (**Fig. 16-6**) can occur. After a hyphema clears, traumatic cataracts and iris damage become more apparent (**Figs. 16-7** and **16-8**).

Epidemiology

• Traumatic hyphemas are most common in young active men, with a male-to-female ratio of approximately 3:1. In general, the risk of complications such as rebleeding, uncontrolled intraocular pressure, or corneal blood staining increases with the size of the hyphema. Patients with sickling hemoglobinopathies, however, are an exception. These patients are at an increased risk of developing complications regardless of the size of the hyphema.

• Rebleeding occurs in up to 35% of patients. The majority of rebleeding episodes take place within 2 to 5 days of the initial injury. Rebleeding is often larger than the original hyphema and more prone to complications.

Pathophysiology

• Blunt trauma causes compressive forces that result in the shearing of iris and ciliary body vessels. Tears in the ciliary body result in damage to the major arterial circle of the iris. Penetrating injuries can cause direct damage to blood vessels. Clots plug these damaged blood vessels, and rebleeding occurs as these clots retract and lyse (Fig. 16-2B).

• Intraocular pressure rises acutely as red blood cells, inflammatory cells, and debris obstruct the trabecular meshwork (Fig. 16-1C). Elevated intraocular pressure can also be the result of pupillary block caused by the clot in the anterior chamber. Eight-ball hyphemas often cause this form of pupillary block and can impair aqueous circulation (Fig. 16-5). The impaired aqueous circulation causes a reduction in oxygen concentration in the anterior chamber, resulting in the black appearance of the clot.

• In patients with sickle cell disease or trait, sickling causes the red blood cells to be rigid and easily trapped in the trabecular meshwork, leading to elevated intraocular pressure even in the presence of a small hyphema. Sickle cell patients are subject to vascular occlusion and optic nerve damage at lower intraocular pressures as a result of microvascular compromise.

History and Clinical Examination

• For patients presenting with a traumatic hyphema, a thorough evaluation of the timing and nature of the trauma is important to determine the likelihood of additional injuries and the need for close observation and treatment. Patients may be asymptomatic or have reduced vision, photophobia, and pain. Nausea and vomiting may accompany a rise in intraocular pressure. There may be evidence of orbital trauma or damage to other ocular tissues.

• Slit lamp: Slit-lamp examination may show circulating red blood cells alone or in combination with a layered hyphema in the anterior chamber. When there is elevated intraocular pressure associated with a large hyphema, corneal blood staining can occur (Fig. 16-6). There may be evidence of trauma to other ocular structures such as cataract (Fig. 16-7), phacodonesis, subconjunctival hemorrhage, foreign bodies, lacerations, or iris damage such as sphincter tears, iridodialysis, or traumatic aniridia (Figs. 16-7A and 16-8).

• Gonioscopy: Gonioscopy should be delayed until the risk of rebleeding has passed. When performed 3 to 4 weeks after the initial injury, the angle may appear undamaged or may show residual blood (see Fig. 16-1C) or angle recession (Fig. 16-9). Occasionally, peripheral anterior synechiae or a cyclodialysis cleft (Fig. 16-10A) may be present.

• Posterior pole: The posterior pole may show evidence of blunt or penetrating trauma. Commotio retinae, choroidal ruptures, retinal detachments, intraocular foreign bodies, or vitreous hemorrhage may be present. Scleral depression should be delayed until the risk of rebleeding has passed. A persistent vitreous hemorrhage can also cause elevated intraocular pressures in the form of ghost cell glaucoma. Unlike the typical red blood cells seen in hyphemas, tan-colored ghost cells can be observed in the anterior chamber. Ghost cells are degenerated erythrocytes that clog the trabecular meshwork as they make their way from the posterior segment to the anterior chamber presumably through a break in the anterior hyaloid face.

Special Tests

• B-scan ultrasonography should be performed in any patient in whom there is no view of the posterior pole. Computed tomographic scan of the orbits should be performed if there is clinical suspicion for orbital fractures or intraocular foreign bodies.

• Any black or Hispanic patient or any patient with a positive family history should undergo sickle prep or hemoglobin electrophoresis to determine the presence of sickling hemoglobinopathies.

Treatment

• The affected eye is shielded, and the patient is typically placed on activity restrictions. The patient is asked to keep the head of the bed elevated to allow the blood to settle below the visual axis (Fig. 16-3). The patient is instructed to avoid aspirin and nonsteroidal agents. Topical cycloplegics and steroids are given to treat inflammation and prevent formation of synechiae. Aminocaproic acid, an antifibrinolytic, can be given systemically to prevent rebleeding. Aminocaproic acid may cause postural hypotension, nausea, and vomiting, and should be avoided in pregnant patients and those with cardiac, hepatic, or renal disease.

• Elevated intraocular pressure is treated topically with beta-blockers, alpha-agonists, or carbonic anhydrase inhibitors (CAIs). Miotics and prostaglandin analogs may increase inflammation and are avoided if possible. Oral or intravenous CAIs or hyperosmotic agents may also be given to lower intraocular pressure. However, these systemic agents should be avoided in patients with sickling hemoglobinopathies because CAIs increase the pH of the aqueous and hyperosmotic agents can cause hemoconcentration, resulting in increased sickling.

• Surgical intervention is indicated in patients at risk for corneal blood staining (Fig. 16-6), uncontrolled intraocular pressure, or persistent pain. The timing of surgical intervention for intraocular pressure control depends on the individual patient. In a patient with a healthy optic nerve, an intraocular pressure of 60 mm Hg for 2 days, 50 mm Hg for 5 days, or 35 mm Hg for 7 days requires surgical intervention. Patients with compromised optic nerves or corneal endothelium require earlier intervention, as do patients with sickle cell disease or trait. Surgical intervention is indicated in sickle cell patients with an intraocular pressure greater than 24 mm Hg for more than 24 hours.

• Surgical options to remove the hyphema include anterior chamber washout, clot expression at the limbus, or removal with anterior vitrectomy instrumentation. If possible, clot removal should be performed 4 to 7 days post trauma in order to prevent new bleeding. In some cases, a guarded filtration procedure is performed concurrently to control intraocular pressure.

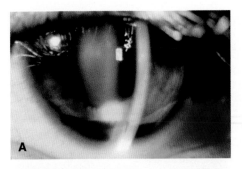
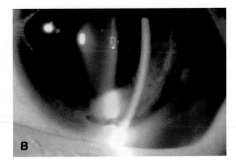
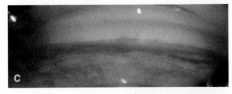

FIGURE 16-1. **Small hyphema. A.** This small hyphema is layering inferiorly in the anterior chamber. Most hyphemas resorb gradually. **B.** The same eye 4 days later has a much smaller clot in the anterior chamber. **C.** This is another eye with persistently elevated pressures 3 weeks after an injury when the layered hyphema was no longer evident on slit-lamp examination. Gonioscopy reveals residual blood in the angle.

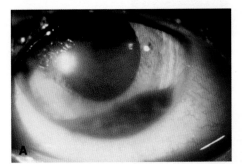
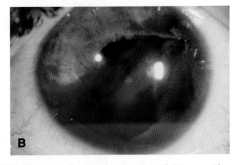

FIGURE 16-2. **Traumatic hyphema with rebleed. A.** Blood layers in the anterior chamber of this eye with a traumatic hyphema. **B.** The same eye rebleeds 24 hours later, demonstrating an increase in the amount of blood in the anterior chamber.

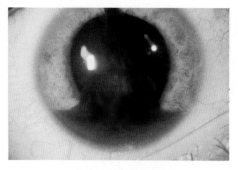

FIGURE 16-3. **Layering hyphema.** The hemorrhage in this new hyphema obscures the visual axis but is beginning to settle into the inferior anterior chamber. Patients are instructed to keep their head elevated to assist this process.

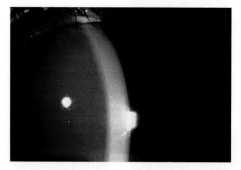

FIGURE 16-4. **Total hyphema.** A total hyphema is present following a baseball injury. The anterior chamber is filled with bright red blood.

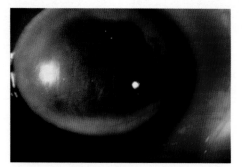

FIGURE 16-5. **Eight-ball hyphema.** An eight-ball hyphema is a total clot of the anterior chamber that gets its black appearance from decreased oxygenation as a result of impaired aqueous circulation.

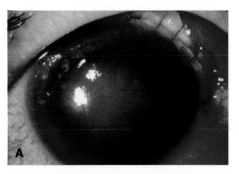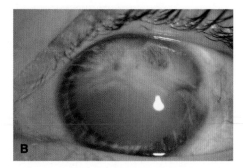

FIGURE 16-6. **Corneal blood staining. A.** Corneal blood staining persists in this eye following surgical evacuation of the hyphema. **B.** A few months after a penetrating eye injury and a total hyphema, this eye has persistent central corneal blood staining with peripheral clearing.

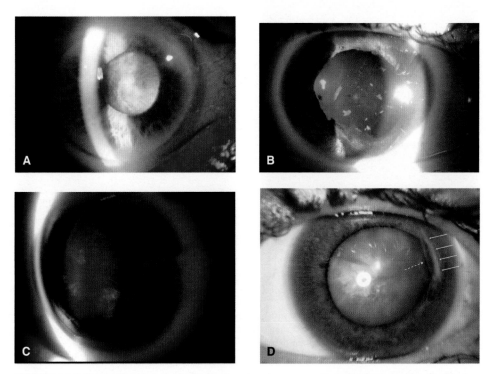

FIGURE 16-7. **Traumatic cataracts. A.** Traumatic cataracts can occur immediately or months after blunt or penetrating eye injuries. This eye has a complete traumatic cataract that developed immediately after a blunt injury but was more evident after the hyphema resolved. **B.** This patient had a large traumatic hyphema associated with high intraocular pressure. The iris sphincter tears, posterior synechiae, and glaukomflecken in the lens became more apparent after his hyphema cleared. **C.** After blunt trauma to the right eye, this patient had significant traumatic mydriasis and a dislocated traumatic cataract with loss of zonules temporally. **D.** This patient had a penetrating injury resulting in a full-thickness corneal laceration (*solid arrows*) with a corresponding defect in the lens (*dashed arrow*) and a diffuse traumatic cataract. The patient developed lens particle glaucoma from the disruption of the lens capsule.

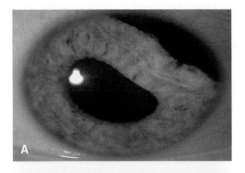

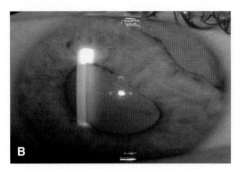

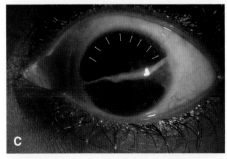

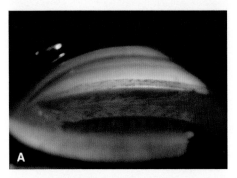

FIGURE 16-8. Iris injury. A. Blunt trauma can cause iridodialysis or tears at the iris root. **B.** Retroillumination highlights the area of iridodialysis in the same patient. **C.** This young patient has traumatic aniridia and aphakia as a result of a penetrating injury through the cornea. The *arrows* point to the edge of the remaining iris.

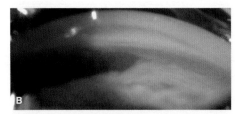

FIGURE 16-9. Angle recession. A. This eye with angle recession shows irregular widening of the ciliary body band on gonioscopy. **B.** This eye has angle recession adjacent to an area of iridodialysis as seen on gonioscopy. The ciliary body processes can be seen through the defect in the iris.

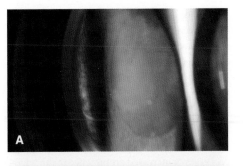

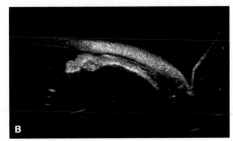

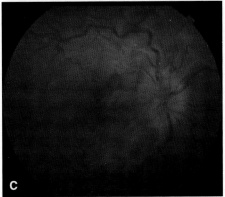

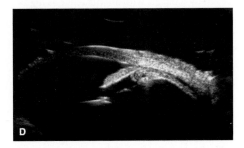

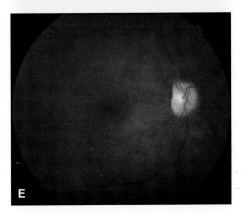

FIGURE 16-10. Cyclodialysis cleft. A. A cyclodialysis cleft appears as a deep angle recess with a gap between the sclera and the ciliary body. **B.** On ultrasound biomicroscopy (UBM), a cyclodialysis cleft can be seen as an abnormal space between the ciliary body and the sclera. **C.** Hypotony maculopathy with disc edema and macular folds is noted here in the same patient. **D.** After direct cyclopexy and suturing of a capsular tension ring into the sulcus, UBM shows closure of the cyclodialysis cleft. **E.** After closure of the cleft, there was improvement in the hypotony maculopathy, with only mild residual macular folds.

ANGLE RECESSION

*A*ngle recession refers to a tear in the ciliary body between the longitudinal and circular muscle layers. Clinically, there is abnormal widening of the ciliary body band on gonioscopy (Fig. 16-9).

Epidemiology

• Angle recession occurs as a result of blunt or penetrating trauma to the anterior segment. The risk of developing angle recession glaucoma is proportional to the extent of ciliary body damage, with an incidence as high as 10% in eyes with greater than 180 degrees of damage. Glaucoma may develop months to years after the original injury.

• Patients who develop angle recession glaucoma may be predisposed to open-angle glaucoma, as evidenced by the fact that up to 50% of them will develop elevated pressures in the contralateral eye.

Pathophysiology

• Angle recession is caused by a tear between the circular and longitudinal muscle layers of the ciliary body. Angle recession glaucoma results from decreased outflow facility. Impaired outflow may occur as a result of direct damage to the trabecular meshwork or as a result of a Descemet-like endothelial proliferation over the trabecular meshwork.

History and Clinical Examination

• Patients present with either a recent or a remote history of trauma in the affected eye. Patients may be asymptomatic or present with pain, photophobia, and reduced vision as a result of elevated intraocular pressure. They may have evidence of visual field loss or an afferent pupillary defect from glaucomatous optic nerve damage. There may also be evidence on examination of damage to other ocular or orbital structures.

• Slit lamp: Slit-lamp examination may show evidence of previous trauma. Corneal blood staining or scarring (Figs. 16-6B and 16-8C), cataract (Fig. 16-7), phacodonesis (Fig. 16-7C), iris sphincter tears, or tears at the iris root (iridodialysis) (Fig. 16-8) may be present.

• Gonioscopy: Gonioscopy demonstrates an irregular widening of the ciliary body band (Fig. 16-9). There may be evidence of torn iris processes or increased prominence of the scleral spur. The normal ciliary body should be roughly even in size around its circumference and not as wide as the trabecular meshwork. Occasionally, peripheral anterior synechiae formation may obscure the full extent of angle recession resulting from the initial trauma. Comparison with the unaffected eye often aids in diagnosis.

• Posterior pole: The posterior pole may show evidence of previous blunt or penetrating trauma. Choroidal ruptures, retinal detachments, or vitreous hemorrhage may be present. Asymmetric optic nerve cupping from elevated intraocular pressure in the affected eye may also be present.

Special Tests

• Visual field testing may demonstrate glaucomatous field loss.

Treatment

• Patients who demonstrate angle recession on gonioscopy following trauma need to be followed indefinitely for the development of glaucoma. If elevated intraocular pressures are found, they are often difficult to control. Initially, they can be treated medically with aqueous suppressants. Hyperosmotics may be added if necessary. Miotics often make angle recession worse, because they decrease uveoscleral outflow in eyes that rely on uveoscleral outflow for intraocular pressure control. Laser trabeculoplasty has limited success in eyes with angle recession. A guarded filtration procedure or implantation of a glaucoma drainage device is often required to control intraocular pressure in these patients.

CYCLODIALYSIS CLEFT

The term *cyclodialysis cleft* refers to a focal detachment of the ciliary body from its insertion at the scleral spur (**Fig. 16-10A** and **B**). It may occur as a result of blunt or penetrating trauma or as a complication of intraocular surgery, and leads to temporary or permanent hypotony.

Epidemiology

● Cyclodialysis clefts that result from blunt or penetrating trauma are less common than angle recession. The presence of a cleft should be considered in any hypotonous eye with a history of trauma or prior intraocular surgery.

Pathophysiology

● Trauma causes a separation of the ciliary body from its attachment to the scleral spur. This allows a direct passage of aqueous from the anterior chamber to the suprachoroidal space, leading to hypotony. Spontaneous or induced closure of the cleft often results in an acute elevation of the intraocular pressure because the primary outflow pathway of aqueous is disrupted.

History and Clinical Examination

● Patients present with a history of trauma or intraocular surgery in the affected eye. They may be asymptomatic or have reduced vision. The affected eye may be hypotonous or have elevated intraocular pressure, pain, photophobia, and redness as a result of spontaneous closure of a previous cleft.

● Slit lamp: Slit-lamp examination may show evidence of previous blunt or penetrating trauma such as corneal scarring or blood staining, cataract, disruption of the zonules supporting the lens (phacodonesis), iris sphincter tears, or tears at the iris root (iridodialysis). Evidence of previous intraocular surgery, such as posterior or anterior intraocular lens placement, may also be present. The affected eye can be hypotonous with corneal folds and a shallow anterior chamber when compared with the contralateral eye.

● Gonioscopy: Gonioscopy demonstrates a deep angle recess with a gap between the sclera and the ciliary body, with the bare white sclera becoming more visible (Fig. 16-10A). This is in contrast to angle recession, which appears as a widened brown or gray ciliary body band. Angle recession may also be present in the affected eye as a result of trauma.

● Posterior pole: Hypotony can result in choroidal effusions, detachments, and folds. H*ypotony maculopathy* refers to choroidal folds that involve the macula and sometimes have accompanying disc edema (**Fig. 16-10C**). Patients can experience markedly reduced vision from this. Evidence of previous trauma may also be present, such as choroidal rupture, posterior vitreous detachment, or macular hole.

Special Tests

● B-scan ultrasonography should be performed in any hypotonous posttraumatic eye with a limited view of the posterior pole in order to rule out occult scleral rupture or retinal detachment. Ultrasound biomicroscopy is a helpful imaging tool in detecting suspected clefts and delineating the extent of the cleft to aid in planning for laser or surgical treatment (Fig. 16-10B). It is also used to follow-up on the spontaneous or surgical closure of a cleft (**Fig. 16-10D**).

Treatment

● Occasionally, medical treatment with atropine may result in cyclodialysis cleft closure. Argon laser and cryotherapy can also be used to treat smaller clefts by inducing scarring between the ciliary body and the sclera. However, larger cyclodialysis clefts with persistent hypotony require surgical closure. Following closure of the cleft, the intraocular pressure often rises dramatically and should be monitored closely. Medical treatment with aqueous suppressants and hyperosmotics may be initiated as necessary. Hypotony maculopathy can be reversed, although residual folds may persist even after normalization of intraocular pressure (**Fig. 16-10E**).

Primary Acute Angle–Closure and Chronic Angle–Closure Glaucoma

Christopher Kai-Shun Leung ■

BACKGROUND

Definition

Angle closure is characterized by iris apposition to the trabecular meshwork. The mechanisms of this anatomic abnormality can be categorized at four structural levels[1]:

- The pupillary margin (e.g., pupillary block)
- The ciliary body (e.g., plateau iris and irido-ciliary cysts)
- The lens (e.g., phacomorphic glaucoma)
- Posterior to the lens (e.g., malignant glaucoma)

Primary angle closure generally refers to the condition of an increase in resistance to the flow of aqueous humor at the pupillary margin (i.e., relative pupillary block).

The clinical course can be classified into three conceptual stages[2]:

1. Primary angle–closure suspects—individuals with narrow angles, usually defined as an angle in which more than

270 degrees of the posterior trabecular meshwork cannot be seen

2. Primary angle closure—defined by the presence of narrow angles combined with peripheral anterior synechiae, elevated intraocular pressure, or a past acute angle–closure attack

3. Primary angle–closure glaucoma—primary angle closure combined with evidence of glaucomatous optic neuropathy

More than half of primary angle–closure glaucoma patients are asymptomatic for many years (chronic angle–closure glaucoma) until an acute angle–closure attack or severe loss of vision occurs. Acute angle closure denotes a specific form of primary angle closure characterized by an acute elevation of intraocular pressure (usually more than 40 mm Hg). Patients complain of having symptoms of ocular pain, nausea, or vomiting, and demonstrate signs of conjunctival injection, corneal epithelial edema, mid-dilated pupil, and shallow anterior chamber.

Pathophysiology

In primary angle closure, the increase in resistance at the pupillary margin raises the pressure gradient between the anterior chamber (anterior to the iris) and the posterior chamber (posterior to the iris) (Fig. 17-1). The iris has a characteristic forward-bowing configuration, leading to narrowing of the angle (primary angle–closure suspect). The adhesion of the peripheral iris to the trabecular meshwork may obstruct the angle and result in elevation of intraocular pressure and formation of peripheral anterior synechiae (primary angle closure). If the degree of relative pupillary block is extensive and the angle is already very narrow, complete obstruction of the angle occurs, and the rise in intraocular pressure would be precipitous, leading to an acute attack (primary acute angle closure). If the degree of relative pupillary block is small and the trabecular meshwork is blocked only in small portions, the intraocular pressure may increase gradually over the years, resulting in chronic progressive degeneration of the optic nerve without development of any symptom (chronic angle–closure glaucoma).

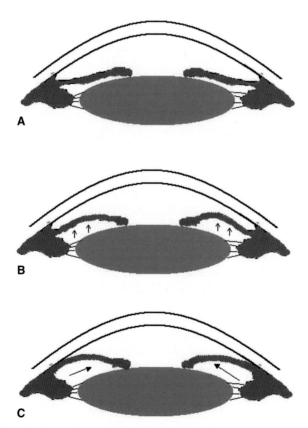

FIGURE 17-1. Pathophysiology of primary angle closure. A drawing of an apposition of the pupillary margin to the anterior surface of the lens (**A**), aqueous pressure developing behind the iris (**B**) (*arrows*) and pushing the iris forward, and iris bombé (**C**) (*arrows*) causing obstruction of the trabecular meshwork.

Epidemiology

Although angle-closure glaucoma represents approximately 25% of glaucoma worldwide, it accounts for nearly half of glaucoma blindness.[3] It is more prevalent in China, India, and Southeast Asia than in Europe and Latin America. A shallow anterior chamber, short axial length, and small corneal diameter are biometric risk factors for primary angle closure. The incidence of acute angle closure has been estimated at approximately 4 to 16 per 100,000 per year in the population aged 30 years and older.[4] In addition to the biometric risk factors for primary angle closure, age more than 60 years, female gender, a positive family history, and a thick and bulky lens impose additional risks for acute attack.

Clinical Examination

Gonioscopy

Gonioscopy is an indispensable technique to visualize the angle structures and detect angle closure. It is important to perform gonioscopy in a completely darkened room using the smallest square of light for a slit beam that sets off the pupil because slit-lamp illumination can stimulate pupillary light reflex and widen the angle (Fig. 17-2). A narrow angle is usually defined as an angle in which more than 270 degrees of the posterior trabecular meshwork cannot be seen. Indentation gonioscopy is useful for differentiating synechial closure from appositional closure. Synechial closure is recognized when there are considerable acquired adhesions between the iris and the corneoscleral junction at the angle. Peripheral anterior synechiae may extend circumferentially, resulting in synechial closure and progressive increase in intraocular pressure (Fig. 17-3). The extent of peripheral anterior synechiae correlates with the risk of developing glaucoma.

Ultrasound Biomicroscopy and Optical Coherence Tomography

Although assessment of the angle with gonioscopy is largely qualitative and subjective, objective and reproducible measurement of the anterior chamber angle can be obtained with cross-sectional imaging devices like the ultrasound biomicroscopy (UBM) and the optical coherence tomography (OCT) (Fig. 17-4). OCT has a number of advantages over UBM for anterior chamber angle imaging. It is a noncontact technique, has a higher image resolution, and is more precise in locating the position of interest for evaluation compared with UBM. UBM, however, has a unique role in visualizing the ciliary body. Commercially available time-domain and spectral-domain models have been developed for anterior chamber angle imaging[5] (Table 17-1). With the development of high-resolution OCT imaging systems, angle structures including the scleral spur, Schwalbe's line, Schlemm's canal, and collector channels can be examined in greater detail (Fig. 17-5). High-speed imaging allows evaluation of the angle in 360 degrees. Visualization of the iris profiles and the angle configurations is enhanced with three-dimensional reconstruction (Fig. 17-6). The latest anterior segment swept-source OCT (CASIA II, Tomey, Nagoya, Japan) provides automatic segmentation of the anterior segment structures and quantification of the anterior chamber angle dimensions in 360 degrees (Fig. 17-7). This new feature would improve the detection of primary angle closure. Examination of the anterior chamber angle with OCT and UBM not only augments the diagnostic performance to detect angle closure, but also improves our understanding in the pathophysiology of primary angle closure.

TABLE 17-1. Comparison of Commercially Available Optical Coherence Tomography (OCT) Systems for Anterior Chamber Angle Imaging

	Visante OCT	SL-OCT	RTVue FD-OCT	Cirrus HD-OCT	CASIA OCT	CASIA II OCT
Manufacturer	Carl Zeiss Meditec	Heidelberg Engineering	Optovue	Carl Zeiss Meditec	Tomey	Tomey
Year available	2005	2006	2006	2007	2009	2016
Light source	Superluminescent diode 1,310 nm	Superluminescent diode 1,310 nm	Superluminescent diode 840 nm	Superluminescent diode 840 nm	Swept-source laser 1,310 nm	Swept-source laser 1,310 nm
Axial resolution (μm)	18	<25	5	5	<10	<10
Scan size	16 mm × 6 mm	15 mm × 7 mm	2 mm × 2 mm (CAM-S) 6 mm × 2 mm (CAM-L)	3 mm × 1 mm	16 mm × 6 mm	16 × 14 mm
Scan speed	2,000 A-scans per second	200 A-scans per second	26,000 A-scans per second	27,000 A-scans per second	30,000 A-scans per second	50,000 A-scans per second
Fixation target	Internal and external	Internal and external	External	Internal and external	Internal and external	Internal and external

CAM-L, cornea-anterior module long; CAM-S, cornea-anterior module short.
Modified with permission from Leung CK, Weinreb RN. Anterior chamber angle imaging with optical coherence tomography. *Eye (Lond)*. 2011;25:261–267.

REFERENCES

1. Ritch R, Liebmann JM, Tello C. A construct for understanding angle closure glaucoma: the role of ultrasound biomicroscopy. *Ophthalmol Clin North Am.* 1995;8:281–293.

2. Foster PJ, Buhrmann R, Quigley HA, et al. The definition and classification of glaucoma in prevalence surveys. *Br J Ophthalmol.* 2002;86:238–242.

3. Quigley HA, Broman AT. The number of people with glaucoma worldwide in 2010 and 2020. *Br J Ophthalmol.* 2006;90:262–267.

4. He M, Foster PJ, Johnson GJ, et al. Angle closure glaucoma in East Asian and European people. Different diseases? *Eye (Lond).* 2006;20:3–12.

5. Leung CK, Weinreb RN. Anterior chamber angle imaging with optical coherence tomography. *Eye (Lond).* 2011;25:261–267.

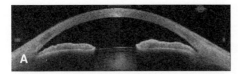

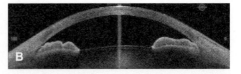

FIGURE 17-2. Effect of illumination on the anterior chamber angle. Anterior segment optical coherence tomography (OCT) images obtained with the Visante OCT (Carl Zeiss Meditec, Dublin, CA) demonstrating narrowing of the angle from light (**A**) to dark (**B**). An appositional closure is detected only in the dark.

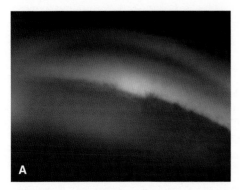

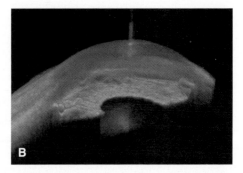

FIGURE 17-3. Peripheral anterior synechiae. A. A gonioscopic view of an eye with extensive peripheral anterior synechiae. **B.** A three-dimensional reconstruction of multiple optical coherence tomography (OCT) B-scans collected from the same eye with a swept-source OCT (Casia OCT, Tomey, Nagoya, Japan).

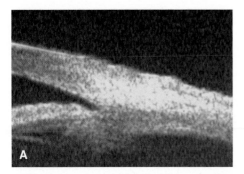
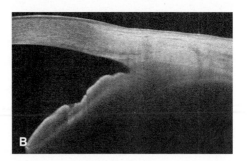

FIGURE 17-4. **Anterior chamber angle imaging with ultrasound biomicroscopy (UBM) and optical coherence tomography (OCT).** Although the ciliary body is better visualized with UBM (**A**), OCT (**B**) provides a higher image resolution of the anterior chamber angle. The UBM and OCT images were obtained with model 840 (Paradigm Medical Industries, Salt Lake City, UT) and a swept-source OCT (Casia OCT, Tomey, Nagoya, Japan), respectively.

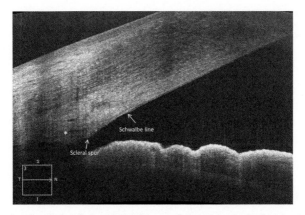

FIGURE 17-5. **Anterior chamber angle imaging with spectral-domain optical coherence tomography (OCT).** Detailed angle structures including the scleral spur, Schwalbe's line, and Schlemm's canal (*) can be visualized with a spectral-domain OCT (Cirrus HD-OCT, Carl Zeiss Meditec, Dublin, CA).

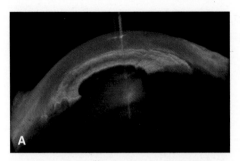 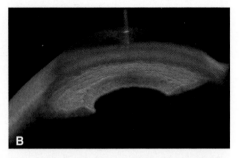

FIGURE 17-6. Three-dimensional visualization of the anterior chamber angle. The Casia OCT (Tomey, Nagoya, Japan) is a swept-source optical coherence tomography with a scan speed of 30,000 A-scans per second. The whole anterior segment can be radially imaged in 64 cross-sections in 1.2 seconds. An open (**A**) and a closed angle (**B**) in a three-dimensional display are illustrated.

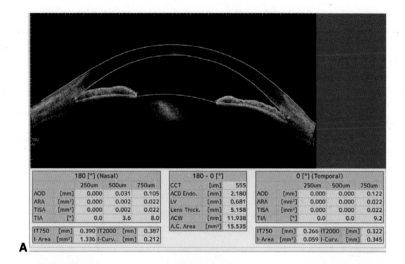

180 [°] (Nasal)	250um	500um	750um
AOD [mm]	0.000	0.031	0.105
ARA [mm²]	0.000	0.002	0.022
TISA [mm²]	0.000	0.002	0.022
TIA [°]	0.0	3.6	8.0
IT750 [mm] 0.390	IT2000 [mm] 0.387		
I-Area [mm²] 1.336	I-Curv. [mm] 0.212		

180 - 0 [°]	
CCT [um]	555
ACD Endo. [mm]	2.180
LV [mm]	0.681
Lens Thick. [mm]	5.158
ACW [mm]	11.938
A.C. Area [mm²]	15.535

0 [°] (Temporal)	250um	500um	750um
AOD [mm]	0.000	0.000	0.122
ARA [mm²]	0.000	0.000	0.022
TISA [mm²]	0.000	0.000	0.022
TIA [°]	0.0	0.0	9.2
IT750 [mm] 0.266	IT2000 [mm] 0.322		
I-Area [mm²] 0.059	I-Curv. [mm] 0.345		

A

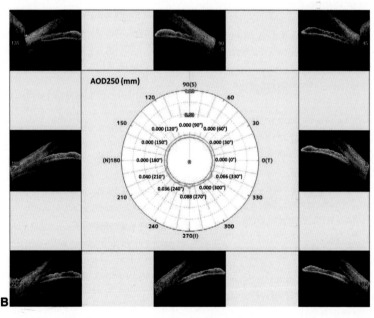

B

FIGURE 17-7. **Anterior segment swept-source optical coherence tomography.** A screen capture from the CASIA II (Tomey, Nagoya, Japan)—the latest anterior segment swept-source optical coherence tomography showing segmentation of the anterior segment structures and quantification of the anterior chamber angle dimensions and other anterior segment parameters (**A**). The angle open distance (mm) at 250 μm away from the scleral spur (AOD250) of an eye with primary angle closure is displayed at 12 angle meridians (**B**). AOD, angle opening distance; ARA, angle recess area; TISA, trabecular iris space area; TIA, trabecular iris angle; CCT, central corneal thickness; ACD, anterior chamber depth; LV, lens vault; ACW, anterior chamber width; AC area, anterior chamber area.

PRIMARY ACUTE ANGLE CLOSURE

Diagnostic Evaluation

• Symptoms of primary acute angle closure range from unilateral blurring and ocular pain to extreme ocular or periocular pain, headache, nausea, vomiting, and diaphoresis. Patients may have a history of subacute angle closure including intermittent attacks of pain and possibly mildly blurry vision, which may be confused with migraine headache. Acute attacks may be precipitated by pharmacologic mydriasis, dim illumination, stress, or prolonged near work.

• Clinical examination shows conjunctival injection, corneal epithelial edema, mid-dilated pupil, a shallow anterior chamber, and often times, the iris in a classic bombé pattern (**Figs. 17-8** to **17-10**). The intraocular pressure may be as high as 80 mm Hg. Mild cell and flare are often present.

• Gonioscopy can be difficult in the presence of the corneal edema. Early in the attack, the optic nerve head can show edema and hyperemia.

• The fellow eye should be examined closely because it will almost always have a shallow anterior chamber with a narrow angle.

Prognosis

• Depending on the level of intraocular pressure and the duration of attack, a variable degree of irreversible ischemic damages can be incurred on the iris, the lens, and the optic nerve, resulting in iris atrophy, glaukom-flecken (flecks of anterior subcapsular opacities representing infarction of anterior lens epithelial cells) (**Fig. 17-11**), and a pale optic nerve head with visual field loss disproportionate to the disc cupping.

• Patients may develop chronic elevation of intraocular pressure and progress to angle-closure glaucoma.

Treatment

• The goals of treatment are to reduce the intraocular pressure and prevent recurrent attack.

• Topical beta-blocker, cholinergic agent, carbonic anhydrase inhibitor, and systemic acetazolamide (i.v. 250 to 500 mg) are usually effective in lowering the intraocular pressure and aborting the attack. An osmotic agent (e.g., i.v. mannitol 1 to 2 g per kg over 45 minutes) may be considered if intraocular pressure control is suboptimal.

• In patients not responsive to medical treatment, argon laser peripheral iridoplasty (ALPI) can be applied from 180 degrees to 360 degrees at the far peripheral iris to pull open the closed angle mechanically. The spot size is usually set at 500 μm with a duration of 0.5 seconds and an energy of 200 to 400 mJ for each application. The optimal energy should be titrated with an end point of visualizing the contraction of the peripheral iris. Charring of the iris with excessive laser energy should be avoided. ALPI alone is a safe and effective alternative in aborting acute angle closure.

• Once the corneal edema has cleared, a laser peripheral iridotomy (LPI) can be performed to prevent recurrent attack. By providing a communicating channel, LPI reduces the pressure gradient between the anterior and the posterior chambers and flattens the iris (**Fig. 17-12**). An LPI should be considered in the fellow eye because of an associated increased risk of developing acute angle closure.

• Patients should be monitored for development of peripheral anterior synechiae, chronic elevation of intraocular pressure, and angle-closure glaucoma in the follow-up visits.

Chronic Angle–Closure Glaucoma

Diagnostic Evaluation

- The diagnosis of primary angle-closure glaucoma requires the detection of primary angle closure together with evidence of glaucomatous optic neuropathy. The eye is usually quiet with a shallow anterior chamber.

- Gonioscopy demonstrates a narrow angle and areas of peripheral anterior synechiae. Patients in an advanced stage may have little trabecular meshwork visible. The optic nerve head may show typical glaucomatous cupping and progressive narrowing of the neuroretinal rim and thinning of the retinal nerve fiber layer similar to open-angle glaucoma.

Treatment

- Preventing acute angle closure and reducing the rate of glaucoma progression are the key objectives in the management of angle-closure glaucoma.

- An LPI can widen the angle and prevent further angle closure. However, the trabecular meshwork may have sustained enough damage that the intraocular pressure will still be elevated despite a patent iridotomy, necessitating continued use of topical medications to lower the intraocular pressure.

- In patients with coexisting cataract, lens removal can widen the angle and lower the intraocular pressure (Fig. 17-13).

Plateau Iris

In plateau iris *configuration,* the iris is displaced anteriorly at its root by large or abnormally positioned ciliary processes. A component of relative pupillary block may also be present, particularly in older individuals. The trabecular meshwork may be occluded if the displacement is anterior enough. Plateau iris *syndrome* is defined by a persistent narrow angle despite a patent LPI. In the complete form, there is occlusion of the trabecular meshwork, and the intraocular pressure increases. In the incomplete form, the upper portion of the filtering trabecular meshwork is open, and the intraocular pressure remains normal.

Diagnostic Evaluation

- Plateau iris typically occurs in the fourth through sixth decades in women.

- Symptoms, as with angle closure secondary to relative pupillary block, are dependent on the rapidity of the angle closure. An acute attack may occur if a component of relative pupillary block exists; the symptoms will mirror those of acute angle closure. In most cases, the angle closes slowly and there are no symptoms until the intraocular pressure is elevated or the visual field loss becomes severe.

- Under slit-lamp examination, the iris is flat, and the central anterior chamber is deep. Compression gonioscopy demonstrates the "double-hump" sign, with the peripheral hump representing a prominent roll of iris pushed forward by the ciliary processes, and the central hump representing the portion of iris over the anterior lens surface (Fig. 17-14).

- UBM is useful for confirming the diagnosis of plateau iris (Fig. 17-15).

Treatment

- No intervention is needed for plateau iris configuration if no obstruction of the trabecular meshwork is occurring. However, an LPI may be indicated if there is an element of relative pupillary block.

- In plateau iris syndrome, an ALPI is useful for opening appositionally closed angle. Typical treatment includes approximately 20 to 30 spots of argon laser placed in the far periphery over 360 degrees. Filtration surgery may ultimately become necessary in some patients.

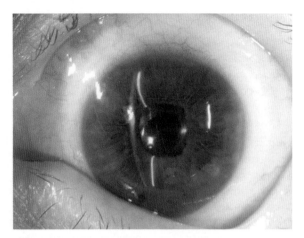

FIGURE 17-8. Iris bombé. A slit-beam photograph showing the appearance of iris bombé. This eye has iris bombé with 360 degrees of posterior synechiae (scarring between the pupillary margin and the anterior surface of the intraocular lens) and secondary pupillary block.

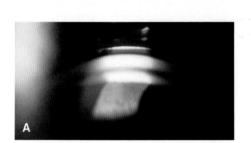
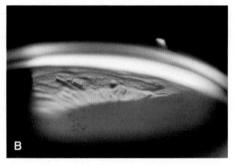

FIGURE 17-9. Primary acute angle closure. A patient with primary acute angle closure and a relatively clear cornea. **A.** The slit-beam photograph of the gonioscopic view shows the steep approach of the iris (iris bombé). **B.** The diffuse illumination of the gonioscopic view of the same eye shows no angle structures (i.e., an occluded angle).

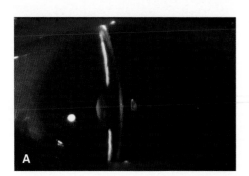
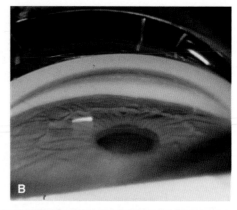

FIGURE 17-10. **Narrow anterior chamber angle. A.** A slit-beam photograph showing a narrow anterior chamber angle. **B.** The gonioscopic view of the same eye showing the absence of angle structures in an eye with normal intraocular pressure. This angle is occludable. (Courtesy of Douglas J. Rhee, MD, Wills Eye Hospital, Philadelphia, PA.)

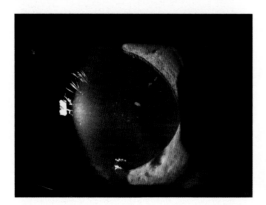

FIGURE 17-11. **Glaukomflecken.** A slit-lamp photograph of an eye 2 months after an acute angle–closure attack shows flecks of anterior subcapsular opacities.

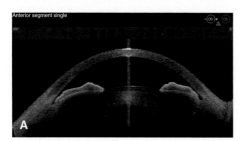
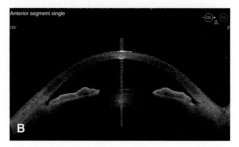

FIGURE 17-12. **Effect of laser peripheral iridotomy (LPI) on the anterior chamber angle.** Optical coherence tomography (OCT) imaging (Visante OCT, Carl Zeiss Meditec, Dublin, CA) of an eye with a narrow angle before (**A**) and after (**B**) LPI. After LPI, the angle is widened, and the iris is flattened.

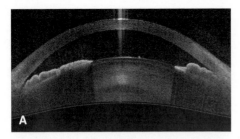 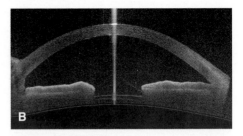

FIGURE 17-13. Effect of lens extraction on the anterior chamber angle. Optical coherence tomography imaging (Casia OCT, Tomey, Nagoya, Japan) of an eye with chronic angle–closure glaucoma before (**A**) and after (**B**) cataract extraction. The angle is widened, and the iris is flattened after cataract extraction.

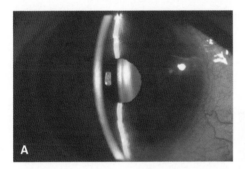 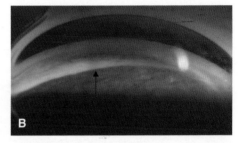

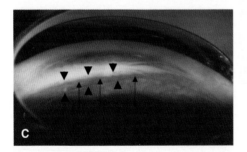

FIGURE 17-14. Plateau iris configuration. A. A slit-beam photograph showing a relatively deep anterior chamber. There is a patent peripheral iridotomy superiorly. **B.** Gonioscopy with no pressure on the cornea; no angle structures are visible. The *black arrow* shows a prominent last iris fold. **C.** Indentation gonioscopy. The *arrows pointing up* shows the same iris fold seen in **B**; the *arrowheads* showing the trabecular meshwork now revealed behind the prominent iris fold. The image is distorted because of the corneal striae induced by the indentation. (Courtesy of Douglas J. Rhee, MD, Wills Eye Hospital, Philadelphia, PA.)

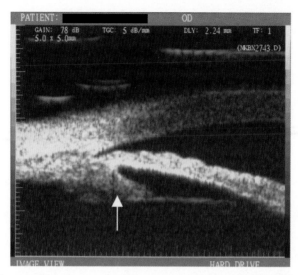

FIGURE 17-15. Ultrasound biomicroscopy of the same eye shown in Figure 17-13. The *arrow* shows the anteriorly displaced ciliary body causing a prominent iris roll directly above it. (Courtesy of Douglas J. Rhee, MD, Wills Eye Hospital, Philadelphia, PA.)

Secondary Angle–Closure Glaucoma

Douglas J. Rhee and Jamie E. Nicholl ■

NEOVASCULAR GLAUCOMA

Neovascular glaucoma (NVG) is a secondary closed-angle form of glaucoma. Initially, a fibrovascular membrane grows over the trabecular meshwork. This is an occluded but open angle. Within a short period of time, the fibrovascular membrane contracts, closing the anterior chamber angle. This often leads to a dramatic elevation of intraocular pressure (IOP), usually greater than 40 mm Hg.

Epidemiology and Pathophysiology

• The exact incidence of all NVGs is not known. NVG can occur as the sequela of several different possible conditions, most commonly, ischemic central retinal vein occlusions and proliferative diabetic retinopathy.

• Other predisposing factors include ischemic central retinal arterial occlusions, ocular ischemic syndrome, branch retinal arterial or vein occlusions, chronic uveitis, chronic retinal detachments, and radiation therapy.

• Some of the best estimates of the incidence of NVG come from studies on central retinal vascular occlusions (CRVOs). Approximately one-third of all CRVOs are ischemic. Between 16% and 60%, depending on the extent of capillary nonperfusion, of ischemic CRVOs will develop neovascularization of the iris. Approximately 20% of eyes with proliferative diabetic retinopathy will develop NVG. Approximately 18% of eyes with central retinal arterial occlusions will develop neovascularization of the iris (Fig. 18-1). Eyes with neovascularization of the iris are at high risk of developing NVG.

History

• Patients may be asymptomatic or may complain of pain, red eye, and reduced vision.

Clinical Examination

• Slit lamp: Corneal edema may be present in the anterior chamber from elevated IOP. The anterior chamber is usually deep with some flare. Hyphema and rare white cells may be present. Fine, nonradial vessels are present on the iris (Fig. 18-1).

• Gonioscopy: If the cornea is clear, gonioscopy may show a vascular net over the angle (NVA) in the early stages (Fig. 18-2).

Later, broad peripheral anterior synechiae occluding some or all of the angles may be seen.

- Posterior pole: Retinal findings are consistent with the underlying pathology.

Management

- Typically, antiglaucoma medical management is not adequate in controlling the IOP.

- The mainstay of initial treatment is immediate anti–vascular endothelial growth factor (anti-VEGF) therapy. Panretinal photocoagulation (PRP) is often still needed.

- If the patient is diagnosed with ischemic retinal disease before the development of NVG, anti-VEGF treatment should be started at the appearance of neovascularization in the angle or the iris. Patients in whom fibrovascular membrane–mediated angle closure is already present, anti-VEGF should be pursued if there is any residual trabecular meshwork exposed. Regression of the NVA can result in some opening of the angle. Typically, regression of neovascularization of the iris (NVI)/NVA will occur within 24 to 72 hours.

- Surgical intervention, to lower the IOP, may be required if anti-VEGF treatment/PRP fails. As the mechanism is a mechanical closing of the angle, trabecular meshwork bypass procedures are not indicated. Options include trabeculectomy with an antifibrotic agent, a glaucoma drainage implant device, and/or cyclodestructive procedures. Anti-VEGF treatments are a useful adjunct to the aforementioned glaucoma procedures.

BIBLIOGRAPHY

Anchala AR, Pasquale LR. Neovascular glaucoma: a historical perspective on modulating angiogenesis. *Semin Ophthalmol.* 2009;24:106–112.

Chan CK, Ip MS, Vanveldhuisen PC, et al; SCORE Study Investigator Group. SCORE Study report #11: incidences of neovascular events in eyes with retinal vein occlusion. *Ophthalmology.* 2011;118:1364–1372.

Chappelow AV, Tan K, Waheed NK, et al. Panretinal photocoagulation for proliferative diabetic retinopathy: pattern scan laser versus argon laser. *Am J Ophthalmol.* 2012;153:137–142.

Ciftci S, Sakalar YB, Unlu K, et al. Intravitreal bevacizumab combined with panretinal photocoagulation in the treatment of open angle neovascular glaucoma. *Eur J Ophthalmol.* 2009;19:1028–1033.

Diabetic Retinopathy Study Research Group. Preliminary report on effects of photocoagulation therapy. *Am J Ophthalmol.* 1976;81:383.

Eid TM, Radwan A, el-Manawy W, et al. Intravitreal bevacizumab and aqueous shunting surgery for neovascular glaucoma: safety and efficacy. *Can J Ophthalmol.* 2009;44:451–456.

Ghosh S, Singh D, Ruddle JB, et al. Combined diode laser cyclophotocoagulation and intravitreal bevacizumab (Avastin) in neovascular glaucoma. *Clin Experiment Ophthalmol.* 2010;38:353–357.

Hayreh SS, Podhajsky P. Ocular neovascularization with retinal vascular occlusion II. Occurrence in central and branch retinal artery occlusion. *Arch Ophthalmol.* 1982;100:1585.

Kwon J, Sung KR. The effect of preoperative intravitreal bevacizumab on the surgical outcome of neovascular glaucoma at different stages. *J Ophthalmol.* 2017:7672485.

Laatikainen L, Kohner EM, Khoury D, et al. Panretinal photocoagulation in central retinal vein occlusion: a randomized controlled clinical study. *Br J Ophthalmol.* 1977;61:741.

Liu L, Xu Y, Huang Z, Wang X. Intravitreal ranibizumab injection combined trabeculectomy versus Ahmed valve surgery in the treatment of neovascular glaucoma: an assessment of efficacy and complications. *BMC Ophthalmol.* 2016;16:65.

Magargal LE, Brown GC, Augsburger JJ, et al. Efficacy of panretinal photocoagulation in preventing neovascular glaucoma following ischemic central retinal vein obstruction. *Ophthalmology.* 1982;89:780.

Miki A, Oshima Y, Otori Y, et al. One-year results of intravitreal bevacizumab as an adjunct to trabeculectomy for neovascular glaucoma in eyes with previous vitrectomy. *Eye (Lond).* 2011;25:658–659.

Netland PA, Ishida K, Boyle JW. The Ahmed glaucoma valve in patients with and without neovascular glaucoma. *J Glaucoma.* 2010;19:581–586.

Park UC, Park KH, Kim DM, et al. Ahmed glaucoma valve implantation for neovascular glaucoma after vitrectomy for proliferative diabetic retinopathy. *J Glaucoma.* 2011;20:433–438.

Shazly TA, Latina MA. Neovascular glaucoma: etiology, diagnosis and prognosis. *Semin Ophthalmol.* 2009;24:113–121.

Sidoti PA, Dunphy TR, Baerveldt G, et al. Experience with the Baerveldt glaucoma implant in treating neovascular glaucoma. *Ophthalmology.* 1995;102:1107–1118.

Takihara Y, Inatani M, Kawaji T, et al. Combined intravitreal bevacizumab and trabeculectomy with mitomycin C versus trabeculectomy with mitomycin C alone for neovascular glaucoma. *J Glaucoma.* 2011;20:196–201.

Tolentino M. Systemic and ocular safety of intravitreal anti-VEGF therapies for ocular neovascular disease. *Surv Ophthalmol.* 2011;56:95–113.

Yalvac IS, Eksioglu U, Satana B, et al. Long-term results of Ahmed glaucoma valve and Molteno implant in neovascular glaucoma. *Eye (Lond).* 2007;21:65–70.

Yildirim N, Yalvac IS, Sahin A, et al. A comparative study between diode laser cyclophotocoagulation and the Ahmed glaucoma valve implant in neovascular glaucoma: a long-term follow-up. *J Glaucoma.* 2009;18:192–196.

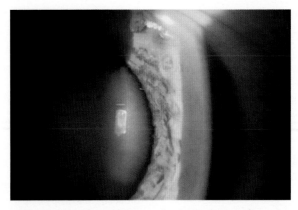

FIGURE 18-1. Neovascularization of the iris. Neovascularization of the iris (fine, noncircular vessels) is seen near the papillary border extending onto the iris.

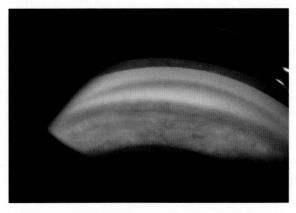

FIGURE 18-2. Neovascularization of the angle. A gonioscopic photograph showing neovascularization (fine, nonradial vessels) over the trabecular meshwork before the fibrovascular membrane has contracted causing peripheral anterior synechiae.

IRIDOCORNEAL SYNDROMES

The iridocorneal endothelial (ICE) syndrome is a group of secondary angle–closure glaucomas with overlapping features. There are three entities within this syndrome:

- Essential iris atrophy (**Figs. 18-3 to 18-5**)
- Chandler syndrome (**Fig. 18-6**)
- Cogan-Reese syndrome (iris nevus; **Fig. 18-7**)

Epidemiology

- ICE syndrome is rare; the exact incidence is not known. Typically, it affects middle-aged women in one eye.

Pathophysiology

- All three entities of the ICE syndrome share a common pathophysiology. The corneal endothelium grows abnormally over the anterior chamber angle covering the iris, which gives the iris the characteristic findings. Initially, the anterior chamber angle is open but occluded. Over time, the endothelial membrane contracts, secondarily closing the angle and distorting the pupil and the iris.

History

- Patients are usually asymptomatic in the early stages. Later, the patient may notice reduced vision in one eye and irregular appearance of the iris. As the IOP rises, the patient may have pain or a red eye, or both.

Clinical Examination

- Slit lamp: The cornea has a fine, beaten-metal appearance in the endothelial layer unilaterally. There are iris abnormalities that are more specific to the separate entities:
  - Essential iris atrophy—There are areas of iris thinning along with a displaced and distorted pupil as the endothelial membrane contracts, pulling on the iris.
  - Chandler syndrome—The changes in the iris are nearly identical to those of essential iris atrophy, but there is a greater degree of corneal edema, and the corneal findings are more apparent.
  - Cogan-Reese syndrome—The iris has a flattened appearance with small nodules of normal iris tissue poking through holes in the endothelial layer, giving the appearance of a mushroom patch.

- Gonioscopy: Early in the disease process, gonioscopy may show a normal-appearing anterior chamber angle. Later, broad and irregular peripheral anterior synechiae occluding some or all of the angles may be seen.

- Posterior pole: The appearance of the posterior pole is normal, aside from some degree of glaucomatous optic nerve cupping as the IOP rises.

Management

- Typically, medical management is not adequate in controlling the IOP.

- Surgical intervention is usually required. Options include trabeculectomy with an antifibrotic agent, a glaucoma drainage implant device, and cyclodestructive procedures.

- Corneal transplantation is helpful once the corneal edema has significantly affected the patient's vision.

BIBLIOGRAPHY

Alvarado JA, Underwood JL, Green WR, et al. Detection of herpes simplex viral DNA in the iridocorneal endothelial syndrome. *Arch Ophthalmol.* 1994;112:1601–1609.

Alvim PT, Cohen EJ, Rapuano CJ, et al. Penetrating keratoplasty in iridocorneal endothelial syndrome. *Cornea.* 2001;20:134–140.

Anderson NJ, Badawi DY, Grossniklaus HE, et al. Posterior polymorphous membranous dystrophy with overlapping features of iridocorneal endothelial syndrome. *Arch Ophthalmol.* 2001;119:624–625.

Doe EA, Budenz DL, Gedde SJ, et al. Long-term surgical outcomes of patients with glaucoma secondary to the iridocorneal endothelial syndrome. *Ophthalmology.* 2001;108:1789–1795.

Groh MJ, Seitz B, Schumacher S, et al. Detection of herpes simplex virus in aqueous humor in iridocorneal endothelial (ICE) syndrome. *Cornea.* 1999;18:359–360.

Grupcheva CN, McGhee CN, Dean S, et al. In vivo confocal microscopic characteristics of iridocorneal endothelial syndrome. *Clin Experiment Ophthalmol.* 2004;32:275–283.

Hirst LW. Bilateral iridocorneal endothelial syndrome. *Cornea.* 1995;14:331.

Hooks JJ, Kupfer C. Herpes simplex virus in iridocorneal endothelial syndrome. *Arch Ophthalmol.* 1995;113:1226–1228.

Huang T, Wang Y, Ji J, et al. Deep lamellar endothelial keratoplasty for iridocorneal endothelial syndrome in phakic eyes. *Arch Ophthalmol.* 2009;127:33–36.

Kupfer C, Kaiser-Kupfer MI, Datiles M, et al. The contralateral eye in the iridocorneal endothelial (ICE) syndrome. *Ophthalmology.* 1983;90:1343–1350.

Lanzl IM, Wilson RP, Dudley D, et al. Outcome of trabeculectomy with mitomycin-C in the iridocorneal endothelial syndrome. *Ophthalmology.* 2000;107:295–297.

Lobo AM, Rhee DJ. Delayed interval of involvement of the second eye in a male patient with bilateral Chandler's syndrome. *Br J Ophthalmol.* 2012;96:134–135, 146–147.

Olawoye O, Teng CC, Liebmann JM, et al. Iridocorneal endothelial syndrome in a 16-year-old. *J Glaucoma.* 2011;20:294–297.

Price MO, Price FW Jr. Descemet stripping with endothelial keratoplasty for treatment of iridocorneal endothelial syndrome. *Cornea.* 2007;26:493–497.

Shields MB. Progressive essential iris atrophy, Chandler's syndrome, and the iris nevus (Cogan-Reese) syndrome: a spectrum of disease. *Surv Ophthalmol.* 1979;24:3–20.

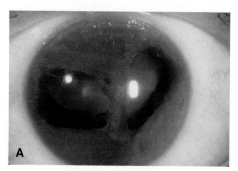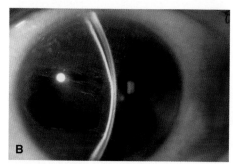

FIGURE 18-3. Essential iris atrophy. A. Essential iris atrophy showing pulling and distortion of the pupil. **B.** A slit-beam photograph of the same eye.

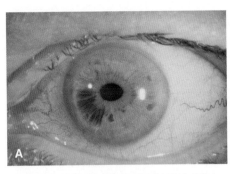
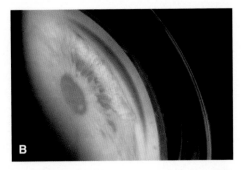

FIGURE 18-4. **Essential iris atrophy. A.** Another example of essential iris atrophy. **B.** A gonioscopic view of the same eye, showing peripheral anterior synechiae.

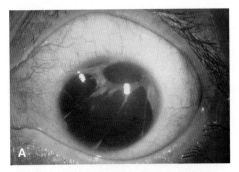
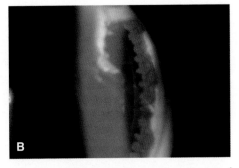

FIGURE 18-5. **Essential iris atrophy. A.** An extreme example of essential iris atrophy. **B.** A gonioscopic view of the same eye, showing peripheral anterior synechiae.

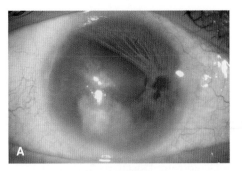
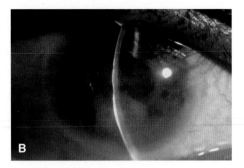

FIGURE 18-6. **Chandler syndrome. A.** The iris findings are similar to those of essential iris atrophy except that the corneal findings are more prominent. **B.** A slit-beam photograph of the same eye.

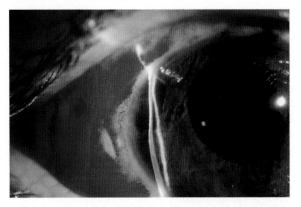

FIGURE 18-7. **Advanced iris nevus syndrome.** A slit-lamp photograph of an individual with an advanced stage of iris nevus syndrome. The temporal aspect of the iris (clock hours 8 to 9) shows loss of the normal crypts of the iris. The small brown dots are tufts of normal iris tissue poking through the abnormal corneal endothelial membrane. From clock hours 9 to 11, the membrane has retracted, causing stretch tears in the iris. The subconjunctival hemorrhage is a result of this patient's recent guarded filtration surgery.

AQUEOUS MISDIRECTION SYNDROME (MALIGNANT GLAUCOMA)

This syndrome usually occurs following penetrating surgery of the eye, although it has certainly been reported following laser procedures.

Epidemiology

● In 1951, Chandler reported the incidence of malignant glaucoma to be 4% of eyes undergoing glaucoma surgery.

● Since then, filtering surgery has undergone some changes, and it is the impression of many clinicians that malignant glaucoma occurs less frequently in modern times.

Pathophysiology

● It is believed that the intervention in the eye changes the direction of aqueous humor flow. Instead of moving forward around the pupil, the aqueous goes into the vitreous. This causes a flattening of the anterior chamber angle and a relatively high or frankly high IOP (Fig. 18-8). Relatively high can be considered greater than 8 mm Hg.

● Typically, a flat anterior chamber is the result of overfiltration causing hypotony and choroidal detachments. One would not expect an IOP greater than 10 mm Hg with a flat anterior chamber. Sometimes, the pressure can be overtly elevated (more than 30 mm Hg).

History

● Typically, there is a recent history of eye surgery. The patient has blurry vision from anterior movement of the iris or lens complex, but this may be difficult to distinguish from normal postoperative blurring of vision.

● Unless the IOP is frankly elevated, there is usually no pain.

Clinical Examination

● Slit lamp: The anterior chamber is evenly narrow. There is no iris bombé. If a glaucoma-filtering procedure has been performed, the bleb is usually low with no evidence of wound leak. The IOP is as discussed earlier. Corneal edema may be present if the IOP is markedly elevated, or if there is lens–corneal contact.

● Gonioscopy: Usually, gonioscopy is not possible secondary to obvious ICE contact.

● Posterior pole: The hallmark of the disease is that there are no choroidals.

Special Studies

● Ultrasound biomicroscopy can be quite helpful. It will typically show flattening of the ciliary body processes and no anterior choroidals.

Management

● Often, the episode can be treated medically with topical cycloplegics and aqueous suppressants. Surgical intervention may be required if medical management fails.

● The key component to resolving the attack is disruption of the anterior hyaloid face. Sometimes, this can be done using lasers if the anterior hyaloid face can be visualized peripheral to the lens or intraocular lens implant.

● If this is not possible, a pars plana vitrectomy may be required. During this procedure, the retinal surgeon must be aware of the need to break the anterior hyaloid face.

BIBLIOGRAPHY

Chandler PA. Malignant glaucoma. *Am J Ophthalmol.* 1951;34:993.

Nielsen NV. The prevalence of glaucoma and ocular hypertension in type 1 and 2 diabetes mellitus: an epidemiological study of diabetes mellitus on the island of Falster, Denmark. *Acta Ophthalmol Scand.* 1983;27:662.

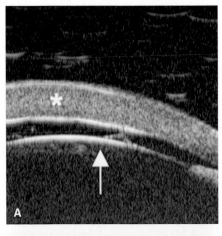

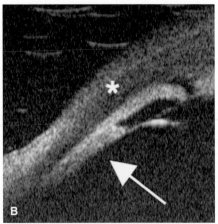

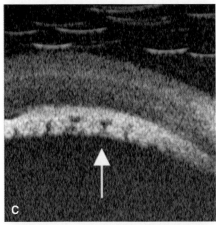

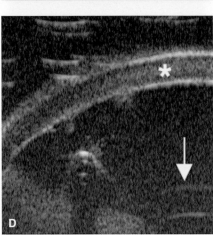

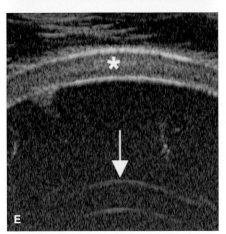

FIGURE 18-8. Aqueous misdirection following glaucoma drainage device implantation. A–C. An ultrasound biomicroscopy of a patient with aqueous misdirection syndrome following a glaucoma drainage device implantation procedure. In panels **A** and **B**, the *star* indicates the cornea. **A.** The *arrow* shows the anterior lens capsule; this central view shows a shallow anterior chamber with an iridocorneal endothelial (ICE) touch to the papillary margin. **B.** The *arrow* shows the flattened ciliary body processes diagnostic of aqueous misdirection syndrome; this view of the angle also shows the ICE touch. **C.** A magnified view of the flattened ciliary processes. Appearance after limited vitrectomy. The *arrow* points to a representative ciliary process seen in a longitudinal cross section view using ultrasound biomicroscopy. **D** and **E.** The same patient following limited vitrectomy with disruption of the anterior hyaloid face. The *star* indicates the cornea, whereas the *arrow* indicates the anterior capsule of the lens. **D.** Deepening of the anterior chamber angle; the tube can be seen lying flat on the iris. Aqueous misdirection following glaucoma drainage device implantation. **E.** A central view showing the deep anterior chamber.

Glaucoma Secondary to Elevated Venous Pressure

Douglas J. Rhee, Ribhi Hazin, and Louis R. Pasquale ∎

INTRODUCTION

This group of disorders shares a common mechanism of disease—glaucoma is the result of an elevation of episcleral venous pressure causing elevated intraocular pressure (IOP). Most cases can be attributed to carotid-cavernous sinus (CS) fistulas, CS thrombosis, dural arteriovenous (AV) shunts, superior vena cava syndrome, Sturge-Weber syndrome (SWS), thyroid ophthalmopathy, orbital obstructive lesions, or orbital varices.

CAROTID-CAVERNOUS FISTULA

Carotid-cavernous fistula (CCF) describes the potentially blinding AV communication between the carotid artery or its branches and the CS.

Classification

• CCF is classified as either a *direct* CCF in which highly pressurized blood from the carotid artery is directly shunted into the venous CS or an *indirect* CCF, which develops as a result of communication between smaller, low-pressure arterial branches and veins of the CS.[1]

• Direct CCFs tend to be "high flow" and typically arise in the setting of trauma, whereas indirect CCFs tend to be "low flow" and typically arise congenitally, during pregnancy, or spontaneously in postmenopausal women.[1]

Pathophysiology

• Individuals with diseases like Ehlers-Danlos syndrome, collagen deficiency syndromes, or other conditions that weaken the integrity of vessel walls may be at increased risk for spontaneous development of CCFs.

• CCFs alter ocular hemodynamics in a way whereby the high-flow, high-pressure profile of the carotid artery is transmitted to orbital and ocular structures to produce a constellation of ocular signs and symptoms. These signs and symptoms are directly proportional to the degree of abnormal communication between arterial and venous blood in the CS.

- This form of venous hypertension yields the classic clinical triad for CCF:

  - Unilateral exophthalmos, which may be pulsatile in high-flow direct CCFs

  - Ocular or cephalic bruit, which is more audible in high-flow CCFs

  - Injection and chemosis of the conjunctiva, which is more pronounced in high-flow CCFs.[1]

Clinical Presentation

- Patients with direct CCF have more pronounced complaints of headaches, diplopia, epistaxis, and visual loss than patients with indirect CCFs.[1,2]

- Indirect fistulas are associated with a myriad of clinical findings that are more subacute or chronic in nature. The presentation of the indirect CCF may include ocular redness and swelling that can be initially construed as an ocular infection. Visual acuity and color vision can be compromised in a gradual manner. There can be extraocular muscle imbalance related to compression of the third and/or sixth cranial nerve in the CS. The proptosis in indirect fistulas is usually more subtle and typically not pulsatile in nature.

Diagnostic Evaluation

- A slit-lamp examination will often reveal arterialized and tortuous, corkscrew conjunctival vessels (Fig. 19-1) and a shallow anterior chamber. The corkscrew appearance distinguishes this condition from episcleritis, where the vessels have a crossing pattern, or scleritis, where there is a deep violaceous hue to ocular surface tissues.

- The IOP is often elevated, and wide mires can be appreciated while the IOP is measured.

- On gonioscopy, the filtration apparatus, that is, angle, may be appositionally closed if choroidal engorgement is present, and blood reflux may be noted where the angle is open. The fundus may exhibit an impending retinal venous occlusive picture with tortuous vessels and intraretinal hemorrhage. The elevated IOP in patients with CCF is often refractory to medical therapy.[3]

- Orbital imaging with computed tomography or magnetic resonance imaging will reveal enlargement of the extraocular muscles and engorgement of the superior ophthalmic vein (Fig. 19-2). With contrast, enhancement of CS will be evident. Carotid angiography is often diagnostic in revealing the exact fistula site.

Management

- The treatment for both direct and indirect CCFs is the same: Endovascular embolization using balloons or detachable coils or stenting for both types of fistulas is typically definitive in resolving most signs and symptoms (Fig. 19-3).

- A more conservative approach is adopted for indirect CCFs because spontaneous regression can occur. However, in patients with indirect CCF where there is evolution to progressive ocular and orbital congestion with compromise of vision and intractably elevated IOP, definitive closure is indicated.[1,4]

- Filtration surgery is to be avoided in eyes with CCFs if at all possible.

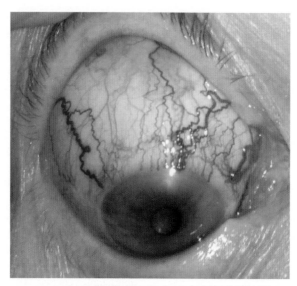

FIGURE 19-1. **Carotid-cavernous fistula.** Arterialization of conjunctival vessels in a 78-year-old patient with a spontaneous indirect carotid-cavernous fistula before endovascular embolization with a detachable coil. (Courtesy of Dr. Peter Veldman.)

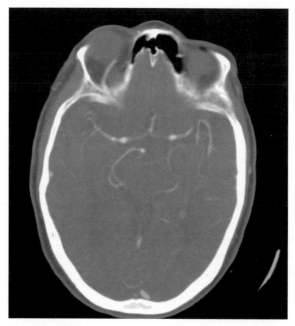

FIGURE 19-2. **Carotid-cavernous fistula.** A magnetic resonance angiography of the patient in Figure 19-1 revealing an enlarged right superior ophthalmic vein. (Courtesy of Dr. Peter Veldman.)

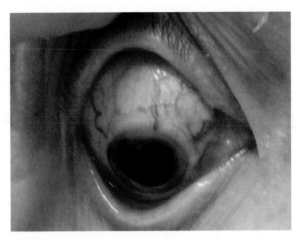

FIGURE 19-3. Carotid-cavernous fistula. An improved clinical appearance of the patient in Figure 19-1 with a marked reduction of conjunctival arterialization following endovascular embolization with a detachable coil. (Courtesy of Dr. Peter Veldman.)

STURGE-WEBER SYNDROME

SWS describes the congenital neurocutaneous condition characterized by a triad of neuropsychiatric, dermatologic, and ophthalmologic manifestations. It is often referred to as the "fourth phacomatosis," but unlike the other phacomatoses, it has no known inheritance pattern.

Etiology

● During development, there is an abnormal vascular plexus adjacent to the neural tube. This vascular nexus fails to regress and is dragged to various surface ectodermal and neuroectodermal locations during development. These loci of aberrant vascular tissue contribute to the clinical manifestations in SWS.

Visual Loss

● The most important cause of vision loss in SWS is the development of glaucoma. As many as 30% to 70% of individuals with SWS develop glaucoma, with 60% of cases reported at birth or in infancy and 40% reported in adolescence or young adulthood.[1]

● When glaucoma is present in the first year of life, the signs (including buphthalmos) and symptoms of congenital glaucoma are often present. If glaucoma does not develop by adulthood, it is generally unlikely to develop later on, unless there is some other predisposition to another type of glaucoma.

● Patients with glaucoma frequently have an episcleral vascular malformation that can be quite subtle (Fig. 19-4). As pointed out by Aggarwal and associates,[2] on gonioscopy, the eye with glaucoma will often have reduced visibility of the scleral spur and the ciliary body band (Fig. 19-5).

● Elevated episcleral venous pressure secondary to the episcleral vascular

malformation appears to be the most common cause of glaucoma in SWS patients.[3] The eye with glaucoma will also often have iris heterochromia (with the darker iridis on the side with the facial vascular malformation).

● Eyes with or without glaucoma may harbor a choroidal vascular malformation, giving the retina a "tomato ketchup" appearance.

● Other causes of visual loss in SWS include serous retinal detachment from large choroidal vascular malformations and homonymous hemianopia.

Clinical Presentation

● Clinically, patients with SWS often exhibit a facial vascular malformation or "port-wine stain" that arises secondary to AV malformations in the skin. These skin lesions do not necessarily respect a strict dermatomal distribution (Fig. 19-6).

● In some patients, the port-wine stain can hypertrophy with age. Sometimes, such hypertrophy can make measurement of IOP challenging. Although the characteristic "port-wine stain" in SWS is typically unilateral, it can be bilateral as well.[4]

Management

● Pulsed dye laser photocoagulation is successful in mitigating the cosmetic effects of cutaneous port-wine lesions, and it does not contribute to clinically significant changes in IOP in SWS patients.[1]

● Medical therapy can be effective in managing SWS-induced glaucoma, but surgical intervention is often warranted. In instances of glaucoma occurring in infancy, goniotomy should be considered.

● Trabeculectomy is possible in children over 3 years of age and in adults.[3] Traditional glaucoma drainage devices (e.g., Baerveldt or Ahmed) are also excellent treatment options.

• Although prophylactic posterior sclerotomy is often recommended to prevent perioperative choroidal hemorrhage in SWS patients requiring trabeculectomy, Eibschitz-Tsimhoni and colleagues reported that in 17 consecutive patients with either SWS or a related condition (Klippel-Trenaunay-Weber syndrome), performance of trabeculectomy without prophylactic sclerotomy did not result in choroidal hemorrhage or effusion, requiring further surgical intervention.[5]

• Cyclodestruction can also be considered in uncontrolled glaucoma, depending on the clinical scenario.

REFERENCES

1. Sharan S, Swamy B, Taranath DA, et al. Port-wine vascular malformations and glaucoma risk in Sturge-Weber syndrome. *J AAPOS*. 2009;13(4):374–378.
2. Aggarwal NK, Gandham SB, Weinstein R, et al. Heterochromia iridis and pertinent clinical findings in patients with glaucoma associated with Sturge-Weber Syndrome. *J Pediatr Ophthalmol Strabismus*. 2010;47:361–365.
3. Patrianakos TD, Nagao K, Walton DS. Surgical management of glaucoma with the Sturge-Weber syndrome. *Int Ophthalmol Clin*. 2008;48(2):63–78.
4. Quan SY, Comi AM, Parsa CF, et al. Effect of a single application of pulsed dye laser treatment of port-wine birthmarks on intraocular pressure. *Arch Dermatol*. 2010;146(9):1015–1018.
5. Eibschitz-Tsimhoni M, Lichter PR, Del Monte MA, et al. Assessing the need for posterior sclerotomy at the time of filtering surgery in patients with Sturge-Weber syndrome. *Ophthalmology*. 2003;110(7):1361–1363.

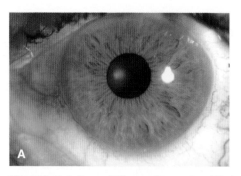 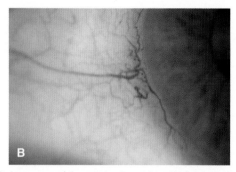

FIGURE 19-4. Sturge-Weber syndrome. A and **B.** A slit-lamp view of the episcleral vascular malformation of a 49-year-old man with Sturge-Weber syndrome and late-onset glaucoma. Note that the episcleral malformation can be subtle and construed as episcleritis if it were unaccompanied by a port-wine stain. A lower magnification slit-lamp view. A higher magnification view of the inferonasal limbal area showing terminal end bulbs at the limbus differentiating these as abnormal vessels.

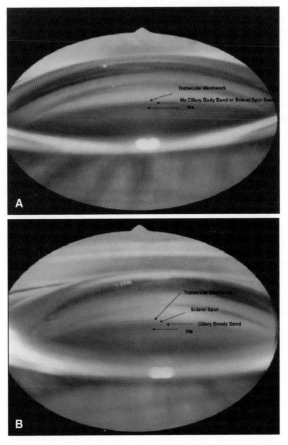

FIGURE 19-5. Sturge-Weber syndrome. A and **B.** A typical appearance of the drainage angle in Sturge-Weber syndrome with reduced visibility of the scleral spur and the ciliary body band. Note the reduced visibility of the ciliary body band, the scleral spur, and the irregular border of the peripheral iris. A gonioscopy of the anterior chamber angle of the contralateral eye of the same patient showing the normal landmarks. (From Aggarwal NK, Gandham SB, Weinstein R, et al. Heterochromia iridis and pertinent clinical findings in patients with glaucoma associated with Sturge-Weber syndrome. *J Pediatr Ophthalmol Strabismus.* 2010;47:361–365, with permission.)

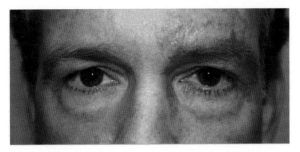

FIGURE 19-6. Sturge-Weber syndrome. An angiomatosis involving the periocular skin and the episclera in the same patient as in Figure 19-4. Note that the periocular involvement does not follow a strict dermatomal distribution.

IDIOPATHIC ELEVATED EPISCLERAL VENOUS PRESSURE

Description

• Idiopathic elevated episcleral venous pressure (IEEVP) is a diagnosis of exclusion. An extensive history, clinical examination, and complete diagnostic evaluation including radiologic testing should be undertaken to detect any primary causes such as those listed in the introduction of this chapter.

Clinical Presentation

• Patients with IEEVP have dilated, tortuous episcleral vessels, with onset occurring subacutely typically in the third or fourth decade of life. The dilated vessels can be unilateral or bilateral, usually with asymmetry even in bilateral cases (Fig. 19-7).[1]

• Patients may have blood in Schlemm canal, which is a generalized sign of elevated episcleral venous pressure (Fig. 19-8), but this finding is not necessary to establish the diagnosis.

Management

• This is similar to the other entities in this chapter. Medical management may not be sufficient, and surgery may therefore be needed. Laser trabeculoplasty is not generally effective. These eyes are prone to choroidal effusions at IOPs that are not considered typically hypotonous, and so aggressive target IOPs should be made with caution. Trabeculectomy and deep sclerectomy offer the benefit of resistance that can be modified during the postoperative period.

REFERENCE

1. Rhee DJ, Gupta M, Moncavage M, et al. Idiopathic elevated episcleral venous pressure and open angle glaucoma. *Br J Ophthalmol.* 2009;93:231–234.

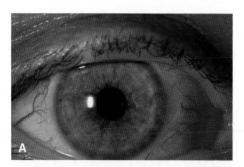
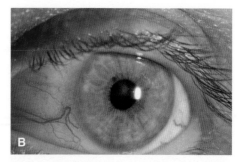

FIGURE 19-7. **Idiopathic elevated episcleral venous pressure. A** and **B.** A bilateral case of idiopathic elevated episcleral venous pressure with greater involvement of the left eye. Images of the individual eyes.

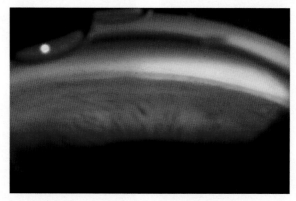

FIGURE 19-8. **Elevated episcleral venous pressure.** Blood in Schlemm canal.

OTHER CAUSES OF ELEVATED EPISCLERAL VENOUS PRESSURE

• Although the cases of most patients can be explained by the differential diagnosis listed in the introduction, an AV malformation distal to the venous drainage of the eye can cause an elevated IOP (**Fig. 19-9**).

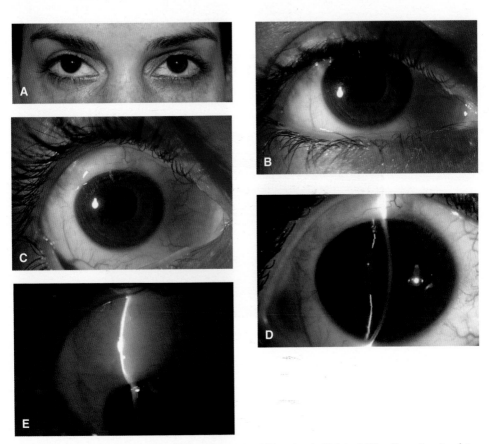

FIGURE 19-9. A–G. Arteriovenous (AV) malformation. This patient had bilateral AV malformations involving the trochlear arteries that were discovered using computed tomography angiography. The left side had greater involvement and received a trabeculectomy. An external photograph showing involvement of both eyes but with greater involvement of the left eye. A view of the right eye with the lid raised showing engorgement of episcleral veins. Images of the left eye following trabeculectomy surgery with ExPress shunt (Alcon, Ft. Worth, TX) and Ologen (Aeon Astron, Netherlands) implants.

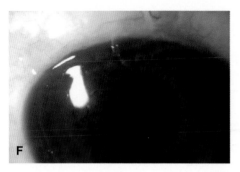
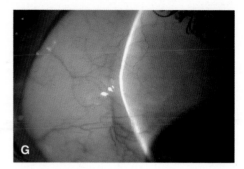

FIGURE 19-9. (*continued*)

Section III ■ Glaucoma Management

Introduction to Glaucoma Management

Douglas J. Rhee ■

WHAT IS THE GOAL OF TREATMENT?

We currently understand the pathophysiology of glaucoma to be a progressive loss of ganglion cells resulting in visual field damage that is related to intraocular pressure (IOP). The goal of treatment is to delay or halt the ganglion cell loss and prevent symptomatic visual loss while attempting not to cause untoward side effects.

Although many clinicians now feel that there are several factors involved in the pathogenesis of glaucoma, the only rigorously proven method of treatment is the lowering of IOP.

HOW DO WE LOWER INTRAOCULAR PRESSURE IN GLAUCOMA?

Glaucoma was first thought of as a surgical disease. The first filtration procedure (not iridectomy) was suggested by Louis de Wecker (1832 to 1906) in 1869. Although the miotic effects of eserine and pilocarpine had been

reported in the early 1860s, they were not used for treatment until later. Adolf Weber (1829 to 1915) first introduced these agents as medical treatments of glaucoma in 1876. The first study comparing the two available forms of glaucoma treatment, eserine and iridectomy, was performed at Wills Eye Hospital in 1895 by Zentmayer et al. This study showed that both treatments were equivalent and that a patient's visual status could be maintained for periods ranging from 5 to 15 years on chronic medical treatment.

The debate over the best initial therapy continues today. Most clinicians use medications as the initial treatment for glaucoma. In the United States, two large studies were performed to compare medical treatment with laser trabeculoplasty (Glaucoma Laser Trial [GLT] and the Selective Laser Trabeculoplasty [SLT] Med Study) and medical treatment with trabeculectomy (Collaborative Initial Glaucoma Treatment Study [CIGTS]). At 2-year follow-up in the GLT, eyes that received argon laser trabeculoplasty (ALT) showed a lower mean IOP (between 1 and 2 mm Hg) than eyes started on timolol but showed no difference in visual field or acuity. At 7 years, eyes that received ALT had a greater reduction in IOP (1.2 mm Hg) and a greater sensitivity in the visual field (0.6 dB). Prospective randomized controlled trials (e.g., SLT/MED study and Nagar et al.) showed equivalence between SLT and prostaglandin analogues at 1-year follow-up. These results seem to indicate that laser trabeculoplasty is at least as good as contemporary medical treatment for glaucoma.

Results from the CIGTS study show no difference in visual field outcomes despite a lower IOP in the surgical group. One exception noted in CIGTS was that initial surgery led to less visual field progression than initial medicine in patients with advanced field loss at enrollment. Patients with diabetes had more visual field loss over time if treated initially with surgery. Smoking was also found to influence final pressure–lowering responses. We do not understand why these differences exist in different subgroups. Overall, visual acuity and local eye symptoms seem to be worse in the surgical group. However, the CIGTS results do not unequivocally support changing the current paradigm of medical treatment as initial treatment.

In recent years, there has been an explosion of innovation for the surgical treatment of glaucoma. New minimally invasive techniques have emerged. Long-term prospective randomized trials comparing these techniques to trabeculectomy are yet to occur, but case-controlled trials, cohort studies, and trials comparing to phacoemulsification cataract surgery seem to show great safety results. Newer generation devices and techniques attempt to build upon the high degree of safety and improve IOP reduction. The placement of these minimally invasive procedures/implants is yet to be resolved, but their safety profile would argue for involvement earlier than trabeculectomy.

The subsequent chapters in this section describe the different therapies commonly utilized for glaucoma.

WHAT MAY THE FUTURE HOLD?

At this time, the predominant treatments are palliative, that is, they do not directly interrupt a known pathophysiologic mechanism of disease. Although lowering the IOP through these other means, for example, enhancing uveoscleral outflow, decreasing aqueous secretion, creating fistulas with or without stents, etc., have been shown to slow the progression of visual field loss, most patients experience a continuation of the pathophysiologic process(es), resulting in a continuous escalation of treatments to keep the IOP under control. The promise of disease-modifying therapy in which a known pathophysiologic mechanism is interrupted holds the promise of potentially inhibiting the constant escalation of treatment. Several disease-modifying strategies and potentially regenerative treatments are being explored in laboratory models and early-stage clinical studies. It is an exciting time in glaucoma management.

IOP-dependent mechanisms: As our understanding of the pathophysiology of Primary Open-Angle Glaucoma (POAG) increases, we hope to develop treatments that directly interrupt the disease mechanism. At the time of publication, new medication classes, such as rho kinase (ROCK) inhibitors and adenosine receptor agonists, are moving through clinical trials. ROCK inhibitors affect cell cytoskeleton and lower IOP through the trabecular meshwork; suggestive evidence to the effect that dysregulation of cell cytoskeleton and tissue rigidity is a primary pathophysiologic mechanism of POAG exists. The most convincing pathophysiologic POAG mechanism is dysregulation of extracellular matrix homeostasis within the juxtacanalicular region likely mediated through transforming growth factor beta-2. Adenosine agonists may work by increasing extracellular matrix turnover in the juxtacanalicular region and lower IOP.

Non–IOP-dependent treatments to slow disease progression remain elusive. Some suggestive data indicate that brimonidine could have an additional benefit beyond IOP reduction. Additional rigorous clinical trial evidence is still needed.

Regenerative treatments to replace retinal ganglion cells and reverse visual field damage seemed like distant science fiction. Recent successes in very early-stage laboratory models lead to hope that restoring visual damage from glaucoma is an attainable goal.

BIBLIOGRAPHY

AGIS Investigators. The Advanced Glaucoma Intervention Study (AGIS): 7. The relationship between control of intraocular pressure and visual field deterioration. *Am J Ophthalmol.* 2000;130:429–440.

Bergea B, Bodin L, Svedbergh B. Impact of intraocular pressure regulation on visual fields in open-angle glaucoma. *Ophthalmology.* 1999;106:997–1005.

Bhorade AM, Wilson BS, Gordon MO, et al; Ocular Hypertension Treatment Study Group. The utility of the monocular trial: data from the ocular hypertension treatment study. *Ophthalmology.* 2010;117:2047–2054.

Collaborative Normal-Tension Glaucoma Study Group. Comparison of glaucomatous progression between untreated patients with normal-tension glaucoma and patients with therapeutically reduced intraocular pressures. *Am J Ophthalmol.* 1998;126:487–497.

Glaucoma Laser Trial Research Group. The Glaucoma Laser Trial (GLT): 2. Results of argon laser trabeculoplasty versus topical medicines. *Ophthalmology.* 1990;97:1403–1413.

Glaucoma Laser Trial Research Group. The Glaucoma Laser Trial (GLT) and glaucoma laser trial follow-up study: 7. Results. *Am J Ophthalmol.* 1995;120:718–731.

Janz NK, Wren PA, Lichter PR, et al; CIGTS Study Group. The Collaborative Initial Glaucoma Treatment Study: interim quality of life findings after initial medical or surgical treatment of glaucoma. *Ophthalmology.* 2001;108:1954–1965.

Katz LJ, Steinmann WC, Kabir A, Molineaux J, Wizov SS, Marcellino G; for the SLT/Med Study Group. Selective laser trabeculoplasty versus medical therapy as initial treatment of glaucoma: a prospective, randomized trial. *J Glaucoma.* 2012;21:460–468.

Krupin T, Liebmann JM, Greenfield DS, Ritch R, Gardiner S; Low-Pressure Glaucoma Study Group. A randomized trial of brimonidine versus timolol in preserving visual function: results from the low-pressure glaucoma treatment study. *Am J Ophthalmol.* 2011;151:671–681.

Lichter PR, Musch DC, Gillespie BW, et al; CIGTS Study Group. Interim clinical outcomes in the Collaborative Initial Glaucoma Treatment Study comparing initial treatment randomized to medications or surgery. *Ophthalmology.* 2001;108:1943–1953.

Mao LK, Steward WC, Shield MB. Correlation between intraocular pressure control and progressive glaucomatous damage in primary open-angle glaucoma. *Am J Ophthalmol.* 1991;111:51–55.

Musch DC, Gillespie BW, Lichter PR, et al; CIGTS Study Investigators. Visual field progression in the Collaborative Initial Glaucoma Treatment Study: the impact of treatment and other baseline factors. *Ophthalmology.* 2009;116:200–207.

Nagar M, Ogunyomade A, O'Brart DPS, Howes F, Marshall J. A randomized, prospective study comparing selective laser trabeculoplasty with latanoprost for the control of intraocular pressure in ocular hypertension and open glaucoma. *Br. J Ophthalmol.* 2005;89:1413–1417.

Realini TD. A prospective, randomized, investigator-masked evaluation of the monocular trial in ocular hypertension or open-angle glaucoma. *Ophthalmology.* 2009;116:1237–1242.

Zentmayer W, Posey WC. A clinical study of 167 cases of glaucoma simplex. *Arch Ophthalmol.* 1895;24:378–394.

Medical Management

Malik Y. Kahook and Douglas J. Rhee ■

INTRODUCTION

Medical treatment of glaucoma began in the late 1800s with the use of eserine and pilocarpine. In the United States, glaucoma treatment is typically begun with topical medications. The short-term goal of medications is to lower intraocular pressure (IOP). The long-term goals are to prevent symptomatic visual loss while minimizing the side effects from the treatments.

DESCRIPTION AND PHYSIOLOGY

Unless there are extreme circumstances, such as an IOP higher than 40 mm Hg or an impending risk to central fixation, treatment is started using a so-called one-eyed therapeutic trial. Typically, one type of drop is started in only one eye with reexamination in 3 to 6 weeks to check for effectiveness. Effectiveness is determined by comparing the difference in IOP in the two eyes before therapy with the difference in IOP after initiating therapy. For example, if IOP is 30 mm Hg OD (*oculus dexter*; in the right eye) and 33 mm Hg OS (*oculus sinister*; in the left eye) before treatment, and, following treatment of the right

eye, IOP is 20 mm Hg OD and 23 mm Hg OS, the drug is not having any effect. If the IOP after starting treatment is 25 mm Hg OD and 34 mm Hg OS, then the drug is having an effect.

It should be noted that the monocular trial when instituting medical therapy has been the topic of intensive studies over the past few years. Realini has reported that the monocular drug trial is of little clinical value in patients being treated with latanoprost. Bhorade and colleagues came to a similar conclusion in their study of prostaglandin analogues. Regardless, it is common practice to initiate medical therapy once glaucomatous optic neuropathy is diagnosed, and a firm understanding of the limited number of glaucoma therapeutics is necessary to choose the best therapy for each individual patient.

There are several different classes of medications. All medications work to lower IOP through varying pharmacologic mechanisms. IOP is determined by the balance between secretion and drainage of aqueous humor. All medications either decrease secretion or increase outflow. In the subsequent sections, the mechanism of action, common side effects, and contraindications for the different classes of medications are presented. **Table 21-1** lists the medications within each class that are available in the United States as of 2010 to 2011.

The side effects and contraindications described in this chapter are not a complete listing. I recommend that all clinicians read the package insert before prescribing any medication. The figures show sample bottles of medications available in the United States.

TABLE 21-1. Pharmacologic Agents Organized by Pharmacologic Class

Medication*	Available Strengths
Alpha Agonists	
Apraclonidine (*Iopidine*)	0.5%, 1%
Brimonidine (*Alphagan*)	0.1% (with purite), 0.15%, 0.2%
Beta-Blockers	
Betaxolol (*Betoptic*)	0.5%
Carteolol (*Ocupress*)	1%
Levobunolol (*Betagan*)	0.25%, 0.5%
Metipranolol (*OptiPranolol*)	0.3%
Timolol hemihydrate (*Betimol*)	0.25%, 0.5%
Timolol maleate (*Timoptic*)	0.25%, 0.5%
Carbonic Anhydrase Inhibitors—Oral	
Acetazolamide (*Diamox*)	125–500 mg
Methazolamide (*Neptazane, Glauctabs*)	25–50 mg
Carbonic Anhydrase Inhibitors—Topical	
Brinzolamide (*Azopt*)	1%
Dorzolamide (*Trusopt*)	2%
Hyperosmolar Agents	
Glycerin (*Osmoglyn*)	50% solution
Isosorbide (*Ismotic*)	4% solution
Mannitol (*Osmitrol*)	5%–20% solution
Miotics	
Physostigmine (*Eserine*)	0.25%
Pilocarpine hydrochloride (*Pilocarpine, Pilocar*)	0.25%, 0.5%, 1%, 2%, 4%, 6%
Pilocarpine nitrate (*Pilagan*)	1%, 2%, 4%
Prostaglandins	
Bimatoprost (*Lumigan*)	0.01%, 0.03%
Latanoprost (*Xalatan*)	0.005%
Travoprost (*Travatan*)	0.004%
Unoprostone isopropyl (*Rescula*)	0.15%
Sympathomimetic Agents	
Dipivefrin (*Propine*)	0.1%
Epinephrine (*Epifrin*)	0.5%, 1%, 2%
Combination Medications	**Available Formulations**
Dorzolamide/Timolol (*Cosopt*)	2%/0.5%
Brimonidine/Timolol (*Combigan*)	0.2%/0.5%
Brinzolamide/Brimonidine (Simbrinza)	1%/0.2%

* Trade names available in the United States are indicated in *italics.*

ALPHA AGONISTS

Mechanism of Action

• Activation of alpha-2 receptors in the ciliary body inhibits aqueous secretion (Fig. 21-1).

Side Effects

• Local irritation, allergy (Fig. 21-2), mydriasis, dry mouth, dry eye, hypotension, and lethargy

Contraindications

• Monoamine oxidase inhibitor use. Brimonidine is not to be used in children younger than 2 years; it has been associated with apnea in children.

Comments

• Apraclonidine is for short-term use and prophylaxis of postlaser IOP spikes.

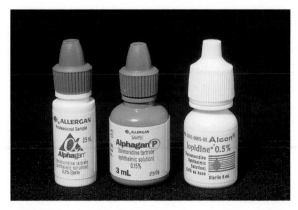

FIGURE 21-1. Alpha agonists. All trade-name alpha agonists available in the United States at the time of publication. From left to right: Alphagan (Allergan; Irvine, CA), Alphagan-P (Allergan; Irvine, CA), and Iopidine 0.5% (Alcon; Fort Worth, TX). Note: Iopidine 1% is not shown.

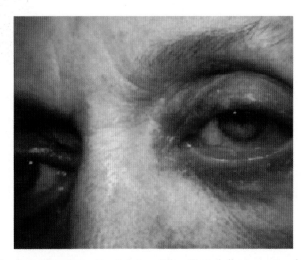

FIGURE 21-2. Allergic reaction from chronic brimonidine. Typical allergic reaction from brimonidine is a follicular conjunctivitis that occurs months to years after chronic use. The prevalence is dose related to the concentration of brimonidine, with lower concentrations having lower prevalence of allergic reactions. This is an extreme case in which an ectropion occurred as a result of periorbital skin excoriation and fibrosis. These findings resolved spontaneously over a few weeks of discontinuing the medication.

BETA-BLOCKERS

Mechanism of Action

● Blockade of the beta receptors in the ciliary body reduces IOP by decreasing aqueous humor production (**Fig. 21-3**).

Side Effects

● Local: blurred vision, corneal anesthesia, and superficial punctate keratitis

● Systemic: bradycardia or heart block, bronchospasm, fatigue, mood change, impotence, reduced sensitivity to hypoglycemic symptoms in insulin-dependent diabetics, worsening of myasthenia gravis

Contraindications

● Asthma, severe chronic obstructive pulmonary disease, bradycardia, heart block, congestive heart failure (CHF), myasthenia gravis

Comments

● Some medications are considered nonselective, whereas some are relatively cardioselective (**Table 21-2**). The relatively cardioselective medications may have fewer pulmonary side effects.

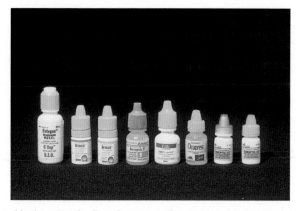

FIGURE 21-3. **Beta-blockers.** Nearly all single-agent, trade-name beta-blockers available in the United States at the time of publication; Betagan 0.25% and Betoptic are missing. From left to right: Betagan 0.5% (Allergan; Irvine, CA), Betimol 0.25% and 0.5%, respectively (Santen; Tampere, Finland), Betoptic-S (Alcon; Fort Worth, TX), OptiPranolol (Bausch & Lomb; Claremont, CA), Ocupress (Novartis; Atlanta, GA), and Timoptic XE 0.25% and 0.5%, respectively (Merck; Whitehouse Station, NJ).

TABLE 21-2. Relative Receptor Selectivity of the Various Beta-Blocker Medications

Drug	Relative Specificity of the Receptor Effect
Betaxolol	Relatively cardioselective
Carteolol	Nonselective; has intrinsic sympathomimetic activity
Levobunolol	Nonselective (long half-life)
Metipranolol	Nonselective (*white* top)
Timolol hemihydrate	Nonselective
Timolol maleate	Nonselective

CARBONIC ANHYDRASE INHIBITORS

Mechanism of Action

- Inhibition of the enzyme carbonic anhydrase decreases aqueous production in the ciliary body. When given parentally, carbonic anhydrase inhibitors (CAIs) will also cause dehydration of the vitreous (Figs. 21-4 and 21-5).

Side Effects

- Local (with topical therapy): bitter taste
- Systemic
  - With topical therapy: diuresis, fatigue, gastrointestinal upset, Stevens–Johnson syndrome, theoretical risk of aplastic anemia
  - With systemic therapy: hypokalemia and acidosis, renal stones, paresthesias, nausea, cramps, diarrhea, malaise, lethargy, depression, impotence, unpleasant taste, aplastic anemia, Stevens–Johnson syndrome

Contraindications

- Sulfa allergy, hyponatremia or hypokalemia, recent renal stones, thiazide diuretics, digitalis use

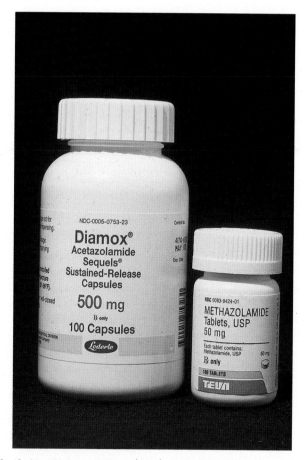

FIGURE 21-4. Oral carbonic anhydrase inhibitors (CAIs). The oral CAIs available in the United States at the time of publication. From left to right: Diamox (Lederle; PA) and methazolamide (generic made by Copley Pharmaceutical; Canton, MA). Other companies have manufactured these medications in their generic forms in recent years.

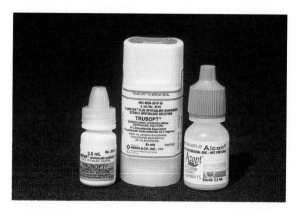

FIGURE 21-5. Topical carbonic anhydrase inhibitors (CAIs). All single-agent, trade-name topical CAIs available in the United States at the time of publication. From left to right: Trusopt, old and new bottle, respectively (Merck; Whitehouse Station, NJ), and Azopt (Alcon; Fort Worth, TX).

HYPEROSMOLAR AGENTS

Mechanism of Action

- These agents dehydrate the vitreous and decrease intraocular fluid volume by osmotically drawing fluid into the intravascular space. The agents are given orally or intravenously.

Side Effects

- Mannitol: CHF, urinary retention in men, backache, myocardial infarction, headache, and mental confusion
- Glycerin: vomiting; less likely to produce CHF than mannitol, otherwise similar to mannitol
- Isosorbide: same as glycerin except that it is perhaps safer in diabetic patients

Contraindications

- CHF, diabetic ketoacidosis (glycerin), subdural or subarachnoid hemorrhage, preexisting severe dehydration

MIOTICS

Mechanism of Action

- Direct-acting cholinergics stimulate muscarinic receptors, and indirect-acting cholinergics block acetylcholinesterase (**Table 21-3**). Miotics cause pupillary muscle constriction, which is believed to pull open the trabecular meshwork to increase trabecular outflow (**Fig. 21-6**).

Side Effects

- Direct-acting cholinergic
  - Local: brow ache, breakdown of the blood/aqueous barrier, angle closure (increases pupillary block and causes the lens/iris diaphragm to move anteriorly), reduced night vision, variable myopia, retinal tear or detachment, and possibly anterior subcapsular cataracts
  - Systemic: rare
- Indirect-acting cholinergic
  - Local: retinal detachment, cataract, myopia, intense miosis, angle closure, increased bleeding post surgery, punctal stenosis, increased formation of posterior synechiae in chronic uveitis
  - Systemic: diarrhea, abdominal cramps, enuresis, and increased effect of succinylcholine

Contraindications

- Direct cholinergic: peripheral retinal pathology, central media opacity, young patient (increases myopic effect), uveitis
- Indirect cholinergic: succinylcholine administration, predisposition to retinal tear, anterior subcapsular cataract, ocular surgery, uveitis

TABLE 21-3. Mechanism of Action of Various Miotic Agents

Drug	Notes
Echothiophate iodide	Indirect; avoid in phakic patients
Physostigmine	Indirect; avoid in phakic patients
Demecarium bromide	Indirect
Acetylcholine	Direct; used during surgery
Carbachol	Direct/indirect
Pilocarpine hydrochloride	Direct
Pilocarpine nitrate	Direct

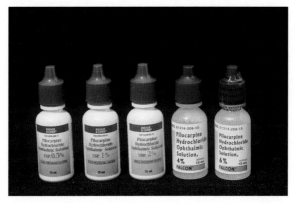

FIGURE 21-6. Pilocarpine strengths. The various strengths of pilocarpine, from 0.5% to 6%.

PROSTAGLANDINS

Mechanism of Action

● Prostaglandin $F_2\alpha$ analogues increase uveo-scleral outflow by increasing extracellular matrix turnover in the ciliary body face (Fig. 21-7).

Side Effects

● Local: increase in melanin pigmentation in iris (Fig. 21-8), blurred vision, and eyelid redness; cystoid macular edema and anterior uveitis have been reported.

● Systemic: systemic upper respiratory infection symptoms, backache, chest pain, and myalgia.

Contraindications

● pregnancy; consider not using in inflammatory conditions

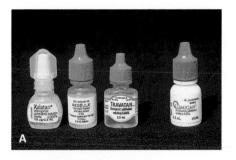

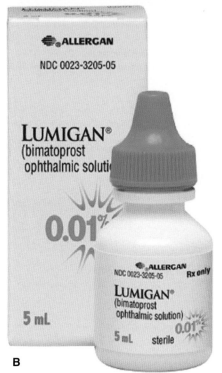

FIGURE 21-7. **Prostaglandin agonists. A.** All prostaglandin agonists available in the United States at the time
of publication. From left to right: Xalatan 0.005% (Pfizer;
New York, NY), Rescula (Sucampo Pharmaceuticals, Inc.,
Bethesda, MD) is no longer in the US market, and Travatan
0.004% (Alcon; Fort Worth, TX). Separated from the rest
of the group is the medication Lumigan 0.03% (Allergan;
Irvine, CA), which is chemically similar to the other drugs
but is considered a prostamide. **B.** A more recent version
of Lumigan (Allergan; Irvine, CA) contains a lower dose of
bimatoprost (0.01%) than the original formulation.

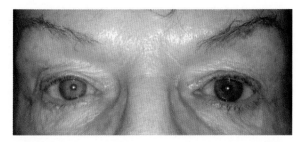

FIGURE 21-8. **Prostaglandin analogue–induced heterochromia.** This patient had been treated monocularly in
the left eye with a prostaglandin analogue, which resulted in a darker iris in the treated eye.

SYMPATHOMIMETIC AGENTS

Mechanism of Action

- In the ciliary body, the response is variable (beta stimulation increases aqueous production, but alpha stimulation decreases aqueous production); in the trabecular meshwork, beta stimulation causes increased trabecular outflow and increased uveoscleral outflow; overall effect lowers IOP (**Fig. 21-9**).

Side Effects

- Local: cystoid macular edema in aphakia (more likely with epinephrine than dipivefrin), mydriasis, rebound hyperemia, blurred vision, adrenochrome deposits, and allergic blepharoconjunctivitis
- Systemic: tachycardia/ectopy, hypertension, headache

Contraindications

- Narrow angles, aphakia, pseudophakia, soft lenses, hypertension, and cardiac disease

Comments

- Dipivefrin requires 2 to 3 months to obtain the full effect. Epinephrine has mixed alpha- and beta-agonist activity.

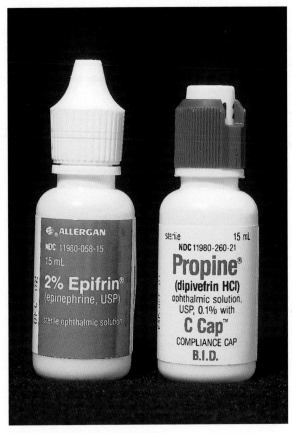

FIGURE 21-9. Sympathomimetic agents. Historically utilized sympathomimetic agents from left to right: Epifrin (Allergan; Irvine, CA) and Propine (Allergan; Irvine, CA).

COMBINATION AGENTS

Three combination agents are currently available: Cosopt, which combines the beta-blocker timolol (0.5%) with the topical CAI dorzolamide; Combigan, which combines the beta-blocker timolol (0.5%) with brimonidine (0.2%); and Simbrinza, which combines brinzolamide (1%) with brimonidine (0.2%). The mechanisms of action, side effects, and contraindications for each component of these combination medications apply as explained in detail (**Fig. 21-10**).

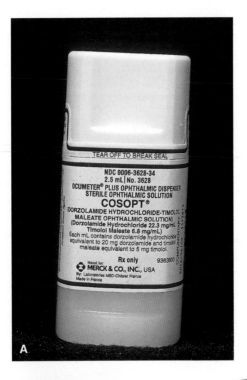

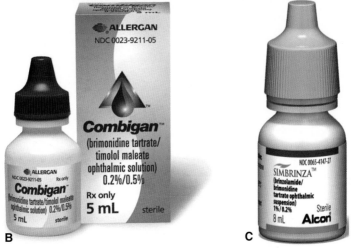

FIGURE 21-10. **Combination agents. A.** The combination agent Cosopt (Merck; Whitehouse Station, NJ). **B.** The combination agent Combigan (Allergan, Irvine, CA). **C.** Simbrinza bottle (Novartis).

TECHNIQUE OF DROP INSTILLATION

Self-administration

In the upright position, drops can be administered in many ways. A two-handed method is briefly described here. First, the patient should tilt the head back, so that he or she is looking upward. With the nondominant hand, the patient uses the thumb and the forefinger to hold open both upper and lower lids. With the dominant hand, the drop bottle is held over the eye, and a drop is administered (Fig. 21-11).

If tremor or generalized weakness makes this technique difficult, an alternate technique using one hand can be utilized. First, the patient should tilt the head back, so that he or she is looking upward. The dominant hand holds the drop bottle so that it rests gently on the bridge of the nose. The tip of the drop bottle should be over the eye. Squeezing the bottle will administer the drop. This technique allows the patient's nose to help brace the bottle and assist the aim of the drop (Fig. 21-12).

Punctal Occlusion

Often, excess drops will drain into the tear drainage system and then into the nose. Absorption of the drug through the nasal mucosa can greatly increase the systemic effect of the medication. This increased systemic absorption does not typically enhance the drug's ocular effects because most drugs penetrate the cornea well and in sufficient quantity to supersaturate the intraocular receptors. However, the increased systemic absorption usually increases the likelihood of undesired systemic side effects.

Manual punctal occlusion minimizes the drug's access to the nasal mucosa. To perform this maneuver, the patient simply holds a finger over the common canaliculi (angle of the nose) (Fig. 21-13).

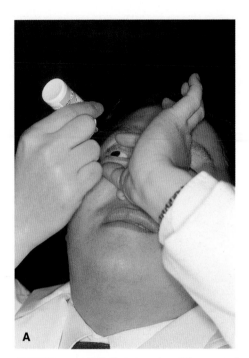 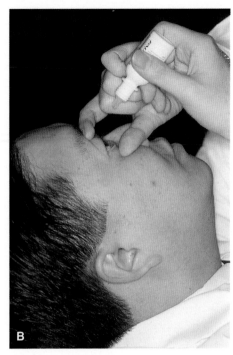

FIGURE 21-11. Self-administration of drops: two-handed method. The two-handed method for self-administration of the topical drop. **A.** Frontal view. **B.** Lateral view.

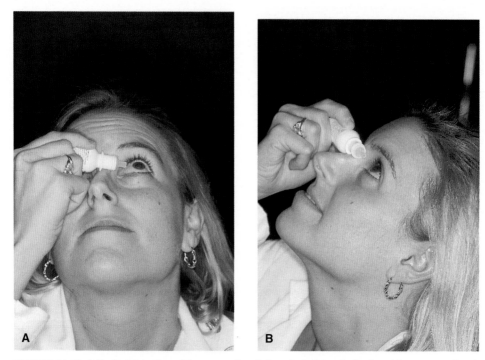

FIGURE 21-12. Self-administration of drops: one-handed method. Using the bridge of the nose to aid with steadiness of the hand for self-administration of the topical drop. **A.** Frontal view. **B.** Lateral view.

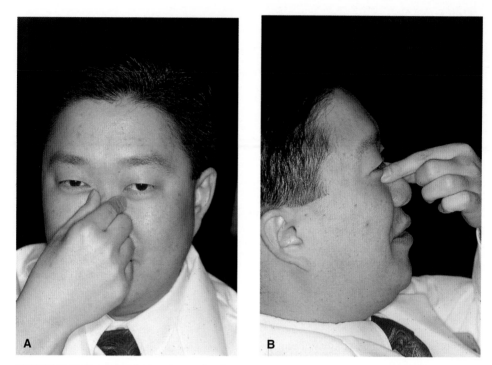

FIGURE 21-13. Punctal occlusion. A punctal occlusion to minimize systemic absorption of topically administered medications through the nasolacrimal system. **A.** Frontal view. **B.** Lateral view.

Laser Trabeculoplasty

L. Jay Katz and Daniel Lee ■

INDICATIONS

- For uncontrolled open-angle glaucoma, either primary or secondary, laser trabeculoplasty has proven to be helpful in lowering the intraocular pressure. Primary open-angle glaucoma, normal-tension glaucoma, pigmentary glaucoma, and pseudoexfoliative glaucoma are the most amenable for getting a good response.

- In juvenile glaucoma and secondary glaucomas, such as traumatic, neovascular, and inflammatory glaucomas, results with laser trabeculoplasty are typically poor.

- A clear media and a good view of the trabecular meshwork are required. Eyes with hazy corneas or extensive peripheral anterior synechiae may prevent proper treatment application with the laser.

- Mastery of gonioscopy and accurate identification of the angle structures are essential for a proper laser trabeculoplasty.

BIBLIOGRAPHY

Van Buskirk EM. Pathophysiology of laser trabeculoplasty. *Surv Ophthalmol.* 1989;33:264–272.

ARGON LASER TRABECULOPLASTY

Technique

- A Goldmann, Latina, or Ritch gonioscopic lens is placed on the anesthetized cornea with a viscous coupling solution. Lens placement is facilitated by asking the patient to look upward and gently inserting the inferior rim of the lens in the lower fornix. Once the lens is in contact with the globe, the patient is asked to look forward (Fig. 22-1). If there is poor visibility of the trabecular meshwork, asking the patient to move his/her gaze toward the mirror may further improve visualization.

- Since the introduction of argon laser trabeculoplasty (ALT) in 1979 by Witter and Wise, there has been remarkably little alteration of the technique. A 50-μm spot size is applied to the trabecular meshwork with up to 1,000 mW of energy, enough to cause minimal blanching of the pigment. The least amount of energy is employed to attain the tissue end point (Fig. 22-2).

- The laser spot is aimed at the junction of the pigmented and nonpigmented trabecular meshwork. Either a single treatment session of the entire 360 degrees with up to 100 applications or two sessions of 180 degrees each with 50 shots may be performed.

● A topical alpha-agonist (apraclonidine or brimonidine) is given pre- and postlaser treatment to minimize the possibility of a transient intraocular pressure spike (Fig. 22-3). A topical corticosteroid is prescribed four times daily for a week to prevent postlaser inflammation.

● After the treatment, the patient is examined 1 hour later to measure the eye pressure. If a pressure spike occurs, it is treated with glaucoma medications such as oral carbonic anhydrase inhibitors or oral hyperosmotic agents. The patient is reexamined at 1 week and again 1 month after the treatment. At the last visit, a determination is made as to whether the laser therapy was beneficial.

Mechanism of Action

● Theories have been offered, but none verified, as to how laser therapy lowers the eye pressure. The extent of pigmentation of the trabecular meshwork seems to be critical for the success of laser trabeculoplasty. Heavier pigmentation is generally a positive predictor of success. The thermal burn with the argon laser has been shown histologically to result in crater formation with associated disruption of trabecular beams and fibrinous exudates and lysis of trabecular endothelial cells.

● The mechanical theory of argon trabeculoplasty states that laser burns to the trabecular meshwork causes tissue contraction and tightening of the trabecular ring, resulting in a mechanical stretch over the intervening tissue and the widening Schlemm canal.

● The cellular theory suggested that the laser stimulated the trabecular endothelial cells to duplicate, migrate, and repopulate the trabecular meshwork (Fig. 22-4). These cells are thought to be instrumental in maintaining the intratrabecular spaces free of excess extracellular matrix components and debris that have been implicated in the increased resistance to outflow seen in glaucomatous eyes.

Efficacy

● Intraocular pressure is typically reduced 20% to 30% below baseline levels with ALT. Not all eyes are responsive to laser trabeculoplasty. Positive predictors of a favorable response include heavy pigmentation of the trabecular meshwork, age (older patients), and diagnosis (pigmentary glaucoma, primary open-angle glaucoma, and exfoliation syndrome).

● There is an apparent waning of the effect of ALT over time. In long-term studies of 5 to 10 years, ALT failure ranged from 65% to 90%. Retreatment after a previous 360-degree application of ALT is at best a short-term benefit, with failure at 1 year up to 80%. Because there is structural alteration of the outflow system with ALT, repeat treatment may lead to a paradoxical persistent elevation of intraocular pressure. Repeat argon laser application to the angle structures in animals was used by Gaasterland to create an experimental open-angle glaucoma model. If a prompt reduction in intraocular pressure is needed, or a relatively large reduction in pressure is desired (e.g., more than a 30% lowering below baseline pretreatment intraocular pressure), then ALT may not be a good choice. Medication or filtering surgery is more likely to achieve those objectives.

● The current treatment paradigm for glaucoma in the United States is medication first, then ALT, and, finally, filtering surgery. This regimen is only a guideline, and treatment needs to be individualized for each patient to provide optimum care.

■ Studies have reexamined the sequencing of treatments for open-angle glaucoma. In the Glaucoma Laser Trial, ALT was compared with medication as the first step in the treatment of newly diagnosed primary open-angle glaucoma. After 2 years, 44% of eyes with ALT alone were controlled, as opposed to only 20% with timolol alone being adequately treated. In a subsequent paper, with a mean follow-up of 7 years, ALT alone was adequate control for 20% of eyes, and timolol alone for 15%. Although there were methodologic flaws in the design for this study, there was intriguing support to at least consider ALT as initial therapy for certain patients.

BIBLIOGRAPHY

Damji KF, Shah KC, Rock WJ, et al. Selective laser trabeculoplasty argon laser trabeculoplasty: a prospective randomised clinical trial. *Br J Ophthalmol.* 1999;83:718–722.

Feldman RM, Katz LJ, Spaeth GL, et al. Long-term efficacy of repeat argon laser trabeculoplasty. *Ophthalmology.* 1991;98:1061–1065.

Glaucoma Trial Research Group. The Glaucoma Laser Trial 2. Results of argon laser trabeculoplasty versus topical medicines. *Ophthalmology.* 1990;97:1403–1413.

Glaucoma Trial Research Group. The Glaucoma Laser Trial (GLT) and glaucoma laser trial follow-up study: 7. Results. *Am J Ophthalmol.* 1995;120:718–731.

Katz LJ. Argon laser trabeculoplasty. *Annu Ophthalmic Laser Surg.* 1992;1:103–110.

Kramer TR, Noecker RJ. Comparison of the morphologic changes after selective laser trabeculoplasty and argon laser trabeculoplasty in human eye bank eyes. *Ophthalmology.* 2001;108:773–779.

Wise JB. Long-term control of adult open angle glaucoma by argon laser treatment. *Ophthalmology.* 1981;88:197–202.

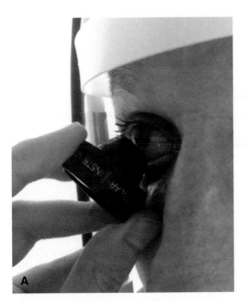
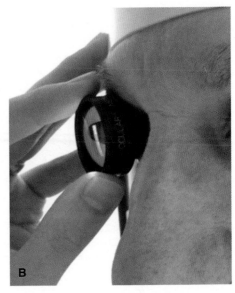

FIGURE 22-1. Lens placement. A. Placement of the lens is facilitated by asking the patient to look upward and gently placing the lens in the inferior fornix. **B.** Once the lens is in contact with the eye, the patient is asked to look in the primary position.

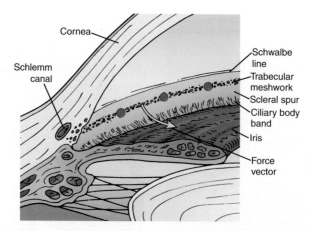

FIGURE 22-2. Tissue response to laser treatment. The "ideal" tissue response is minimal bubble formation and mild blanching of the trabecular meshwork. The laser is aimed at the junction of the pigmented and nonpigmented trabecular meshwork. (Reprinted with permission from Katz LJ. Argon laser trabeculoplasty. *Annual Ophthalmic Laser Surg.* 1992;1:103–110.)

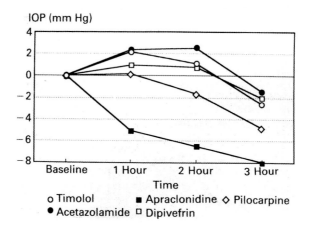

FIGURE 22-3. Effects of postlaser medication administration. Blunting of the postlaser intraocular pressure spike after argon laser trabeculoplasty with apraclonidine is compared with other glaucoma medications.

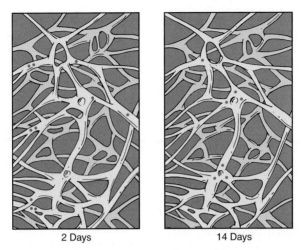

2 Days   14 Days

FIGURE 22-4. **Argon laser trabeculoplasty (ALT): One proposed mechanism of action.** The cellular theory states that ALT stimulates the replication of trabecular endothelial cells that promote aqueous outflow. (Reprinted with permission from Van Buskirk EM. Pathophysiology of laser trabeculoplasty. *Surv Ophthalmol.* 1989;33:264–272.)

SELECTIVE LASER TRABECULOPLASTY

Technique

- The use of a pulsed-frequency doubled neodymium (Nd):YAG laser for trabeculoplasty was introduced in 1998 by Latina. In contrast to the continuous-wave argon laser, laser energy is selectively absorbed by pigmented tissue, reducing collateral thermal effects. The fixed spot size of 400 μm dwarfs the typical 50-μm spot size used with ALT (Fig. 22-5). Therefore, the spacing between laser spots with the selective laser trabeculoplasty (SLT) is much more compact and almost confluent (Fig. 22-6). The spot size with SLT is so large that the entirety of the angle is covered with the aiming beam. The variables in applying the laser are the number of shots (50 to 60), the extent of the angle treated (180 to 360 degrees), and the power (up to 0.8 J).

- The power end point is determined by the tissue reaction with the initial laser application. Blanching of the pigmented trabecular meshwork with slight bubble vaporization is ideal. If there is a great deal of bubble formation, then the power is adjusted downward. The use of low power is strongly recommended in heavily pigmented angles as seen in pigmentary glaucoma.

Mechanism of Action

- Scanning electron microscopy highlights the difference between argon laser application, with the "melting" of trabecular beams, and the selective laser, with little, if any, observable structural alteration (Fig. 22-7). Therefore, the mechanical stretching theory is not applicable for the selective laser effect on the intraocular pressure. In vitro cultures of trabecular meshwork cells were irradiated by Latina with either argon or selective laser. Argon laser application damaged both pigmented and nonpigmented cells.

In contrast, the selective laser targeted only the pigmented cells. Recruitment of macrophages into the outflow system has been demonstrated in animal models and in human eyes. These macrophages may release chemical mediators that regulate the outflow rate. Elevated interleukin levels detected following laser application have been postulated to improve aqueous outflow.

- Recently, Alvarado described a junction disassembly in Schlemm canal cells when they were exposed to laser-irradiated Schlemm canal cells and trabecular meshwork cells. This same junction disassembly was demonstrable with prostaglandin analogue treatment as well. In both cases, endothelial cell junction disassembly was associated with a congruous increase in the conductivity. Alvarado concluded that the intraocular pressure–lowering effects of SLT and prostaglandin analogues share a common mechanism of action affecting the barrier properties of Schlemm canal cells.

Efficacy

- Comparative trials have confirmed that ALT and SLT have equivalent efficacy in lowering the intraocular pressure in eyes that have failed medical therapy. Studies suggest that initial therapy with SLT before any glaucoma medication use lowers the intraocular pressure by 24% to 35% below baseline levels. Positive predictors of success include higher baseline intraocular pressure and the 2-week postlaser pressure response. Like ALT, SLT's efficacy wanes over time, on average failing somewhere between 6 months and 3 years.

- Because there is minimal structural damage with SLT, repeat SLT is generally thought to be safe. Early studies show that retreatment yields significant ($\geq$20%) intraocular pressure reduction. Also, in eyes that have received previous ALT, SLT has been shown to be successful in lowering intraocular pressure.

SLT has also been shown to be effective in PXF glaucoma, pigmentary glaucoma, juvenile open-angle glaucoma, and secondary pseudophakic glaucoma.

BIBLIOGRAPHY

Alvarado JA, Iguchi R, Juster R, et al. From the bedside to the bench and back again: predicting and improving the outcomes of SLT glaucoma therapy. *Trans Am Ophthalmol Soc.* 2009;107:167–181.

Alvarado JA, Iguchi R, Martinez J, et al. Similar effects of selective laser trabeculoplasty and prostaglandin analogs on the permeability of cultured Schlemm canal cells. *Am J Ophthalmol.* 2010;150(2):254–264.

Damji KF, Shah KC, Rock WJ, et al. Selective laser trabeculoplasty argon laser trabeculoplasty: A prospective randomised clinical trial. *Br J Ophthalmol.* 1999;83:718–722.

Hodge WG, Damji KF, Rock W, et al. Baseline IOP predicts selective laser trabeculoplasty success at 1 year post-treatment: Results from a randomized clinical trial. *Br J Ophthalmol.* 2005;89:1157–1160.

Hong BK, Winer JC, Martone JF, et al. Repeat selective laser trabeculoplasty. *J Glaucoma.* 2009;18(3):180–183.

Jindra LF. SLT as primary treatment. *Ophthalmol Manag.* 2004;8(11):77–78.

Johnson PB, Katz LJ, Rhee DJ. Selective laser trabeculoplasty: predictive value of early intraocular pressure measurements for success at 3 months. *Br J Ophthalmol.* 2006;90:741–743.

Kramer TR, Noecker RJ. Comparison of the morphologic changes after selective laser trabeculoplasty and argon laser trabeculoplasty in human eye bank eyes. *Ophthalmology.* 2001;108:773–779.

Lai JSM, Chua JKK, Tham CCY, et al. Five-year follow up of selective laser trabeculoplasty in Chinese eyes. *Clin Exp Ophthalmol.* 2004;32(4):369–372.

Latina MA, Sibayan SA, Shin DH, et al. Q-Switched 532-nm Nd:YAG laser trabeculoplasty (selective laser trabeculoplasty). *Ophthalmology.* 1998;105:2082–2090.

Lee R, Hutnik CM. Projected cost comparison of selective laser trabeculoplasty versus glaucoma medication in the Ontario Health Insurance Plan. *Can J Ophthalmol.* 2006;1(4):449–456.

Nagar M, Shah N, Kapoor B. Selective laser trabeculoplasty in pseudophakic glaucoma. *Ophthalmic Surg Lasers Imaging.* 2010;9:1–2.

Spaeth GL, Baez KA. Argon laser trabeculoplasty controls one third of cases of progressive, uncontrolled, open angle glaucoma for 5 years. *Arch Ophthalmol.* 1992;110:491–494.

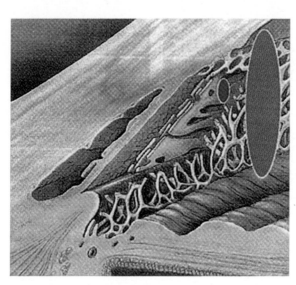

FIGURE 22-5. Comparison of argon and selective laser spots. Comparative size of the argon laser spot (50 μm) versus the Nd:YAG selective laser spot (400 μm). (Courtesy of Michael S. Berlin, MD, Associate Clinical Professor, University of California–Los Angeles; Jules Stein.)

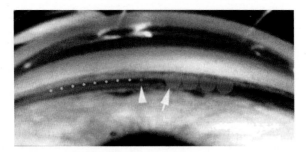

FIGURE 22-6. Comparison of spacing of laser spots. Spacing of the argon laser versus the close application of the selective laser. The triangle indicates an approximate 50-μm spot size with argon laser trabeculoplasty versus the 400-μm spot size of selective laser trabeculoplasty (*right arrow*). (Courtesy of Michael S. Berlin, MD, Associate Clinical Professor, University of California–Los Angeles, Jules Stein.)

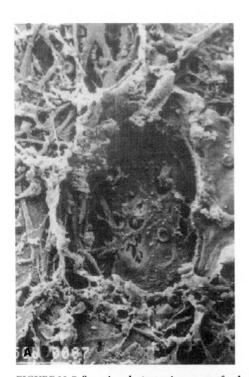
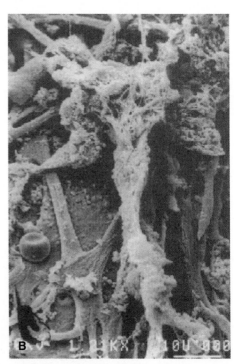

FIGURE 22-7. Scanning electron microscopy of cadaver eyes treated with argon or selective laser. A. Argon burn resulted in coagulative melting of the trabecular beam. A high magnification view showing the curling of the collagen caused by the thermal damage. **B.** The selective laser did not cause any significant structural alteration. By contrast, fracturing of a single collagen beam is visible without significant collateral thermal damage. (Reprinted with permission from Kramer TR, Noecker RJ. Comparison of the morphologic changes after selective laser trabeculoplasty and argon laser trabeculoplasty in human eye bank eyes. *Ophthalmology.* 2001;108:773–779.)

SELECTIVE LASER TRABECULOPLASTY AS INITIAL TREATMENT

- Many practitioners today still adhere to the treatment paradigm of medications as first-line therapy, followed by laser trabeculoplasty, and then possibly surgery. Yet, comparisons in the literature between medications and laser trabeculoplasty demonstrate equivalent efficacy in reducing intraocular pressure.

- Furthermore, several economic studies have indicated that laser trabeculoplasty is significantly more cost-effective than treatment with medication.

- The choice of initial treatment should be tailored to each individual patient. In light of medication cost, side effects, and poor adherence, SLT should be considered earlier, if not first, in the treatment strategy for open-angle glaucoma.

BIBLIOGRAPHY

Cantor LB, Katz LJ, Cheng JW, et al. Economic evaluation of medication, laser trabeculoplasty and filtering surgeries in treating patients with glaucoma in the US. *Curr Med Res Opin.* 2008;24(10):2905–2918.

Katz LJ, Steinmann WC, Kabir A, Molineaux J, Wizov SS, Marcellino G. Selective laser trabeculoplasty versus medical therapy as initial treatment of glaucoma: a prospective, randomized trial. *J Glaucoma.* 2012;21(7):460–468.

Taylor HR. Glaucoma: where to now? *Ophthalmology.* 2009;116(5):821–822.

Deep Sclerectomy Surgery for Glaucoma

Konrad S. Palacios, José I. B. Sanchis, and Konrad W. S. Wenyon ■

INTRODUCTION

Nonpenetrating glaucoma surgery, such as deep sclerectomy, has become more popular among surgeons in Europe,[1] primarily because of its safety. Deep sclerectomy was described by Epstein and Krasnov in the late 1950s and subsequently revised by Fyodorov and others. Deep sclerectomy involves creating two partial-thickness scleral flaps with the second, deeper flat at 90% depth. During the procedure, the inner flap is removed, creating an intrascleral lake. The procedure is termed "nonpenetrating" because the inner wall of Schlemm canal, trabecular meshwork, and Descemet membrane remains intact. Filtration across the outer flap is allowed to create a conjunctival bleb. A dual mechanism of action is proposed with both enhanced uveoscleral outflow through the area of uvea exposed during the inner dissection and the formation of the conjunctival bleb. Other names for deep sclerectomy include nonpenetrating trabeculectomy and external trabeculectomy.

STUDIES

- In 1984, Zimmerman reported a retrospective study showing comparable results between the trabeculectomy (without antimetabolites) and nonpenetrating trabeculectomy in terms of intraocular pressure (IOP) control, but with lower postoperative complications such as shallow anterior chamber, uveitis, hyphema, and loss of vitreous; in their study, trabeculectomy ($n = 86$) controlled the IOP of 70% of patients (with or without medications), whereas nonpenetrating trabeculectomy ($n = 71$) similarly controlled the IOP in 84% of patients with a mean follow-up of 1.7 years.[2]

- In a prospective study in which patients ($n = 39$) were randomized to receive deep sclerectomy in one eye and trabeculectomy in the other, El Sayyad et al. reported success rates (i.e., IOP < 21 mm Hg) of 92.3% and 94.9% at 1 year ($p = 0.9$) for deep sclerectomy and trabeculectomy, respectively; serious complications were more prevalent with trabeculectomy.[3] In El Sayyad's study, both groups were treated with postoperative 5-fluorouracil (5-FU) subconjunctival injections at the discretion of the investigators.

- The results of deep sclerectomy are improved when combined with an implant. The implant is designed to maintain the suprachoroidal space (i.e., intrascleral bleb) avoiding the closure of the sclerectomy. The implants can be absorbable or nonabsorbable.

  ▪ In a case series of 105 eyes with an average follow-up of 64 months, Shaarawy et al., using absorbable implants of collagen, reported a success rate of 91% (IOP < 21 mm Hg with or without medications) at 96 months; half of the eyes underwent laser goniopuncture with a mean time to goniopuncture at 21 months, and 23% received postoperative 5-FU injections.[4] They reported no incidence of flat anterior chamber or endophthalmitis.[4]

  ▪ Using the nonabsorbable T-Flux implant (IOL TECH Laboratories, France), Jungkim et al.[5] reported a case series of 35 eyes with 12-month follow-up demonstrating a lowering of IOP from 33 mm Hg to a approximately 15 mm Hg with an average of 0.1 antiglaucoma medications. Ates et al.[6] reported similar results in a small case series of 25 eyes.

  ▪ The advantages of other methods using cheaper materials, like viscoelastic, show some long-term validity.[7] It has been over 50 years since trabeculectomy was popularized; we are familiar with its advantages, disadvantages, and success rate but trabeculectomy comes with a price, and this is its complications. Most of the complications are related to excessive filtration, especially in the early postoperative period, such as flat anterior chamber, hypotony, choroidal detachment, and cataract formation. With trabeculectomy, complications occur in 10% to 18% of patients. The

well-guarded dissection in deep sclerectomy reduces the complications related to overfiltrations.[8]

- An important point exists when analyzing the results of nonpenetrating surgery. Deep sclerectomy is highly dependent on the technical skills of the surgeon, which can show large differences when results from different authors are compared. Deep sclerectomy has a long learning curve during which the surgical time is longer and the initial outcomes might not be very satisfactory.

  ▪ Dahan and Drusedau reported the results including patients from the learning curve, during which time perforations into the anterior chamber were 1 in 3, necessitating converting to a standard trabeculectomy. They also mention that as the manual technique improves, the perforation rate drops to 1 in 20.[9]

  ▪ In our personal experience, the first 20 cases were converted to penetrating trabeculectomies for different reasons. Deep sclerectomy is not a simple surgery; on the contrary, time is needed to learn it properly, but once it is mastered, it is elegant, secure, and comfortable for the patients in most of the cases.

  ▪ One of the surgeons with more expirience in Europe is André Mermoud and his group. They presented the results of 52 patients with Deep sclerectomy follow up for 10 years with a initial IOP around 26 mm Hg; 89% of them had an IOP < 21 with or without medication, 61% of them need goniopuncture during the follow-up.[10]

REFERENCES

1. Baudouin C, Rouland JF, Le Pen C. Change in medical and surgical treatments of glaucoma between 1997 and 2000 in France. *Eur J Ophthalmol*. 2003;13(suppl 4): S53–S60.

2. Zimmerman TJ, Kooner KS, Ford VJ, et al. Trabeculectomy vs nonpenetrating trabeculectomy: a retrospective study

of two procedures in phakic patients with glaucoma. *Ophthalmic Surg.* 1984;15:734–740.

3. El Sayyad F, Helal M, El-Kholify H, et al. Nonpenetrating deep sclerectomy versus trabeculectomy in bilateral primary open angle glaucoma. *Ophthalmology.* 2000;107:1671–1674.

4. Shaarawy T, Mansouri K, Schnyder C, et al. Long-term results of deep sclerectomy with collagen implant. *J Cataract Refract Surg.* 2004;30:1225–1231.

5. Jungkim S, Gibran SK, Khan K, et al. External trabeculectomy with T-Flux implant. *Eur J Ophthalmol.* 2006;16:416–421.

6. Ates H, Uretmen O, Andaç K, et al. Deep sclerectomy with nonabsorbable implant (T-Flux): preliminary results. *Can J Ophthalmol.* 2003;38:482–488.

7. Ravinet E, Bovey E, Mermoud A. T-flux implant versus Healon GV in deep sclerectomy. *J Glaucoma.* 2004;13:46–50.

8. Drolsum L. Conversion from trabeculectomy to deep sclerectomy. Prospective Study of the first 44 cases. *J Cataract Refract Surg.* 2003;29:1378–1384.

9. Dahan E, Drusedau M. Non penetrating filtration surgery for glaucoma: control by surgery only. *J Cataract Refract Surg.* 2000;26:696–701.

10. Bissig A, Rivier D, Zaninetti M, Shaarawy T, Mermoud A, Roy S. Ten years follow-up after deep sclerectomy with collagen implant. *J Glaucoma.* 2008; 17: 680–686.

SURGICAL TECHNIQUE

● The surgery can be done with any type of local anesthesia; the authors prefer sub-Tenon and peribulbar anesthesia. If the procedure is to be combined with phacoemulsification, it will also benefit from intracameral anesthesia.

   ■ For sub-Tenon anesthesia, we use a mixture of Lidocaine 5% plus Bupivacaine 0.75%, 1.5 mL of each for a total volume of 3 mL. We use around 1.5 mL of this and keep the rest in case we need complementary anesthesia.

   ■ We also use drops of topical anesthesia and begin with a buttonhole in the conjunctiva/Tenon (**Fig. 23-1A**) in the inferotemporal quadrant introducing an 18-gauge Angiocath (**Fig. 23-1B**); usually after the infusion of the anesthetic, we have

a chemosis (**Fig. 23-1C**) that helps with the initial conjunctival dissection.

● Nonpenetrating surgery should be performed in the superior quadrant of the globe; the reason is that filtration surgery has been associated with infections when it is done at the inferior quadrant.

   ■ To have a better exposure of the superior surgical field a traction suture can be used to rotate the globe inferiorly. A 5-0 black silk for the superior rectus or a corneal traction suture of 7-0 or 8-0 (**Fig. 23-2A**) black silk or vicryl can be used. The authors prefer the corneal traction suture (**Fig. 23-2B**).

● The conjunctival flap can be initiated at the limbus (**Fig. 23-3A**) or the fornix (**Fig. 23-3B** and **C**); authors prefer a limbus base with an L-shaped incision that is a modification of the Dahan incision (inverse L) (**Fig. 23-3D**). This is made using a Westcott scissors and a nontoothed utility forceps. It is important to extend the dissection in the subconjunctival space at either the nasal or the temporal side to the main incision. The sclera can be cleaned of any adhesions with the use of a scarifier.

   ■ Bleeding vessels should be lightly cauterized (**Fig. 23-4A**), or another option is to use the scarifier (**Fig. 23-4B**); the technique is the same as that of trabeculectomy.

● The superficial scleral flap measures 5 × 5 mm, and the measurements can be done with a caliper (**Fig. 23-5A** and **B**) or with a marker. For example, the Huco Vision has two different makers. One is the (Dahan) double-ended T-Flux trapezoidal marker that measures 5 × 5 × 2 mm at one end and a smaller 3.3 × 3 × 1 mm at the other end (**Fig. 23-5C** and **D**). Another is the (Mermoud) nonpenetrating glaucoma surgery double-ended marker that is 4 × 5 mm at one end and 4 × 4 mm at the other end. Authors prefer the trapezoidal maker, but there are no differences if the flap is square (Fig. 23-5E and F) or trapezoidal (Fig. 23-5G and H).

■ It is important to dissect the flap far anteriorly into the cornea, enough to ensure that we will be able to create a wide trabeculodescemetic window. The flap thickness should be between one-half and one-third of the sclera.

● The second or deep scleral flap (Fig. 23-6A) is the critical part, and it should have a total depth of 90% to 99% of scleral thickness; one tip is to start the dissection far back away from the limbus and progressively deepen in order to get the desired depth (Fig. 23-6B). As we get closer to the clear cornea, more care has to be taken. The reason is that the trabeculodescemetic membrane is very thin and can break easily just by a little excess of pressure; the dissection can be made more safely with a spatula (Fig. 23-6C). A diamond knife is too sharp and makes it very easy to perforate the trabeculodescemetic membrane. There is a diamond knife designed for dissecting this membrane, which is the Dahan Diamond Schlemm canal opener knife. Personally, authors prefer a 45-degree-angled steel knife.

● During the dissection when we start observing the change in color between the sclera and the clear cornea, it is better to do small cuts at the sides of the flap (Fig. 23-7A). We need to get far anterior into the clear cornea before we amputate the deep scleral flap (Fig. 23-7B). If the surgeon is working alone, a tip is to use an additional stitch to fix the superior scleral flap and to get a better view of the surgical field (Fig. 23-7C).

● The trabeculodescemetic membrane (Fig. 23-8A and B) is the key point of the surgery, and therefore, special care must be taken to prepare for it. The first and most important step is to get the right depth.

The second step is to peel the Schlemm canal (Fig. 23-8C), and sometimes when we have done a very deep dissection, it will be already removed. After this, we can dilate the temporal and nasal sides of Schlemm canal, and this maneuver can be done with a spatula (Fig. 23-8D). Authors prefer the Mermoud predescemetic spatula (Huco Vision SA) or a scraper; the one shown in the figure is the Dahan trabecular meshwork scraper (Fig. 23-8E). When the canal is properly dilated, the aqueous humor will flow abundantly.

● The position where the implants are left is the space left after removing the second scleral flap. The implants are then cover by the superior scleral flap. There are two types, the absorbable implants such as the aquaflow collagen glaucoma drainage device (Staar Surgical, Monrovia, CA) (Fig. 23-9A), which has a complete resorption within 6 to 9 months, and the SKGEL (Corneal, Paris, France) (Fig. 23-9B) made of reticulated sodium hyaluronate. The nonabsorbable implants, like T-Flux (Carl Zeiss Meditec Company, La Rochelle, France) (Fig. 23-9C), have a T shape, and the superior haptics are inserted into the Schlemm canal after they have been dilated. The body will rest in the scleral bed and can be fixated with a 10-0 nylon suture.

● One of our favorite implants is the Esnoper V-2000 (AJL Ophthalmic S.A., Álava, Spain) (Fig. 23-10A). This implant has a trapezoidal shape with longitudinal striations (Fig. 23-10B) that enhance the flow of the aqueous humor into the suprachoroidal space. There is a new modification of the Esnoper, called Esnoper Clip (Fig. 23-10C), which has two portions one goes into the suprachoroidal space and the other into the scleral lake. When both portions are in place, there is a U shape leaving the trabeculodescemetic window clear for a future goniopuncture; the results at 1 year shown by

Loscos are a reduction from 26 mm Hg down to 15 mm Hg, with an important decrease in drops.[1] Both Esnopers can be fixated with suture or by introducing the posterior part into the suprachoroidal pocket, as described by Muñoz.[2] He reported a further decrease in IOP of 2 mm Hg at more than 1 year after the year of surgery. All of these implants are colorless, but they can be tinted with fluorescein, as has been described by us.[3]

● This technique involves making an incision in the scleral bed about 2 or 3 mm posterior to the trabeculodescemetic membrane with very small cuts to expose the suprachoroidal space (**Fig. 23-11A** and **B**); this space is dilated with a spatula (**Fig. 23-11C**), and we place part of the implant inside that pocket (**Fig. 23-11D**). A tip for the use of these implants, colorless as they are (**Fig. 23-11E**), is to tint them with fluorescein (personal technique) (**Fig. 23-11F**); this is especially helpful during the learning process. If everything is successful—good dissection with the correct thickness and depth, implant in place, and appropriate aqueous humor filtration (**Fig. 23-11G**)—we should be able to observe a formed anterior chamber if no ruptures of the membrane have occurred. We can now close the superficial flap without the suture using Muñoz technique[1] (**Fig. 23-11H**)

or using a 10-0 nylon suture (**Fig. 23-11I**). The conjunctiva can be closed with a running suture of 8-0 Vicryl (Ethicon) (**Fig. 23-11J**), particularly if it is a limbus-based conjunctival flap, or with a 10-0 nylon if it is fornix based.

● We also like to use antimetabolites like Mitomycin C 0.05 mg per mL for 1.0 to 1.5 minutes or 5-FU at 50 mg per mL for 3 minutes. We apply it by cutting two small pieces of sponge that are introduced in the dissected conjunctival pockets (**Fig. 23-12A**) and under the superficial scleral flap (**Fig. 23-12B**); after the elapsed time, the area should be irrigated with sufficient saline solution or with balanced salt solution (**Fig. 23-12C**).

REFERENCES

1. Loscos-Arenas J, Parera-Arranz A, Romera-Romera P, Castellvi-Manent J, Sabala-Llopart A, de la Cámara-Hermoso J. Deep sclerectomy with a new nonabsorbable uveoscleral implant (Esnoper Clip): 1 year outcomes. *J Glaucoma.* 2015;24:421–425.

2. Muñoz G. Nonstitch suprachoroidal technique for T-flux implantation in deep sclerectomy. *J Glaucoma.* 2009;18(3):262–264.

3. Schargel K, Placeres-Daban J, Garcia-Conca V, Belda JI, Aguirre Balsalobre F. Improving the visualization of non-absorbable T-Flux⁻ implants in deep sclerectomy. Colouring technique. *Arch Soc Esp Oftalmol.* 2014;89(6):226–228.

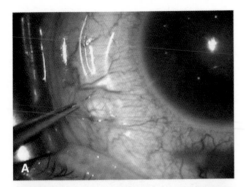

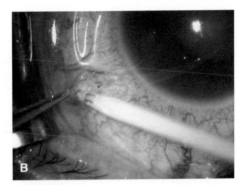

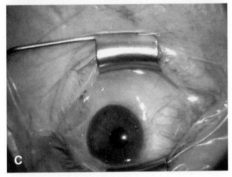

FIGURE 23-1. **Sub-Tenon anesthesia. A.** Incision in the conjunctiva for sub-Tenon anesthesia, better in the inferior temporal or nasal. **B.** Teflon cannula, 18 gauge. A mixture (1 to 1.5 mL) of Lidocaine 5% + Bupivacaine 0.50%. **C.** Chemosis after applying the sub-Tenon anesthesia; it is useful for dissection.

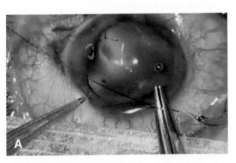

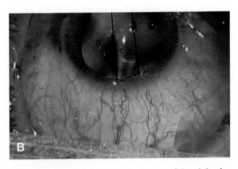

FIGURE 23-2. **Traction suture. A.** Silk suture 7-0 placed in clear cornea at 12 hours. **B.** Rotation of the globe for better presentation of the field.

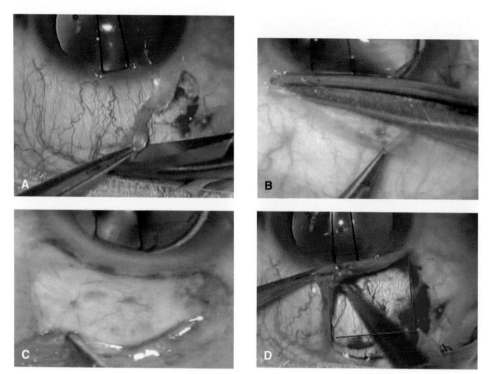

FIGURE 23-3. Initial incisions. A. Limbus-based incision. **B.** Fornix-based incision, first step. **C.** Fornix-based incision, second step. **D.** L-shaped inverses. Dahan describes the L incision, fornix based.

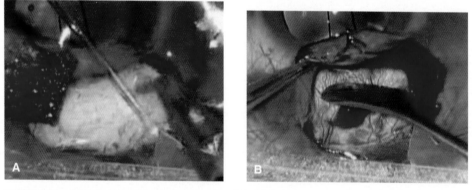

FIGURE 23-4. Scleral preparation. A. Cauterization of the field, diathermy very light. **B.** Scarificator, an instrument used to break the unions at the sclera and the conjunctiva.

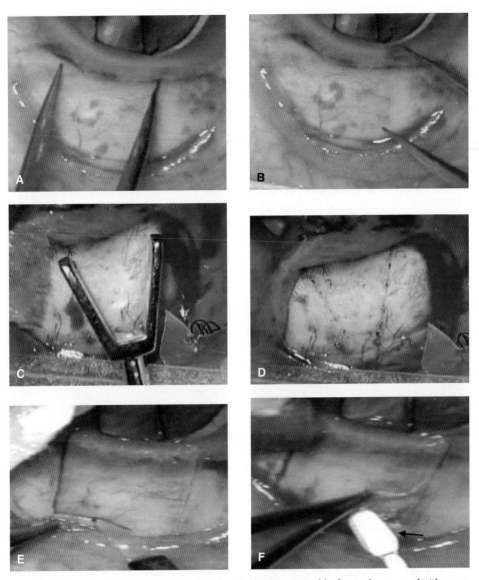

FIGURE 23-5. Creation of the superficial scleral flap. A. The dimension of the flap can be measured with a compass, horizontal. **B.** The dimension of the flap can be measured with a compass, vertical. **C.** Fix trapezoidal marker. **D.** Area marked. **E.** Superficial flap, rectangle in shape, first step. **F.** Superficial flap, rectangle in shape.

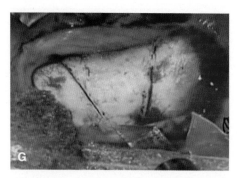

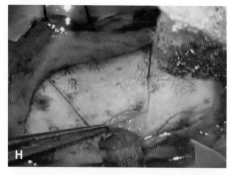

FIGURE 23-5. (*continued*) **G.** Superficial flap, trapezoid in shape, first step. **H.** Superficial flap, trapezoid in shape, 5 × 5 × 2 mm.

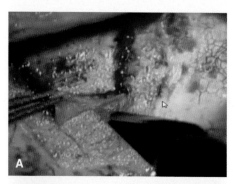

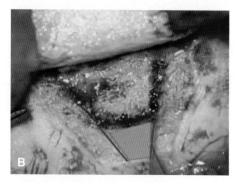

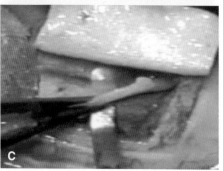

FIGURE 23-6. **Creation of the deep scleral flap. A.** Deep flap 3.3 × 3 × 1 mm. **B.** It is better to start far back until we get the right plane. **C.** When we get close to the trabeculodescemetic membrane, the dissection can be done with a blunt spatula.

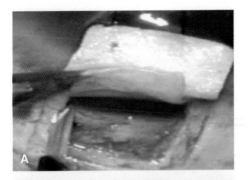

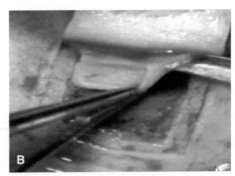

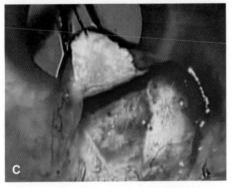

FIGURE 23-7. **Cutting the deep scleral flap. A.** Checking the window, which is the trabeculodescemetic membrane. **B.** Cutting the deep scleral flap. **C.** Fixing the superficial flap with a suture nylon 10-0 or silk 8-0 helps to finish the trabeculodescemetic membrane.

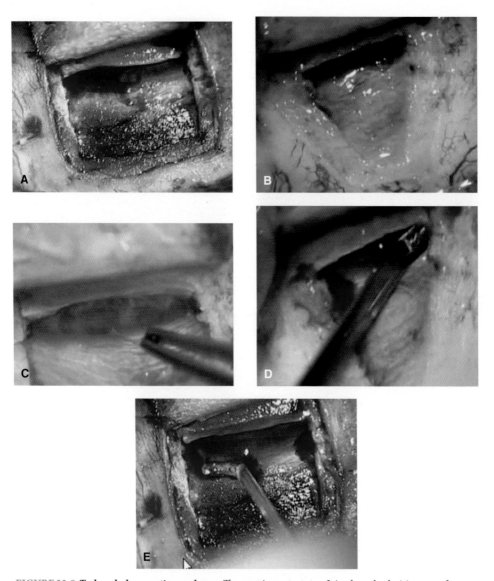

FIGURE 23-8. Trabeculodescemetic membrane. The most important step. It is where the decision to perforate or not perforate is made. **A.** Square flap. **B.** Trapezoidal flap. **C.** Peeling Schlemm canal to enhance filtration. **D.** Dilating Schlemm canal also enhances filtration. **E.** Using the scraping over the trabeculodescemetic membrane will enhance filtration and facilitate peeling of the Schlemm canal.

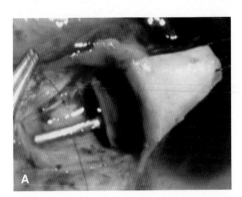

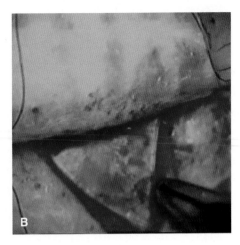

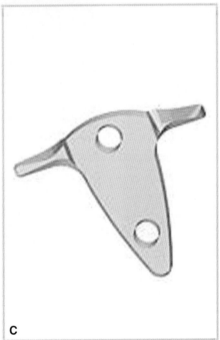

FIGURE 23-9. **Implants. A.** Aquaflow collagen absorbable implant (Staar Surgical Monrovia, CA). **B.** SKGEL (Corneal, Paris, France) made of reticulated sodium hyaluronate. **C.** T-Flux (Carl Zeiss Meditec Company, La Rochelle, France).

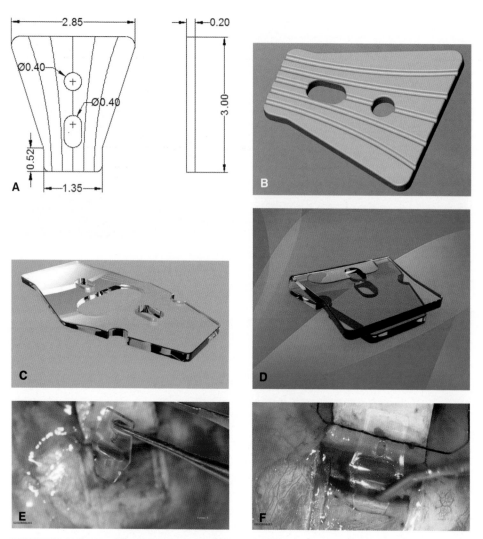

FIGURE 23-10. Esnoper Clip. A. Esnoper V-2000 (AJL Ophthalmic S.A., Álava, Spain) schematic design. **B.** Esnoper V-2000, trapezoid in shape with longitudinal striations. **C.** Esnoper Clip design in an open position, the notch on the internal part works to fix it into the scleral incision. **D.** Esnoper Clip design in a close position, in between both layers is the sclera when the implant is in the correct position. **E.** Esnoper Clip out of the package and into the surgical field must be handled with nontooth forceps. **F.** Esnoper Clip being introduced in the suprachoroidal space.

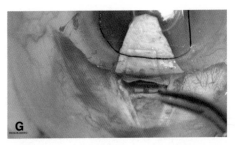
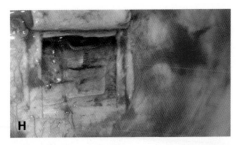

FIGURE 23-10. (*continued*) **G.** Esnoper Clip inserted until the notch, which allows a proper fixation without movement of the implant. **H.** Esnoper Clip put in place; once close to the trabeculodescemetic membrane, the clear U shape area is central for the future need of goniopuncture

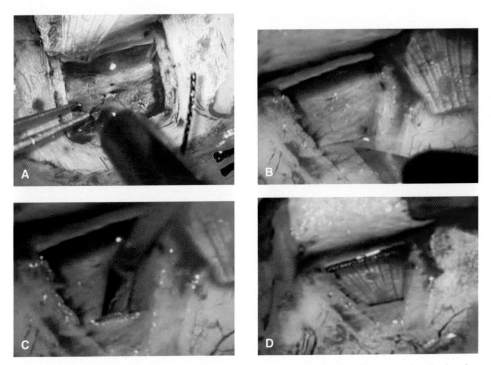

FIGURE 23-11. **Placing an implant. A.** Creating the scleral pocket in a square flap. **B.** Creating the scleral pocket in a trapezoidal flap. **C.** Widen the pocket with a spatula. **D.** Esnoper V-2000 nonabsorbable implant in the scleral bed with the posterior part in the suprachoroidal pocket.

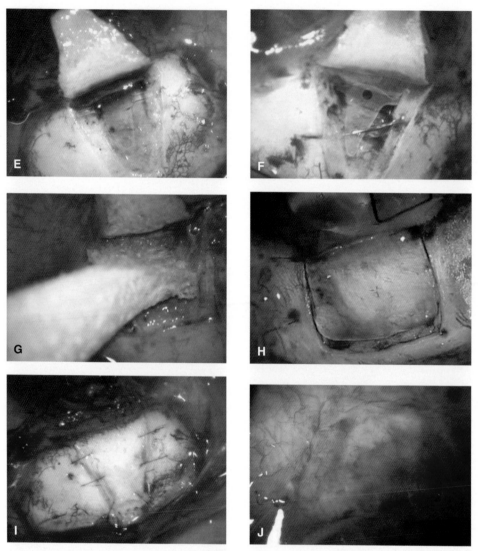

FIGURE 23-11. (*continued*) **E.** T-Flux nonabsorbable colorless implant. **F.** T-Flux after using fluorescein. **G.** Aqueous humor outflow. **H.** Closing the scleral flap, no suture. **I.** Closing the scleral flap with nylon 10-0. **J.** Conjunctival closure with Vicryl 8-0 running suture.

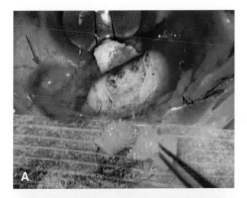

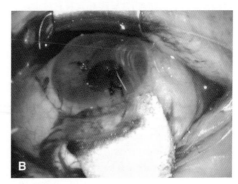

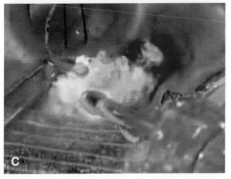

FIGURE 23-12. Using an antimetabolite. A. Sponge soaked in antimetabolites, three fragments, one for each side, nasal and temporal, and the third to leave under the scleral flap. **B.** Sponge soaks in antimetabolite under the scleral flap. **C.** Wash out the antimetabolite with a saline solution of about 250 mL.

POSTOPERATIVE CARE

• The postoperative care of the deep sclerectomy is critical. Some advantages of deep sclerectomy include minimal intraocular inflammation (Fig. 23-13A), and the risk of flat anterior chamber is very low if there is no perforation into the anterior chamber. Now, we are leaving the superior flap unsutured, but in case of doubt or excessive filtration, we place an 8-0 Vicryl suture as a belt over the scleral flap (Fig. 23-13B). This will keep a pressure over the flap that will be slowly reduced due to the absorption of the suture.

• For infection prophylaxis and treatment of inflammation, we use moxifloxacin or ciprofloxacin four times a day for 7 days, dexamethasone also four times a day for 2 weeks, and nonsteroidal anti-inflammatory drugs like topical diclofenac three times a day for 6 weeks. Generally, we see our postoperative patients at 24 hours (Fig. 23-14A) and every week for 1 month (Fig. 23-14B) and every 2 weeks for another month (Fig. 23-14C). The visual acuity is usually very stable, but we prefer not to change the refraction (Fig. 23-14D) until the third month.

• The bleb tends to be diffuse, and as we use antimetabolites in most of our patients, we usually see an avascular bleb in the first 12 weeks (Fig. 23-15A and B). In some patients, the bleb can be very exuberant in the first week, but this is not common; in most of these patients when this happens, the bleb will become diffuse in time (Fig. 23-15C).

• During the next 3 months, it is very important to observe the IOP; if it starts to rise, a gonioscopy is very helpful (Fig. 23-16A); the trabeculodescemetic membrane is so thin that it can break and the implant can enter the anterior chamber (Fig. 23-16B). This is very uncommon and is related to ocular trauma or a technical problem. The trabeculodescemetic membrane can be blocked by the iris

(Fig. 23-16C), and an application of argon laser at the base of the iris with mild power and spots of 500 microns size (gonioplasty) will flatten the iris and pull it away from the membrane; in some patients, topical pilocarpine is enough to pull the iris away from the trabeculodescemetic membrane. If the rise of IOP is not due to a mechanical blockage, goniopuncture can be performed. This consists of using the YAG laser to create small holes through the membrane. Authors believe that it should be done only in case of need where a rise of IOP is not related to mechanical blockage but is due to trabecular pathology.

• The bleb can become encapsulated and can benefit from needling. Bleb needling can be done with topical anesthesia at the slit lamp. The surgeon inserts a 25-gauge needle, fixed on a syringe for stability, into the subconjunctival space at 2 mm from the cyst (Fig. 23-17A). In the first step, we try to break the adhesions between the conjunctiva and the wall of the bleb (Fig. 23-17B). Next, we try to get under the flap; most of our patients have no suture, which helps to lift the flap. Then, we very gently break any subconjunctival synechia. 5-FU injected helps to reduce healing and fibrosis injected, after completing all maneuvers, into the subconjunctival space (Fig. 23-17C). The bleb fibrosis can be observed using the anterior-segment optical coherence tomography (OCT) (Fig. 23-17D and E) to help guide therapy.

• The anterior-segment image, such as can be obtained using spectral domain OCT, is very useful for the postoperative management following deep sclerectomy. The thickness of the trabeculodescemetic membrane and its integrity can be monitored (Fig. 23-18A); also, the implant position (Fig. 23-18B), fibrosis of the bleb (Figs. 23-18C and D). When the bleb has become flat or collapses, one can consider needling to timely resolve this complication (Fig. 23-18E). Microperforations and iris incarceration between other complications can also be seen (**Fig. 23-18F**) with the anterior-segment OCT or ultrasonic biomicroscopy.

CONCLUSION

- This chapter is not intended as a comprehensive review of the literature. Deep sclerectomy is a complex surgery with a significant learning curve. Furthermore, there are differences in each surgeon's technique, making it difficult to compare results between surgeons, but the IOP is typically in the high teens in most of the meta-analyses.[1] What seems to be clear is that trabeculectomies lower[2] the IOP more than deep sclerectomies do but with more complications.[3,4]

- There are many unanswered questions about the implants, such as whether they are absorbable or not, their ability to enhance filtration and improve results, and so on. For many surgeons, they do improve results. The concept of keeping the virtual space or a lake improves the results.[5,6,7,8,9] For some others, they do not change the long-term results.[10,11] Deep sclerectomy seems to work in primary and secondary open angle glaucoma as pseudoexfoliation,[12,13] uveitic,[14] and in some traumatic patients with hyphema (personal experience).

- In most of the published articles, with deep sclerectomy, the rate of complication is comparatively very low, and there is no flat anterior chamber, less incidence of cataract, and less choroidal hemorrhage. Because of the low rate of complications in early and late postoperative periods, deep sclerectomy can be done early in mild to moderate glaucomas of different types.

REFERENCES

1. Hondur A, Onol M, Hasanreisoglu B. Nonpenetrating glaucoma surgery: meta-analysis of recent results. *J Glaucoma*. 2008;17:139–146.
2. Chiselita D. Non-penetrating deep sclerectomy versus trabeculectomy in primary open angle glaucoma surgery. *Eye*. 2001;15:197–201.
3. Lachkar Y, Neverauskiene J, Jeanteur-Lunel MN, et al. Nonpenetrating deep sclerectomy: 6 year retrospective study. *Eur J Ophthalmol*. 2004;14:26–36.
4. Khary HA, Green FD, Nassar MK, et al. Control of intraocular pressure after deep sclerectomy. *Eye*. 2006;20:336–340.
5. Sanchez E, Schnyder CC, Sickenberg M, et al. Deep sclerectomy: results with and without collagen implant. *Int Ophthalmol*. 1997;20:157–162.
6. Karlen ME, Sanchez E, Schnyder CC, et al. Deep sclerectomy with collagen implant: medium term results. *Br J Ophthalmol*. 1999;83:6–11.
7. Dahan E, Ravinet E, Ben-Simon GJ, et al. Comparison of the efficacy and longevity of nonpenetrating glaucoma surgery with and without a new nonabsorbable hydrophilic implant. *Ophthalmic Surg Laser Imaging*. 2003;34:1–7.
8. Shaarawy T, Nguyen C, Schnyder C, et al. Comparative study between deep sclerectomy with and without collagen implant: long term follow up. *Br J Ophthalmol*. 2004;88:95–98.
9. Bissig A, Rivier D, Zaninetti M, et al. Ten years follow-up after deep sclerectomy with collagen implant. *J Glaucoma*. 2008;17:680–686.
10. Demailly P, Lavat P, Kretz G, et al. Non penetrating deep sclerectomy (NPDS) with or without collagen device (CD) in primary open-angle glaucoma: middle term retrospective study. *Int Ophthalmol*. 1997;20:131–140.
11. Cheng JW, Wei RL, Cai JP, et al. Efficacy and tolerability of nonpenetrating filtering surgery with and without implant in treatment of open angle glaucoma. A quantitative evaluation of the evidence. *J Glaucoma*. 2009;18:233–237.
12. Mendrinos E, Mansouri K, Mermoud A, et al. Long-term results of deep sclerectomy with collagen implant in exfoliative glaucoma. *J Glaucoma*. 2009;18:361–367.
13. Drolsum L. Deep sclerectomy in patients with capsular glaucoma. *Acta Ophthalmol Scand*. 2003;81:567–572.
14. Auer C, Mermoud A, Herbort CP. Deep sclerectomy for the management of uncontrolled uveitic glaucoma: preliminary data. *Klin Monatsbl Auehenheilkd*. 2004;221:339–342.

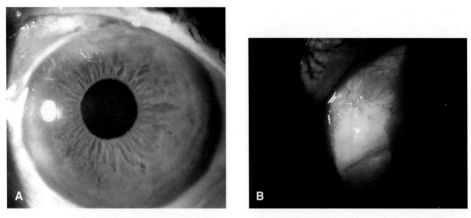

FIGURE 23-13. **Postoperative appearance. A.** Eye 24 hours after a deep sclerectomy and phacoemulsification. **B.** Belt suture over the scleral flap made with Vicryl 8-0.

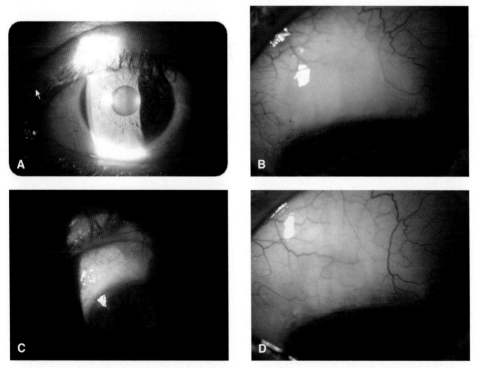

FIGURE 23-14. **Postoperative appearance. A.** Eye 24 hours after a deep sclerectomy. **B.** Eye 1 month after a deep sclerectomy. **C.** Eye 6 weeks after a deep sclerectomy. **D.** Eye 3 months after a deep sclerectomy.

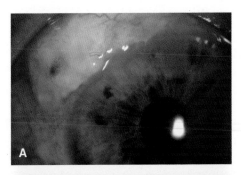

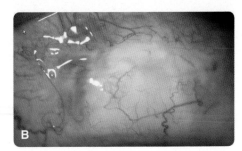

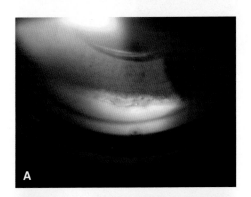

FIGURE 23-15. Postoperative appearance. A. Diffuse bleb. **B.** Avascular bleb. **C.** Enlarged bleb.

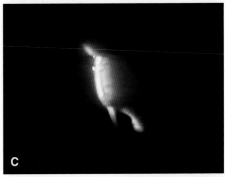

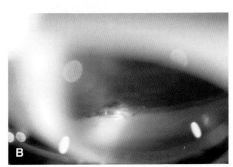

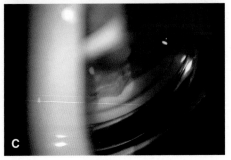

FIGURE 23-16. Postoperative appearance.
A. Trabeculodescemetic membrane, a gonioscopic view.
B. T-Flux haptics and a part of the body in the anterior chamber in an eye with a previous trabeculectomy.
C. Trabeculodescemetic membrane block by the iris, a gonioscopic view.

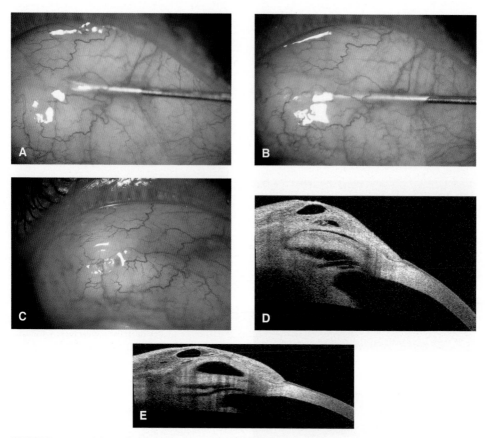

FIGURE 23-17. **Bleb needling. A.** Needling breaking the adhesion between the conjunctiva and the sclera. **B.** Needling trying to get under the superficial flap. **C.** After needling in a 5-fluorouracil (5-FU injection). **D.** Optical coherence tomography (OCT) from the anterior segment before needling. **E.** Anterior-segment OCT after needling, bleb created after the injection of 5-FU.

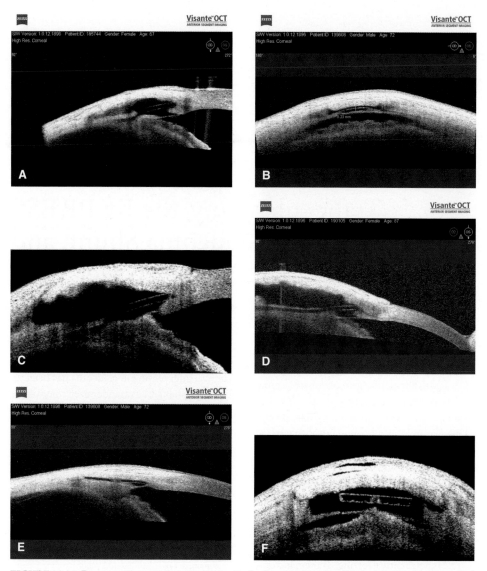

FIGURE 23-18. Postoperative anterior-segment optical coherence tomography. A. Anterior-segment optical coherence tomography (OCT) details of the trabeculodescemetic membrane, implant, and position of the iris can be observed. **B.** A coronal view from the anterior-segment OCT, T-Flux in position, end of the haptics can be seen and measured. **C.** A Visante OCT of a deep sclerectomy big bleb over the implant can be seen. **D.** An anterior-segment OCT with a suprachoroidal view from the implant. **E.** An anterior-segment OCT in a nonfunctioning deep sclerectomy, showing the collapse of the tissue over the surgery. No filtration. **F.** An Esnoper V-2000 nonabsorbable implant coronal view with an iris incarceration after a perforation.

Trabeculectomy, the Ex-PRESS Mini Glaucoma Shunt, and the Xen Gel Stent

Marlene R. Moster and Augusto Azuara-Blanco ■

TRABECULECTOMY

Guarded filtration surgery, or trabeculectomy, lowers the intraocular pressure (IOP) by creating a fistula between the inner compartments of the eye and the subconjunctival space (i.e., filtering bleb; Fig. 24-1). Cairns[1] reported the first series in 1968. A number of techniques are available to assist in establishing and maintaining the function of filtration blebs and avoiding complications (see below).

Trabeculectomy is the most commonly used surgical procedure in patients with glaucoma, but its role is constantly evolving. Trabeculectomy has been compared with initial topical medical treatment as an initial treatment for glaucoma in a large randomized controlled trial.[2] It seems that patients presenting with more advanced disease had slower visual field progression if their primary intervention was surgical rather than medical. Trabeculectomy as the primary surgical intervention in glaucoma has been recently questioned, but a randomized comparative study between trabeculectomy and Baerveldt glaucoma drainage device did not show any difference in mean IOP after 5-year follow-up.[3]

REFERENCES

1. Cairns JE. Trabeculectomy: preliminary report of a new method. *Am J Ophthalmol.* 1968;(66):673–679.
2. Musch DC, Gillespie BW, Lichter PR, Niziol LM, Janz NK; CIGTS Study Investigators. Visual field progression in the Collaborative Initial Glaucoma Treatment Study: the impact of treatment and other baseline factors. *Ophthalmology.* 2009;116(2):200–207.
3. Gedde SJ, Schiffman JC, Feuer WJ, Herndon LW, Brandt JD, Budenz DL; Tube versus Trabeculectomy Study Group. Treatment outcomes in the Tube versus Trabeculectomy (TVT) study after five years of follow-up. *Am J Ophthalmol.* 2012;153(5):789–803.

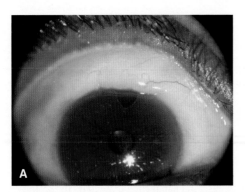 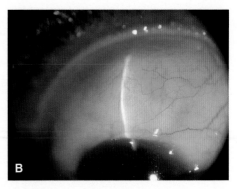

FIGURE 24-1. Trabeculectomy filtering bleb. A slit-lamp view of an eye that underwent trabeculectomy 3 months earlier (**A** and **B**). Note the nonlocalized elevation of the conjunctiva.

SURGICAL TECHNIQUE

• Any type of regional anesthesia (retro-bulbar, peribulbar, and sub-Tenon) can be used. Topical anesthesia is also possible, with topical 2% lidocaine gel, 0.1 mL of intracameral 1% nonpreserved lidocaine (Fig. 24-2), and 0.2 mL of subconjunctival 1% lidocaine injected from the superior temporal quadrant to balloon the conjunctiva over the superior rectus muscle (Fig. 24-3).

• Trabeculectomy should be done at the superior limbus, because inferiorly located blebs are associated with a much higher risk of bleb-associated infections.

• A fixation or traction suture is used to keep the eye in downward position, giving a good area of exposure.

▪ A corneal traction suture in the quadrant of the planned surgery (7-0 or 8-0 black silk or nylon, or 8-0 Vicryl on a spatulated needle) is the preferred option of the authors. The needle is passed through clear, midstromal cornea approximately 2 mm from the limbus for approximately 3 to 4 mm.

▪ Alternatively, a superior rectus traction suture (4-0 or 5-0 black silk on a tapered needle) can be used to rotate the globe inferiorly and bring the superior bulbar conjunctival into view. Using a muscle hook to rotate the globe downward, the conjunctiva and superior rectus are grasped with toothed forceps and the threaded needle is passed through the tissue bundle (Fig. 24-4).

• A limbus-based (Fig. 24-5) or fornix-based (Fig. 24-6) conjunctival flap is made with Westcott scissors and nontoothed utility forceps. A fornix-based flap is more likely to be associated with diffuse blebs.

▪ When forming limbus-based flaps, the conjunctival incision is placed 8 to 10 mm posterior to the limbus. The conjunctival and Tenon wound should be lengthened to approximately 8 to 12 mm cord length. The flap is then extended anteriorly to expose the corneoscleral sulcus.

▪ When making fornix-based flaps, the conjunctiva and Tenon are disinserted. Approximately, a 2-clock-hour limbal peritomy (6 to 8 mm) is sufficient. Blunt dissection is carried posteriorly.

• A scleral flap is then dissected. The scleral flap should completely cover the fistula to provide resistance to the aqueous outflow. The aqueous will flow around the scleral flap.

▪ The differences in the shape or size of the scleral flap probably have little effect on surgical outcome. The flap thickness should be between one-half and two-thirds (Fig. 24-7).

▪ It is important to dissect the flap anteriorly (approximately 1 mm into the clear cornea) to ensure that the fistula is created anterior to the scleral spur and the ciliary body.

• A corneal paracentesis is made before opening the globe (Fig. 24-8) with either a 30- or a 27-gauge needle or a sharp point blade. A block of tissue at the corneoscleral junction is then excised.

▪ Two radial incisions are made first with a sharp blade or knife starting in the clear cornea, and extending posteriorly approximately 1 to 1.5 mm. The radial incisions are made approximately 2 mm apart. The blade or Vannas scissors are used to connect the incisions; thereby, a rectangular piece of tissue is removed (Fig. 24-9).

▪ Alternatively, an anterior corneal incision, parallel to the limbus and perpendicular to the eye, is made to enter into the anterior chamber, and a Kelly or Gass punch is used to excise the tissue.

• A peripheral iridectomy may then be performed. Iridectomy is not necessary in many cases (e.g., pseudophakic eyes with open anterior chamber angle), but recommended in patients with a shallow anterior chamber and an angle-closure glaucoma.

■ The iris is grasped near its root with toothed forceps. It is retracted through the sclerostomy, and an iridectomy is performed with Vannas or DeWecker scissors (Fig. 24-10).

■ The iridectomy should avoid damage to the iris root and the ciliary body so as not to cause bleeding.

● The scleral flap is sutured initially with two interrupted 10-0 nylon sutures (in case of a rectangular flap; Fig. 24-11) or with one suture (in a triangular flap). Slipknots are useful to adjust the tightness of the scleral flap and the rate of aqueous outflow. Additional sutures can be used to better control the outflow.

■ During the suturing of the scleral flap, the anterior chamber is filled through the paracentesis, and the flow around the flap is observed. If flow seems excessive, or the anterior chamber shallows, the slipknots are tightened or additional sutures are placed. If aqueous does not flow through the flap, the surgeon may loosen the slipknots or replace tight sutures with looser ones.

■ In some situations, the scleral flap is tightly closed to avoid hypotony, for example, angle-closure glaucoma and high preoperative IOP. Releasable sutures can be used (Fig. 24-12) instead of interrupted ones. Externalized releasable sutures are easily removed and are effective in cases of inflamed or hemorrhagic conjunctiva or thickened Tenon capsule.

● Conjunctival closure in limbus-based flaps is done with a double or single running suture (Fig. 24-13), with an 8-0 or 9-0 absorbable suture, or with a 10-0 nylon suture. Many surgeons favor a round-body needle.

■ In fornix-based flaps, a tight conjunctival–corneal apposition is needed. Sutures (e.g., mattress 10-0 nylon suture; Fig. 24-14) at the edges of the incision can be used to anchor the conjunctiva to the cornea. Alternatively, the fornix-based flap can be closed with a running modified Condon suture technique. https://eyetube.net/video /closing-the-fornix-based-conjunctival-flap/

● After the wound is closed, a 30-gauge cannula is used to fill the anterior chamber with a balanced salt solution (BSS) through the paracentesis track to elevate the conjunctival bleb and test for leaks (Fig. 24-13). Antibiotics and corticosteroids can be injected in the inferior fornix.

● Patching the eye is individualized, depending on the patient's vision and the anesthesia used.

Intraoperative Application of Antimetabolites

● To reduce postoperative subconjunctival fibrosis, especially important in patients with a high risk for failure, mitomycin C (MMC) (Fig. 24-15) is used. The use of antifibrotic agents is associated with a higher success rate, although the risk of complications may also increase. MMC (0.2 to 0.5 mg per mL solution) or 5-fluorouracil (5-FU; 50 mg per mL solution) is applied for 1 to 5 minutes using soaked cellulose sponges (Fig. 24-16) placed over the episclera. Application under the scleral flap is also possible. The conjunctival–Tenon layer is draped over the sponge, avoiding contact of the MMC with the wound edge.

● After the application, the sponge is removed and the entire area is irrigated thoroughly with BSS. The plastic devices that collect the liquid runoff (Fig. 24-17A) are changed and disposed of according to toxic waste regulations (Fig. 24-17B).

- Alternatively, MMC can be injected sub-conjunctivally. A tuberculin syringe on a 30-gauge needle can be used to inject 0.1 cc of MMC 0.4 mg per cc mixed with 0.1 cc of 1% nonpreserved lidocaine. The total volume is 0.2 cc. The injection is given under tenons/conjunctiva approximately 8 mm from the limbus in the temporal quadrant to avoid a buttonhole.

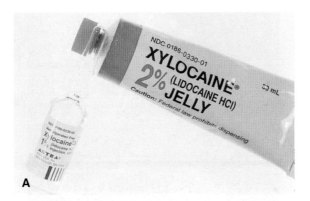

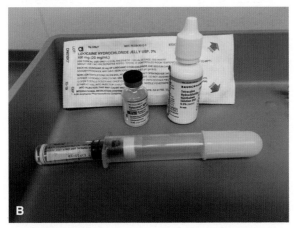

FIGURE 24-2. Topical anesthetic agents. A. Xylocaine 2% gel for topical application and lidocaine 1% nonpreserved for sub-Tenon or subconjunctival injection. **B.** Anesthetic preparations.

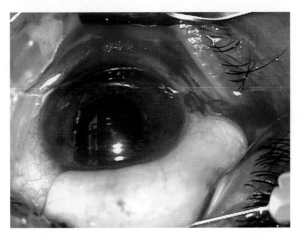

FIGURE 24-3. Ballooning of conjunctiva. Ballooning of the conjunctiva with nonpreserved lidocaine 1% (0.5 mL) using a 30-gauge sharp needle in the direction of the superior rectus muscle.

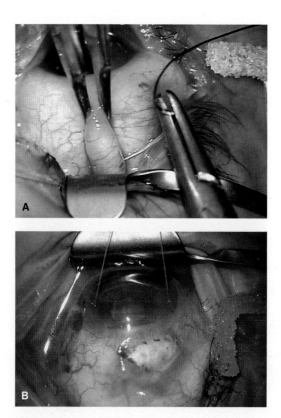

FIGURE 24-4. Traction suture placement. A. Placement of a superior rectus traction suture before a limbus-based trabeculectomy. **B.** Placement of a corneal traction suture for a limbal based conjunctival flap suture.

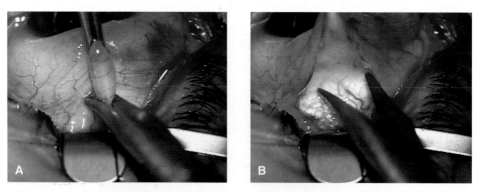

FIGURE 24-5. Limbus-based flap. Developing a limbus-based conjunctival–Tenon flap. **A.** The conjunctiva is grasped with forceps and elevated before the initial cut, and placed approximately 8 to 10 mm posterior to the limbus. **B.** The incision is extended laterally exposing the episclera.

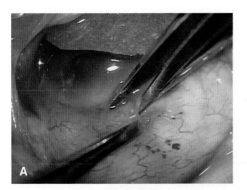
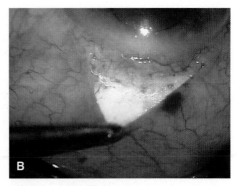

FIGURE 24-6. **A fornix-based flap.** Developing a fornix-based conjunctival–Tenon flap. **A.** The conjunctiva is grasped with forceps and elevated before the initial cut. **B.** The conjunctival incision is done as anteriorly as possible at the limbus, extending 2 to 3 clock hours.

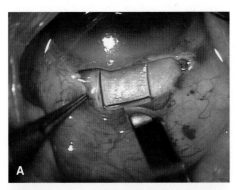
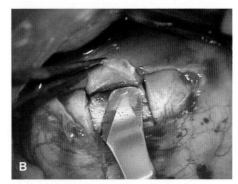

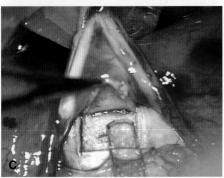

FIGURE 24-7. **A partial-thickness flap.** Developing a one-half to two-thirds partial-thickness scleral trabeculectomy flap with a fornix-based conjunctival flap (**A** and **B**) or with a limbal-based flap (**C**).

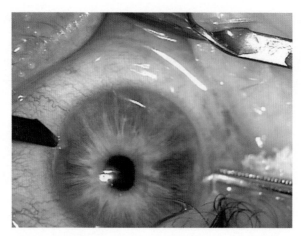

FIGURE 24-8. Corneal paracentesis. A corneal paracentesis is done temporally or nasally before creating the fistula. A sharp knife is used, and a long track is created.

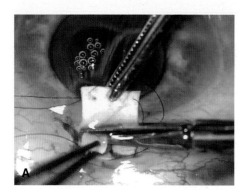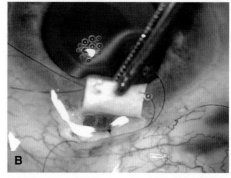

FIGURE 24-9. Removing the internal tissue block. After an initial incision with a sharp knife to enter into the anterior chamber, the fistula can be created with a punch or with Vannas scissors (**A**). The block excised can be corneal and/or limbal (**B**). Note the preplaced scleral flap sutures, used to expedite closure and minimize the time when the eye is hypotonous (**A** and **B**).

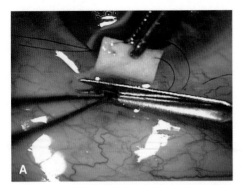 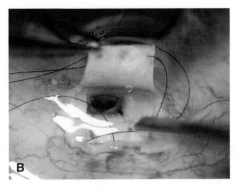

FIGURE 24-10. **Surgical iridectomy.** Surgical iridectomy with Vannas scissors (**A** and **B**) after trabeculectomy block removal. It is important to avoid the iris root when grasping the peripheral iris.

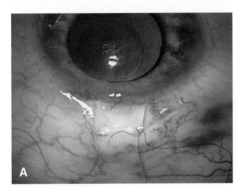 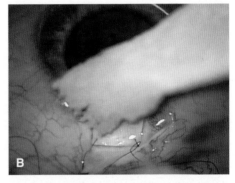

FIGURE 24-11. **Suturing the scleral flap.** There are many different techniques for suturing the scleral flap. In this technique, the surgeon is tying the preplaced interrupted sutures at each corner of the scleral flap (**A**). A slipknot is helpful for adjusting the tightness and the amount of drainage through the flap (**B**).

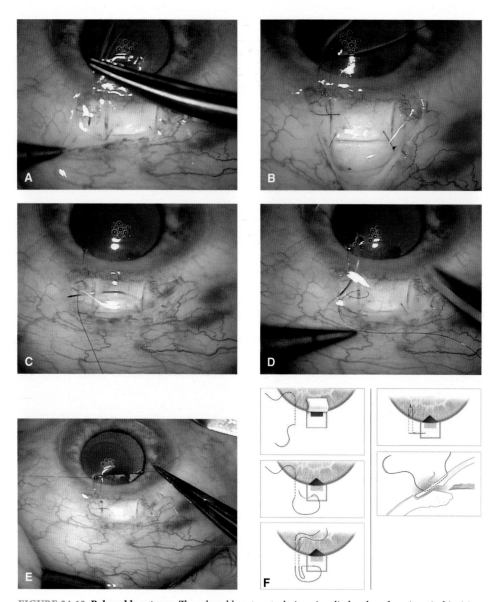

FIGURE 24-12. Releasable sutures. The releasable suture technique in a limbus-based conjunctival incision described by Richard P. Wilson, MD. A 10-0 nylon suture is used. **A** and **B. Step 1:** The suture enters into the cornea 1 mm anterior to the limbus (depth: midstromal) and exits through the sclera adjacent to the flap (going underneath the corneoscleral limbus and the insertion of the conjunctiva). **C. Step 2:** The needle is passed through the scleral flap and sclera adjacent to the flap. **D. Step 3:** The needle enters the sclera and exits through the cornea (direction parallel to step 1). **E. Step 4:** The suture is then tied up securely. **F.** Illustration of the depth of the suture. (Illustrations by Christine Gralapp; adapted with permission of the American Academy of Ophthalmology from Moster MR, Azuara-Blanco A. Focal Points Volume XVIII, number 6. San Francisco, CA: American Academy of Ophthalmology, 2000.)

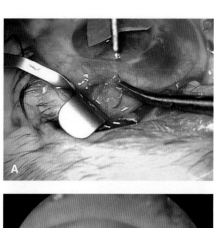

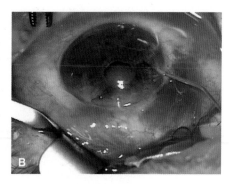

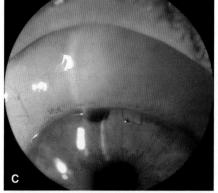

FIGURE 24-13. **Conjunctival closure: limbus-based flap. A.** A running 8-0 Vicryl suture technique is used, closing separately the Tenon layer (first) followed by the conjunctiva. **B.** The watertightness of the wound is confirmed by injecting a balanced salt solution into the anterior chamber and elevating the bleb. **C.** Immediate postoperative appearance of a limbus-based conjunctival–Tenon flap.

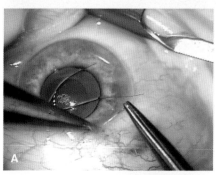

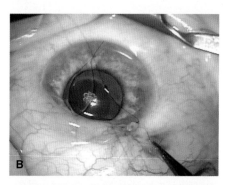

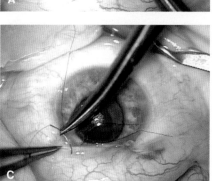

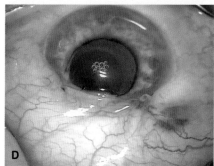

FIGURE 24-14. **Conjunctival closure: fornix-based flap.** Closure of a fornix-based conjunctival–Tenon flap with 10-0 nylon mattress sutures at each corner (**A–D**).

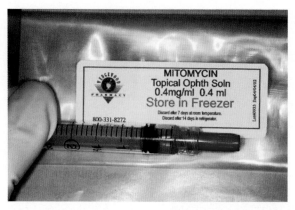

FIGURE 24-15. **Mitomycin C (MMC) solution.** MMC (0.4 mg per mL) as delivered to the operating room.

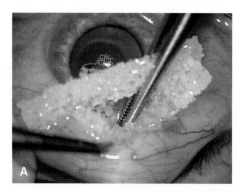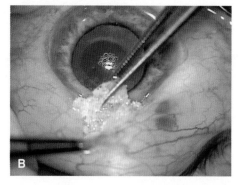

FIGURE 24-16. **Application of mitomycin C (MMC).** Delivery of MMC on a Weck-cell sponge under the conjunctiva and Tenon capsule (**A** and **B**). In this case, large sponges are used. Other surgeons prefer to use multiple small sponges.

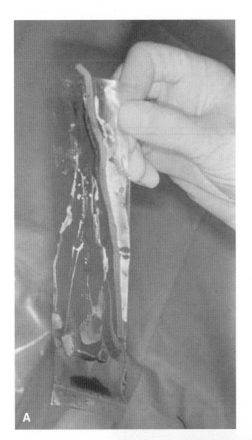

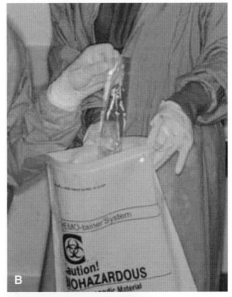

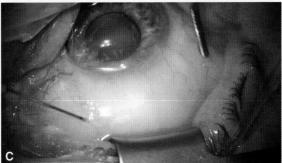

FIGURE 24-17. **Handling of mitomycin C (MMC) sponges. A.** Collection of sponges of MMC and contaminated fluid after irrigation. The number of sponges used and collected should be counted. **B.** Proper disposal of MMC-contaminated materials is mandatory. **C.** Injection of subconjunctival mitomycin-C.

POSTOPERATIVE CARE

- *Topical steroids* (e.g., prednisolone acetate 1%, four times daily) are tapered after 6 to 8 weeks. Some clinicians use topical nonsteroidal anti-inflammatory agents (e.g., 1 to 4 times a day for 1 month). Antibiotics are required for 1 week after surgery and stopped. Postoperative cycloplegics are utilized on an individual basis in patients with shallow anterior chambers or intense inflammation.

- Digital ocular compression applied to the inferior sclera or the cornea through the inferior eyelid, and focal compression with a moistened cotton tip at the posterior edge of the scleral flap, can be useful to elevate the bleb and reduce the IOP in the early postoperative period, especially after laser suture lysis (**Fig. 24-18**).

- Suture lysis and cutting and pulling releasable sutures are necessary when there is a high IOP, a flat filtration bleb, and a deep anterior chamber. Gonioscopy must be performed before the laser treatment to confirm an open sclerostomy, with no tissue or clot occluding its entrance. Suture lysis and cutting and pulling releasable sutures should be done within the first few weeks after surgery, although it may be successful even months after surgery in patients in whom MMC had been used.

- In patients prone to early failure (e.g., vascularized and thickened blebs), repeated subconjunctival applications of 5-FU (5 mg in 0.1 mL solution) and anti–vascular endothelial growth factor (anti-VEGF) therapy (see below) over the first 2 to 3 weeks are recommended.

Anti-VEGF Therapy for Bleb Vascularization

- The use of anti-VEGF agents (bevacizumab and ranibizumab) as an adjunct to trabeculectomy has recently been proposed. The wound-healing process is potentiated through both fibroblast activity and angiogenesis. Therefore, an anti-VEGF agent should reduce new vascular growth and potentially lead to a healthier bleb with less scarring and better long-term IOP control. Anti-VEGF agents may have a synergistic effect with MMC and 5-FU in those patients whose trabeculectomies may fail with the use of MMC or 5-FU alone.

- The use of subconjunctival anti-VEGF (bevacizumab 1 mg) after glaucoma surgery was first reported associated with a bleb needling procedure after a failed trabeculectomy. Many subsequent reports have illustrated the use of both bevacizumab and ranibizumab as subconjunctival or sub-Tenon injections after filtration surgery or at the time of bleb needle revision.

- It has been proposed to use anti-VEGF injections administered proximal to blebs after trabeculectomy at the earliest sign of vascularization, and this is our current practice. Further studies are needed to better understand the dose and route of injection as well as the side-effect profile of bevacizumab.

Bleb Needling

- In patients with subconjunctival–episcleral fibrosis, an external revision or bleb needling can be tried. A 27- or 25-gauge needle is used to cut the edge of the scleral flap and restore aqueous outflow. Entry of the needle tip into the anterior chamber beneath the flap is important but should be undertaken with extreme caution in phakic eyes.

- The outcome may be more favorable if there was a previously well-established filtration bleb before the fistula became occluded. Repeated administration of subconjunctival injections of 5-FU after revision increases the probability of success.

- MMC before or after needling has also been used in conjunction with needling of blebs. We are currently using a 0.1 cc of nonpreserved 1% lidocaine mixed with a 0.1 mL of 0.4 mg per mL MMC at the time of the needling.

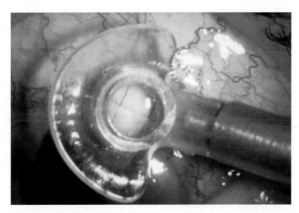

FIGURE 24-18. **Suture lysis.** A Hoskins lens is used to compress the conjunctiva and facilitate the view of the nylon suture. (Courtesy of Richard P. Wilson, MD, Wills Eye Hospital, Philadelphia, PA.)

COMPLICATIONS

● Complications and their management are briefly described in **Table 24-1** (**Figs. 24-19** to **24-29**).

● Transient hypotony is very common after glaucoma surgery, and often well tolerated, but occasionally it may lead to other possible complications, including flat anterior chamber (Fig. 24-19), Descemet membrane folds, choroidal effusions (**Fig. 24-20**), suprachoroidal hemorrhage (**Fig. 24-21**), cataract, macular and optic disc edema, and chorioretinal folds (predominantly in young myopic patients). Hyphema is not rare (**Fig. 24-22**), but often resolves with conservative management.

▪ The initial management of early postoperative hypotony with a formed anterior chamber is conservative with topical steroids and cycloplegics. Intervention is indicated in cases when hypotony is associated with other complications such as persistent low IOP with loss of visual acuity and hypotony maculopathy (**Fig. 24-23**, see below). Treatment should be aimed at correcting the specific cause of hypotony. Most commonly, hypotony is due to overfiltration of a filtering bleb. When there is a flat anterior chamber with lens–corneal touch, immediate surgical intervention is necessary to prevent endothelial damage and cataract formation. Reformation of the anterior chamber with a viscoelastic can be done at the slit lamp or under the operating microscope through the paracentesis made intraoperatively. When there are large appositional choroidal effusions, drainage of the fluid is recommended.

● When overfiltration persists (**Fig. 24-24**), several treatments can be used to induce an inflammatory or healing reaction in the filtering bleb, which modify the morphology of the blebs and increase the IOP. Surgical revision is the most efficacious option.

▪ Palmberg transconjunctival sutures are often helpful to reduce overfiltration (**Fig. 24-25**). Resuturing the scleral flap through the conjunctiva is currently the author's favored option. Suturing the scleral flap can be done through the conjunctiva, as reported by Richman et al.[1] After anesthetic eye drops are instilled, the filtering bleb on the scleral flap is compressed by a cotton tip and released to confirm the site of excess filtration at the scleral flap. Then, using a round, tapered needle with a 10-0 nylon suture, the scleral flap is sutured tightly directly through the conjunctiva. If necessary, an additional suture can be placed and tightened to achieve a watertight closure.

▪ When it is difficult to see the margin of the scleral flap, compression and suturing while observing with a Hoskins lens are helpful. Usually, a slight leakage at the sutured points occurs, especially when the bleb wall is thin. However, it stops spontaneously a few hours or days later because of the decrease in filtration and/or downsizing of the filtering bleb. After the procedure, a topical antibiotic is prescribed. The suture is buried in the conjunctiva spontaneously in 1 week in all cases.

▪ Occasionally, bleb revision for overfiltration must be associated with patch grafting (i.e., in cases of incompetent scleral flap, when resuturing is not possible).

● Late bleb-related infection can be a very severe complication, potentially leading to endophthalmitis (**Fig. 24-26**). It is more common in surgeries supplemented with MMC and in leaking (**Figs. 24-27** to 24-29), avascular, thin, localized filtering blebs.

REFERENCE

1. Richman J, Moster MR, Myeni T, Trubnik V. A prospective study of consecutive patients undergoing full-thickness conjunctival/scleral hypotony sutures for clinical ocular hypotony. *J Glaucoma*. 2014;23:326–328.

TABLE 24-1. Complications of Trabeculectomy

Complication	Treatment
Conjunctival buttonholes	A purse-string suture with a 10-0 or 11-0 needle on a rounded ("vascular") needle
Early overfiltration (**Fig. 24-25**)	If AC is shallow or flat with no lens–cornea touch, use cycloplegics, restriction in activity, and avoidance of Valsalva maneuvers. If there is lens–corneal touch, perform urgent reformation of AC. If complication persists, resuture the scleral flap
Choroidal effusions (**Fig. 24-21**)	Observation, cycloplegics, steroids. Drainage is considered if effusions are appositional and associated with a flat anterior chamber
Suprachoroidal Hemorrhage	
Intraoperative	Prompt closure of eye and gentle reposition of a prolapsed uvea. Intravenous mannitol and acetazolamide
Postoperative	Observation; control IOP and pain. Drain (after 7–10 days) patients with persistent flat AC and intolerable pain
Aqueous misdirection	Initial medical treatment: intensive topical cycloplegic–mydriatic regimen, topical and oral aqueous suppressants, and osmotics
	In pseudophakics: Nd:YAG laser hyaloidotomy or peripheral anterior vitrectomy via AC
	In phakics: phacoemulsification and anterior vitrectomy. Pars plana vitrectomy
Bleb encapsulation (**Fig. 24-30**) Bleb dysesthesia (**Fig. 24-26**)	Initial observation. Aqueous suppressants if IOP is elevated. Consider needling with 5-fluorouracil or a surgical revision. Topical lubrication. Compression sutures (Palmberg)
Late bleb leak (**Fig. 24-29**)	If the leak is not brisk, do an initial observation and give topical antibiotics. If it persists, do a surgical revision (conjunctival advancement or autograft)
Chronic hypotony (**Fig. 24-24**)	If there is reduced vision or maculopathy, perform transconjunctival flap sutures or revision of the scleral flap
Blebitis (**Fig. 24-27**), endophthalmitis	Bleb infection without any intraocular involvement: provide an intensive topical treatment with wide-spectrum fortified antibiotics
	Bleb infection with a mild anterior segment cellular reaction: intensive topical treatment with fortified antibiotics recommended
	Bleb infection with a severe anterior segment cellular reaction or vitreous involvement: vitreous sample and intravitreal antibiotics suggested

AC, anterior chamber; IOP, intraocular pressure.

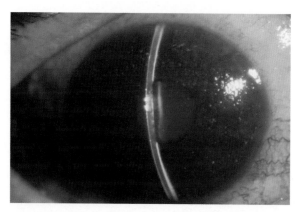

FIGURE 24-19. **Flat anterior chamber.** The anterior chamber is flat (Spaeth Grade II), with iris–cornea touch, but with no lens–cornea touch.

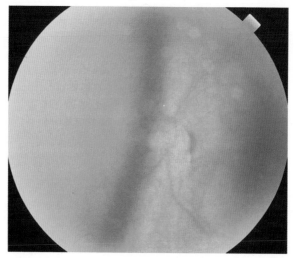

FIGURE 24-20. **Choroidal detachment.** A fundus photograph showing serous choroidal detachment obscuring the optic nerve.

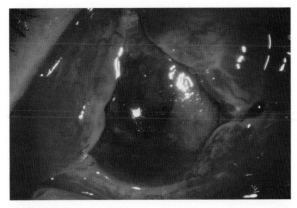

FIGURE 24-21. Suprachoroidal hemorrhage. A slit-lamp photograph of an eye with suprachoroidal hemorrhage; the retina can be seen through the pupil.

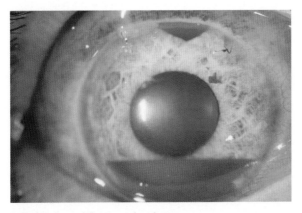

FIGURE 24-22. Hyphema. Hyphema following trabeculectomy.

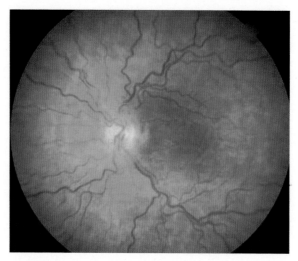

FIGURE 24-23. **Chronic hypotony.** A fundus photograph showing retinal folds and tortuosity of the vessels—so-called hypotony maculopathy.

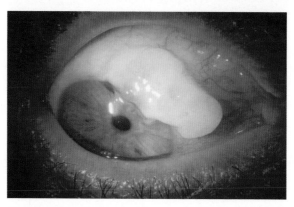

FIGURE 24-24. **Overfiltration.** Overfiltration caused by an exuberant bleb. Note the avascularity of the bleb.

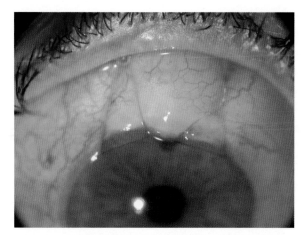

FIGURE 24-25. Palmberg sutures. Transconjunctival sutures can be used to reduce the size of the bleb and treat overfiltration.

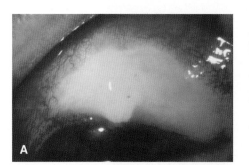

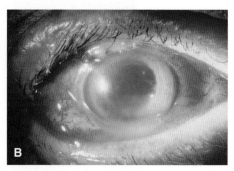

FIGURE 24-26. Bleb-related ocular infection. A. A slit-lamp photograph of a case of blebitis; purulent discharge can be seen on the bleb. **B.** Hypopyon in a patient with blebitis.

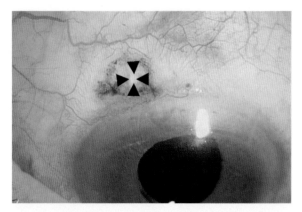

FIGURE 24-27. Conjunctival buttonhole. A conjunctival buttonhole identified several weeks following trabeculectomy with mitomycin C. The *arrowheads* denote the edges of the hole.

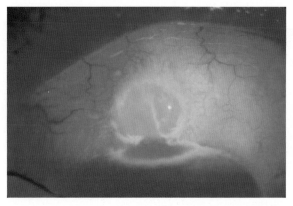

FIGURE 24-28. Late bleb leak. A late bleb leak 3 years following a trabeculectomy surgery. Under cobalt blue light, Seidel test shows aqueous flow from the leak. The bleb is small, localized, and avascular.

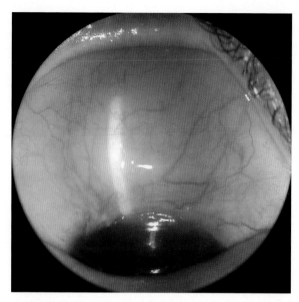

FIGURE 24-29. Encapsulated bleb. Typically, encapsulated blebs are localized and vascularized.

EX-PRESS MINI GLAUCOMA SHUNT

The Ex-PRESS is a small stainless-steel implant that is inserted through the limbus into the anterior chamber under a 4- to 5-mm–wide partial-thickness scleral flap, similar to a standard trabeculectomy flap. There are several models with different shapes and sizes (length ranges from 2.4 to 2.9 mm). The internal lumen diameter varies between 50 μm (most commonly used) and 200 μm.

The appeal of the Ex-PRESS shunt is that it may provide a more uniform, consistent, and reliable postoperative course than does standard trabeculectomy. Noncomparative studies have suggested that the incidence of early hypotony with Ex-PRESS shunt is lower than after trabeculectomy, with similar clinical efficacy.[1]

SURGICAL TECHNIQUE

• The surgical technique for Ex-PRESS implantation is similar to that for standard trabeculectomy. After conjunctival dissection, subconjunctival MMC is usually applied to minimize scarring and bleb failure. Alternatively, the mitomycin can be injected under the conjunctiva/tenons. Then, the scleral flap is lifted, extending the dissection 1 to 2 mm into the cornea. A 27- to 25-gauge needle is bent and inserted at the gray line into the anterior chamber. Lateral movement of the needle should be avoided while creating the entry track. The shunt is then introduced with a disposable inserter on its side, parallel to the iris plane (Fig. 24-30). Once the shunt clears the cornea (a slight "pop" is noted), it is rotated to the 12 o'clock position. It is best to insert the shunt when the IOP is about 20 mm Hg, so the cornea is not indented at the time of placement. The shunt is inserted all the way into the wound, making the plate flush with the scleral bed. Immediate flow is then observed through the lumen.

• Scleral flap closure with adjustable or releasable sutures is similar to that for trabeculectomy. Watertight conjunctival closure is important (see earlier). Postoperative management (topical steroids, use of postoperative 5-FU or anti-VEGF) is similar to that for standard trabeculectomy (Fig. 24-31).

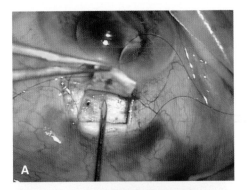

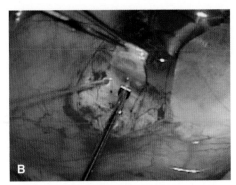

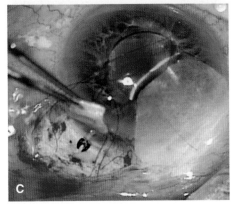

FIGURE 24-30. Ex-PRESS mini-shunt implantation. Surgical technique. A. After the scleral flap is dissected, a needle is used to create the entrance. **B.** The shunt is introduced using a disposable inserter. **C.** The implant is secure, and the scleral flap will be sutured over the implant.

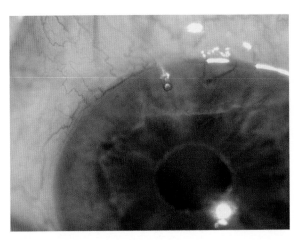

FIGURE 24-31. Ex-PRESS mini-shunt. Postoperative appearance.

XEN GLAUCOMA IMPLANT (AQUESYS XEN GEL STENT [ALLERGAN, DUBLIN])

The Xen glaucoma implant creates an aqueous drainage pathway from the anterior chamber into the subconjunctival space by the introduction of a small gelatin stent (tube) through a small corneal incision and controlled placement of this shunt through the corneoscleral junction. This process mimics the mechanism of trabeculectomy. Before inserting the implant, a 0.1 mL of 2 to 4 mg per mL MMC is injected subconjunctivally and massaged into the subconjunctival space.

Xen is a gelatin tube 6 mm long with a lumen diameter of 45 μm. The implant comes preloaded in a specially designed injector. It can be inserted at the time of cataract surgery or as a stand-alone procedure. The chamber is filled with viscoelastic, and before insertion, the conjunctiva is marked 3 mm from the limbus in two spots to guide the surgeon to the endpoint through the sclera and under the conjunctiva between the two guiding marks. A gonio prism can be used to assure the correct location, but it is not absolutely necessary, because the procedure can be done without one. The inserter is placed in the angle and slowly inserted through the sclera until the needle is visible under the conjunctiva. Then, the inserter releases the gel stent, so that a small portion remains in the anterior chamber (to drain the aqueous) to the longer portion under the superior conjunctiva which forms a low diffuse bleb. The Xen gel stent is done from an internal approach, requires a small incision, and does not require any sutures. However, because it mimics a trabeculectomy, management of the bleb is critical for success. Bleb needling in a significant number of cases is necessary to maintain a low IOP.

The postoperative regimen is similar to that for trabeculectomy but may require fewer outpatient visits. Visual recovery can be faster and the discomfort is less because no major surgical incisions are made to disturb the surface of the eye (Figs. 24-32 and 24-33).

ACKNOWLEDGMENT

The authors thank Dr. K. Mansouri (Consultant Ophthalmologist, Glaucoma Center, Montchoisi Clinic, Lausanne. Switzerland, and Adjoint Associate Professor, Department of Ophthalmology, University of Colorado, Denver, USA) for providing the Xen illustrations.

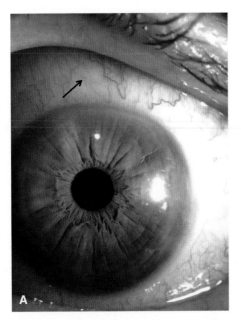
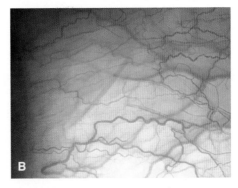

FIGURE 24-32. External subconjunctival appearance of a Xen implant. A. Arrow pointing at the exiting point of the Xen implant, approximately 3 mm posterior to the limbus. **B.** Higher magnification. (Courtesy of Dr. Kaweh Mansouri.)

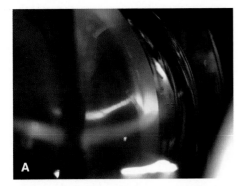
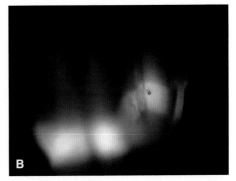

FIGURE 24-33. Xen implants. Gonioscopic internal appearance of two different Xen implants, one with a larger segment within the anterior chamber (**A** and **B**). (Courtesy of Dr. Kaweh Mansouri.)

Glaucoma Drainage Devices

Laura A. Vickers, Nathaniel C. Sears, JoAnn A. Giaconi, and Marlene R. Moster ■

DESCRIPTION

● Glaucoma drainage devices (GDDs) are designed to lower intraocular pressure (IOP). They are also known as aqueous shunts, aqueous shunting devices, or tube shunts.

● Traditionally, they have been used to lower IOP in cases of failed filtration surgery and recalcitrant and complex glaucomas, such as inflammatory, neovascular, and traumatic glaucoma. Increasingly, since the publication of the Tube versus Trabeculectomy Study that compared Baerveldt 350-mm² implants to trabeculectomy with mitomycin-C,[1] some centers are using GDDs as a primary glaucoma surgery.

● All GDDs consist of a silicone tube connected to an episcleral plate (or explant), which is made of various materials in different shapes and surface area sizes depending on the specific model (Figs. 25-1 and 25-2). The plate is placed against the sclera at the globe's equator, while the tube is inserted into the anterior chamber (or, more rarely, through the pars plana). Despite nonreactive materials, a collagenous and fibrovascular capsule (or bleb) develops around

the episcleral plate. Once within the bleb, aqueous flows passively through the wall of the capsule and is reabsorbed by venous capillaries and lymphatics.

● GDDs can be divided into restrictive and nonrestrictive devices.

■ *Nonrestrictive, or nonvalved, devices* permit the free flow of fluid from inside the eye to the episcleral plate. Nonrestrictive shunts in today's market include the various models of the Molteno and Baerveldt GDDs (Fig. 25-1). Resistance to outflow depends on the density of the capsule that forms around the plate.

■ *Restrictive, or valved, devices* incorporate a flow-controlling element within the posterior part of the tube (i.e., valve or membrane) designed to limit fluid flow in an attempt to prevent postoperative hypotony. Restrictive models available are the Ahmed (Fig. 25-2) and Krupin GDDs.

● Thus far, no one GDD model is superior to the others. The Ahmed Baerveldt Comparison Trial was a multicenter, randomized clinical trial comparing the safety and efficacy of the Ahmed FP-7 and Baerveldt 350-mm² implants. At 5-year follow-up, mean IOP was lower in the Baerveldt group on a similar number of glaucoma medications, but that there were also a greater number of early and serious complications in the Baerveldt group compared to the Ahmed group.[2] The Ahmed versus Baerveldt study also compared these two devices. After 5-year follow-up, the Baerveldt group had a significantly lower cumulative probability of failure and required fewer medications than the Ahmed group, but it also experienced more hypotony-related complications.[3]

REFERENCES

1. Gedde SJ, Schiffman JC, Feuer WJ, Herndon LW, Brandt JD, Budenz DL; Tube versus Trabeculectomy Study Group. Treatment outcomes in the Tube versus Trabeculectomy study after five years of follow-up. *Am J Ophthalmol*. 2012;153(5):789–803.
2. Budenz DL, Barton K, Gedde SJ, et al. Five-year treatment outcomes in the Ahmed Baerveldt Comparison Study. *Ophthalmology*. 2015;122(2):308–316.
3. Christakis PG, Kalenak JW, Tsai JC, et al. The Ahmed versus Baerveldt Study: five-year treatment outcomes. *Ophthalmology*. 2016;123(10):2093–2102.

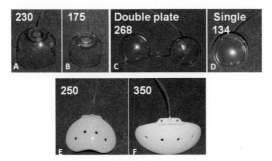

FIGURE 25-1. **Nonrestrictive glaucoma drainage devices.** Models commercially available. **A–D.** Molteno devices. The newer Molteno3 shunts (**A** and **B**) are characterized by a larger, more flexible episcleral plate than the older models (**C** and **D**). Numbers adjacent to the models indicate surface area of the episcleral plate. **E** and **F.** Baerveldt devices, the plates of which are made of barium-impregnated silicone.

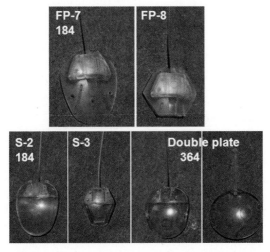

FIGURE 25-2. **Restrictive devices.** Ahmed valves come with a flexible plate (FP models) or a rigid polypropylene plate (S models). The smaller sizes are intended for pediatric eyes. The double-plate model consists of a valved plate connected to a nonvalved plate by an intervening silicone tube that crosses over a rectus muscle (in this figure, the intervening tube is not connecting the two plates on the bottom right).

SURGICAL TECHNIQUE

- Local anesthesia is recommended because some of the surgical steps can be painful without adequate anesthesia. A retrobulbar, peribulbar, or sub-Tenon's injection can be utilized.

- The superotemporal quadrant (Fig. 25-3) is the preferred location for implantation of the first GDD (additional shunts can be implanted in other quadrants). For better exposure of the surgical site, a corneal traction (Fig. 25-4) or superior rectus bridle suture is helpful. The tube should be flushed with balanced salt solution to ensure patency using a 30-gauge cannula.

- Generally, a fornix-based peritomy is used. A 90- to 110-degree conjunctival incision is adequate for single-plate implants. Stevens tenotomy scissors are used to bluntly dissect posteriorly in the quadrant to make room for the plate. The episcleral plate is placed between adjacent rectus muscles with its anterior edge at least 8 mm posterior to the limbus (Fig. 25-5). Nonabsorbable sutures (6-0 to 8-0 nylon, prolene, mersilene) are passed through the fixation holes of the episcleral plate and sutured to the sclera.

- The optimal length of tubing is estimated by laying the tube across the cornea. The tube is then trimmed, bevel up, to extend 2 to 3 mm into the anterior chamber (Fig. 25-6). A corneal paracentesis is made to provide access to the anterior chamber in case of collapse (Fig. 25-7). A 22- or 23-gauge needle is used to create a track into the anterior chamber, parallel to the plane of the iris, starting approximately 1 to 2 mm posterior to the corneoscleral limbus (Fig. 25-8). The tube is then inserted through this track into the anterior chamber with smooth forceps (Fig. 25-9).

- Proper positioning of the tube in the anterior chamber is essential, ensuring that it does not touch the iris, lens, or cornea. The tube may or may not be fixed to the sclera with sutures of 10-0 nylon or prolene (Fig. 25-10). This anterior suture is wrapped tightly around the tube to prevent movement into or out of the anterior chamber, but not so tightly that it occludes the tube lumen. To avoid conjunctival erosion by the tube, processed pericardium, donor sclera or cornea, and, less commonly, fascia lata or dura, are used to cover the anterior scleral portion of the tube (Figs. 25-11 and 25-12). The patch graft is sutured in place using interrupted sutures. Alternatively, a partial-thickness limbal-based scleral flap can be fashioned, and the tube entry is made underneath this flap, so that the sutured flap covers the tube (Figs. 25-13 and 25-14).

- The tube can also be placed through the pars plana (Figs. 25-8 to 25-31) in cases where placement into the anterior chamber is difficult or undesirable. This approach requires a pars plana vitrectomy by a retina surgeon with careful attention to remove the vitreous skirt in the quadrant where the tube will be inserted.

- During the insertion of *nonrestrictive devices*, an additional step is needed to prevent immediate and prolonged postoperative hypotony—occlusion of the tube. This step can be performed before suturing down the episcleral plate, in a number of ways. Absorbable 6-0 to 8-0 Vicryl suture can be tied around the tube so that there is no flow to the plate (Fig. 25-15). Vicryl of this size will dissolve in 4 to 8 weeks, by which time a flow-restrictive capsule will have formed around the plate. Because the tube is completely ligated, several venting slits in the anterior extrascleral portion of the tube can be made with a needle or 15-degree blade to allow some aqueous outflow in the early postoperative period. The amount of aqueous egress can be checked with a 27-gauge cannula on a syringe with saline inserted into the end of the tube. If the pressure cannot be controlled with medication during the period before the ligature dissolves, ablating the Vicryl suture with an argon laser can open the tube (the suture needs to be posterior enough to the patch graft to be seen). Another option is a ripcord suture of 5-0 nylon suture, 3-0 prolene, or 3-0 mersilene placed into the tube, entering from the plate end (Fig. 25-16). An absorbable suture is then tied around the tube and the ripcord suture (Fig. 25-17). The distal end of the ripcord is placed subconjunctivally in the inferior quadrant, where it can be accessed by cutting through the conjunctiva at the slit lamp and pulled weeks after surgery, if IOP needs to be lowered before the Vicryl suture dissolves. The ripcord suture has the advantage of not requiring treatment with an argon laser if early opening of the tube is needed, and allowing lowering of the IOP in the clinic in a more controlled environment. The third option is to tie off the intracameral portion of the tube before inserting it into the anterior chamber (Fig. 25-18). This is generally done with nylon or prolene suture, which can be lysed with the laser if IOP needs to be brought down in the postoperative period. A watertight conjunctival closure completes the procedures.

Postoperative Care

● The postoperative regimen includes a topical antibiotic for 1 to 2 weeks and topical steroids for 2 to 3 months postoperatively. Occasionally, a cycloplegic is used if there is anterior chamber shallowing. Nonsteroidal anti-inflammatory drops can also be used concomitantly.

● With restrictive devices, a hypertensive phase may develop 4 to 16 weeks postoperatively as the capsule forms. Postoperative checks should be scheduled to catch this phase as it develops, because it may

require the reintroduction of hypotensive medications.

● With nonrestrictive, ligated devices, preoperative hypotensive medications must be continued until the tube opens.

● Weekly visits should start around 5 to 6 weeks anticipating ligature opening. Hypotensive medications and inflammatory medications will be adjusted as necessary.

Complications

● Implantation of aqueous tube shunts is associated with a risk of significant postoperative complications.

● Early postoperative complications
  ▪ Hypotony: This is usually the result of excessive aqueous outflow and may lead to complications listed here.
  ▪ Hypotony maculopathy (Figs. 25-19 and 25-20)
  ▪ Flat anterior chamber (Fig. 25-21)
  ▪ Choroidal effusions (Figs. 25-22 to 25-24)
  ▪ Suprachoroidal hemorrhage (Fig. 25-25)
  ▪ Aqueous misdirection (Fig. 25-26)
  ▪ Hyphema
  ▪ Ocular hypertension: High IOP can be related to occlusion of the tube by fibrin (Fig. 25-27), a blood clot, iris, or vitreous. Fibrin or blood may resolve spontaneously. An intracameral injection of tissue plasminogen activator may help dissolve the clot within a few hours but can be associated with severe bleeding. When iris tissue occludes the lumen of the tube, neodymium (Nd):YAG laser iridotomy or argon laser iridoplasty may reestablish the patency of the tube. Vitreous incarceration can be successfully treated with Nd:YAG laser, but an anterior vitrectomy may be necessary to prevent recurrence.

- Late postoperative complications

  - Ocular hypertension: Late failure with increased IOP is usually caused by excessive fibrosis around the plate.

  - Hypotony

  - Conjunctival erosion over the tube (Fig. 25-28) or episcleral plate

  - Corneal edema or decompensation (Fig. 25-29): Corneal decompensation may result from direct contact between the tube and the cornea. When the tube is touching the cornea, repositioning of the tube should be considered, especially in cases where there is a risk of endothelial failure (i.e., cases with focal corneal edema, or after penetrating keratoplasty).

  - Tube retraction, migration, or malposition: Figure 25-30 shows a tube that has eroded through the cornea and is resting on the cornea's surface. Tubes placed in young pediatric eyes are especially prone to changing position within the anterior chamber over time because the cornea and sclera are pliable and do not always hold the tube in place (Fig. 25-31).

  - Cataract

  - Diplopia: Mechanical restriction of the extraocular muscles by the bleb or episcleral plate can cause diplopia. If diplopia is persistent and not responsive to prisms, the shunt may need to be removed or relocated.

  - Retinal detachment: This can occur if the needle pass to secure the episcleral plate goes through full thickness sclera and retina.

  - Endophthalmitis

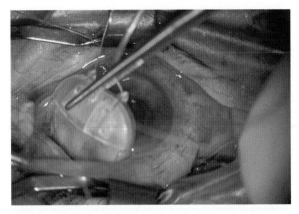

FIGURE 25-3. Superotemporal quadrant. Placement of an Ahmed tube shunt in the superotemporal quadrant of the eye receiving the first glaucoma drainage device.

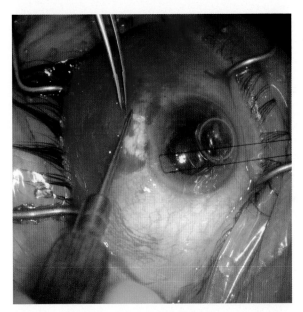

FIGURE 25-4. Traction suture. A superior traction suture of 6-0 silk placed through corneal stroma allows infraduction of the eye for better exposure of the superotemporal quadrant.

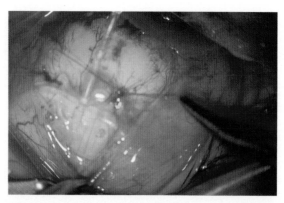

FIGURE 25-5. Scleral fixation. Ahmed tube shunt sewn down to sclera 8–10 mm posterior to the limbus using a nonabsorbable suture.

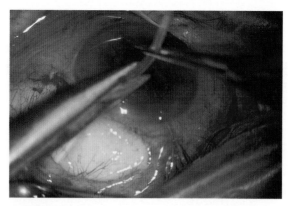

FIGURE 25-6. Tube trimming. Before insertion in the eye, the tube is trimmed to an appropriate length with Westcott scissors so that it will rest 2 to 3 mm long within the anterior chamber. When cut, the bevel should face upward to decrease the risk of iris incarceration into the tube.

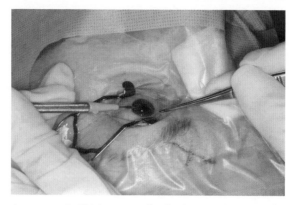

FIGURE 25-7. Corneal paracentesis. This is not considered to be a mandatory step, but in the case of anterior chamber collapse intraoperatively or flat chamber postoperatively, it allows access to reform the anterior chamber.

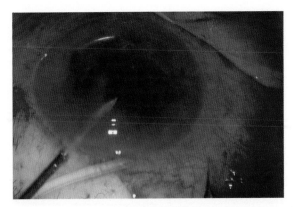

FIGURE 25-8. Track creation. A 23-gauge needle entering the anterior chamber before placement of the tube. This track should be created at the posterior surgical limbus for ideal tube position.

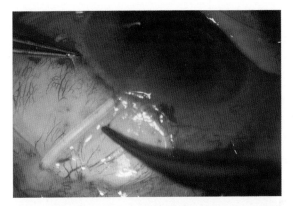

FIGURE 25-9. Tube insertion. Placement of the tube shunt into the anterior chamber.

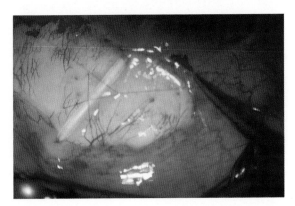

FIGURE 25-10. Tube fixation. Suturing the tube shunt to the sclera with 10-0 nylon. This type of suture can help direct the tube toward a track that is not directly in front of it (i.e., it can change the course of the track, so that it will hold a bend where the suture is placed), or it can be used to help prevent movement of the tube. This is an optional step.

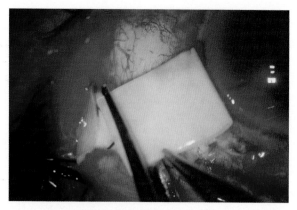

FIGURE 25-11. **Patch graft.** A pericardial patch graft is placed over the tube before suturing it to the episclera at two to four corners.

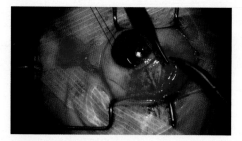

FIGURE 25-12. **Corneal patch graft.** A split-thickness corneal patch graft may be used to cover the tube.

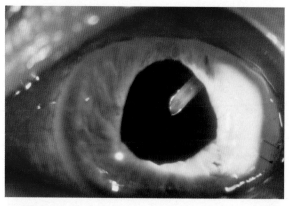

FIGURE 25-13. **Pars plana tube shunt.** The tube enters through the sclerostomy used for pars plana vitrectomy.

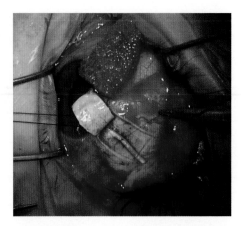

FIGURE 25-14. **Scleral flap.** A partial-thickness scleral flap can be fashioned to cover the tube. A corneal patch graft may be placed on top of the scleral flap. (Courtesy of Dr. Simon K. Law.)

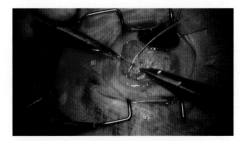

FIGURE 25-15. **Ligature suture.** A 6-0 Vicryl suture may be used to ligate the nonrestrictive Baerveldt tube.

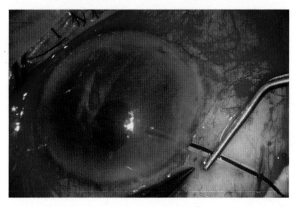

FIGURE 25-16. **Latina or ripcord suture.** The Baerveldt 350-mm^2 tube shunt with prepared ripcord placed in the anterior chamber.

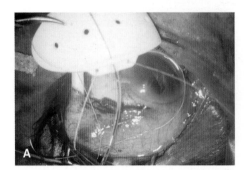

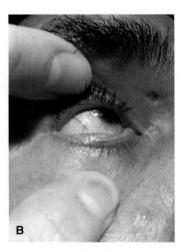

FIGURE 25-17. **Ripcord suture. A.** Ripcord suture easily seen within the lumen of tube. The absorbable Vicryl suture is tied tightly around the tube with ripcord to prevent outflow. **B.** Subconjunctival end of a ripcord is visible in the postoperative eye.

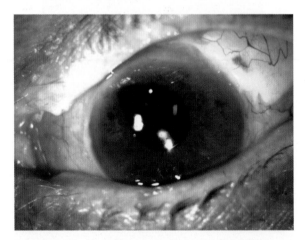

FIGURE 25-18. **Ligature suture.** Nonabsorbable suture ligating intracameral tube.

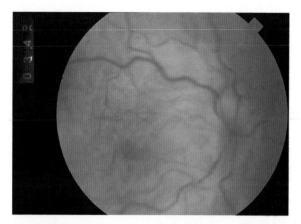

FIGURE 25-19. **Chronic hypotony.** Chronic hypotony with maculopathy and choroidal folds.

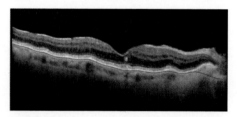

FIGURE 25-20. **Hypotony maculopathy.** An optical coherence tomography image of hypotony maculopathy in a patient with decreased vision and low intraocular pressure.

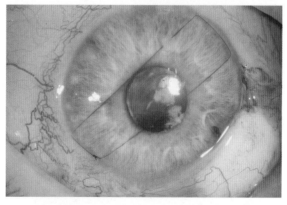

FIGURE 25-21. **Shallow anterior chamber.** Shallow anterior chamber following tube shunt with chamber-maintaining suture holding back the lens implant.

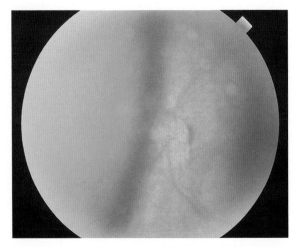

FIGURE 25-22. Choroidal effusion. Fundus photograph showing serous choroidal detachment impinging on the optic nerve.

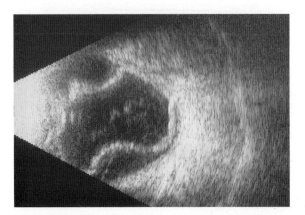

FIGURE 25-23. Choroidal detachment. B-scan ultrasound of serous choroidal detachments.

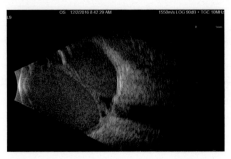

FIGURE 25-24. Choroidal effusion. A B-scan image of large hemorrhagic choroidal effusions after placement of an Ahmed valve.

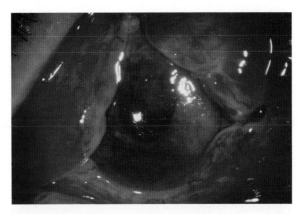

FIGURE 25-25. **Suprachoroidal hemorrhage.** Slit-lamp photograph of an eye with suprachoroidal hemorrhage; the retina can be seen through the pupil.

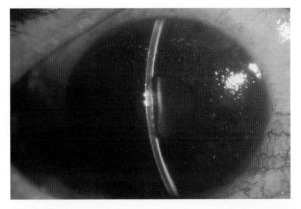

FIGURE 25-26. **Aqueous misdirection.** Slit-lamp photograph of an eye with aqueous misdirection. There is a flat anterior chamber and an elevated intraocular pressure.

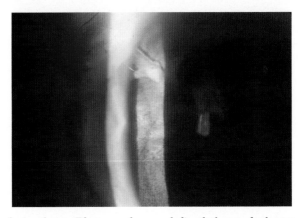

FIGURE 25-27. **Implant occlusion.** Fibrous membrane occluding the lumen of a glaucoma drainage device.

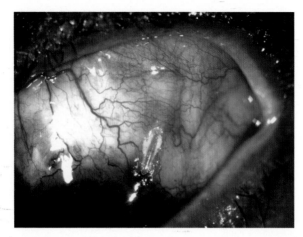

FIGURE 25-28. **Conjunctival erosion.** Erosion of the conjunctiva over the anterior scleral portion of a glaucoma drainage device near the limbus. There is an increased risk of endophthalmitis with this complication. (Courtesy of Simon Law, MD.)

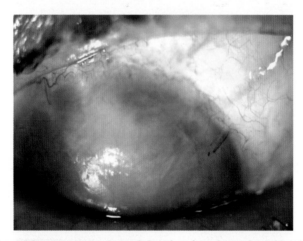

FIGURE 25-29. **Corneal decompensation.** Pericardial patch graft overlying tube visible at limbus in decompensated cornea.

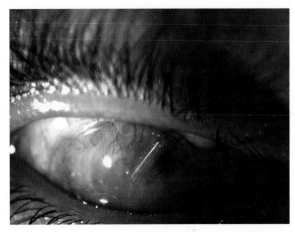

FIGURE 25-30. Tube malposition. Tube erosion through the cornea and resting on the surface of the cornea. (Courtesy of Simon Law, MD.)

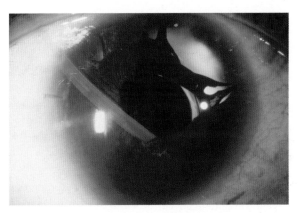

FIGURE 25-31. Implant migration. Migration of the tube shunt anteriorly into the anterior chamber in a 14-year-old patient with congenital cataract and glaucoma.

Schlemm Canal–Based Surgery

Richard A. Lewis and Jacob W. Brubaker ◼

INTRODUCTION

The surgical treatment of elevated intraocular pressure (IOP) at the site of outflow obstruction has long been a goal of glaucoma management. Canal-based surgery is not new. In fact, trabeculectomy was first described as a way to enhance outflow through the excised trabecular meshwork (TM) into the canal. Although further studies revealed that trabeculectomy functioned by directed flow to the subconjunctival space, the search for a safe and effective canal-based surgery did not stop. The current interest in procedures in and around the canal is the result of a number of factors, including the complications that arise in the early and late postoperative period after trabeculectomy. It is also the result of the development of more sophisticated surgical instruments and devices that allowed easier access to the canal. These procedures can now be partitioned into three basic categories.

Canal dilating: ab externo canaloplasty, ab interno canaloplasty, and Visco360

TM ablating: Trabectome, Kahook Dual Blade (KDB), gonioscopy-assisted

transluminal trabeculotomy (GATT), and Trab 360

Canal stenting: iStent

INDICATIONS

• Canal-based procedures have been used successfully in the full spectrum of open-angle glaucomas, from congenital to adult primary open angle including pigmentary and pseudoexfoliation.

• Ab externo procedures require an open angle, whereas ab interno procedures can sometimes be successful in previously closed angles.

• Clear media is necessary for the ab interno–based procedures.

• Ab externo canaloplasty can be performed in the presence of hazy media or scarred cornea.

CANALOPLASTY

The concept of nonpenetrating glaucoma surgery has evolved as an alternative to full- or partial-thickness procedures that rely on subconjunctival flow and a bleb. The complex and unique individual variability of these procedures because of wound healing led to the search for a more direct surgical treatment of glaucoma. The first nonpenetrating procedure to utilize a microcatheter (iTrack, Ellex Medical Lasers Ltd, Adelaide, Australia) to take advantage of the full extent of the canal was canaloplasty, first described in 2007.

Mechanism of Action

● Ultrasound studies of patients with primary open-angle glaucoma (POAG) demonstrate collapse or narrowing of the canal of Schlemm. During the procedure, the canal is dilated, the TM is tensioned, and after removal of the deep scleral flap, a Descemet window is created.

● Canaloplasty is thought to lower IOP primarily by enhancing conventional circumferential outflow through the canal and the collector system. Studies using dyes and viscoelastic have confirmed enhanced intraoperative outflow in this manner. The greater the canal suture tension, the greater the IOP-lowering effect. Whether this continues to function months to years postoperatively has not been validated. Structural dilation of the canal has been demonstrated for at least 2 years (Fig. 26-1).

● Other sites of drainage have been postulated. These include percolation or flow through Descemet window into a "scleral lake." Some patients are noted to have formation of a bleb, suggesting a transscleral flow or a "mini" perforation through the window.

Technique

● After creating a superficial scleral flap with a 4-mm base, a deeper scleral flap is used to access the canal (Fig. 26-2).

● The iTrack microcatheter (Fig. 26-3) is placed in the canal and threaded for the full 360 degrees until it comes out the other end.

● A 10-0 prolene suture is attached to the distal end and the catheter is withdrawn while injecting viscoelastic. The remaining prolene suture is tied tightly, creating tension in the meshwork to enhance outflow into the canal.

● Before suturing the superficial flap and conjunctiva, the deeper scleral flap is excised, leaving a Descemet window to further enhance outflow (Fig. 26-4).

● Blebs are avoided.

Outcomes

● On the basis of the published data, canaloplasty efficacy results are comparable to the published reports of trabeculectomy. Mean IOP at 2 years decreased to 16.2 mm Hg in eyes having canaloplasty alone. In eyes undergoing combined canaloplasty and cataract surgery, IOP decreased to 13.7 mm Hg and medication use decreased to 0.6 and 0.2, respectively

● Studies demonstrate that canaloplasty is safer than trabeculectomy. Hypotony, choroidal detachment, and bleb infections were reported in less than 1% of all cases. The most common side effect is transient hyphema.

BIBLIOGRAPHY

Lewis RA, von Wolff K, Tetz M, et al. Canaloplasty: circumferential viscodilation and tensioning of Schlemm's canal using a flexible microcatheter for the treatment of open-angle glaucoma in adults: interim clinical study analysis. *J Cataract Refract Surg.* 2007;33:1217–1226.

Lewis RA, von Wolff K, Tetz M, et al. Canaloplasty: circumferential viscodilation and tensioning of Schlemm's canal using a flexible microcatheter for the treatment of open-angle glaucoma in adults: two-year interim clinical study results. *J Cataract Refract Surg.* 2009;35: 814–824.

Shingleton B, Tetz M, Korber N. Circumferential viscodilation and tensioning of Schlemm canal (canaloplasty) with temporal clear corneal phacoemulsification cataract surgery for open-angle glaucoma and visually significant cataract: one-year results. *J Cataract Refract Surg.* 2008;34:433–440.

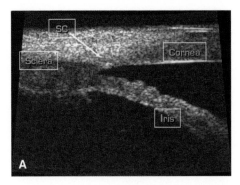
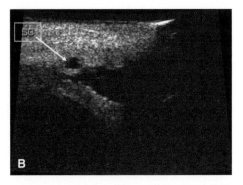

FIGURE 26-1. **Canaloplasty effect.** Ultrasound image of canal preoperatively (**A**) and 2 years postoperatively (**B**). **A.** The collapsed canal in open-angle glaucoma suggests limited flow. **B.** Canaloplasty viscodilates the canal during surgery and facilitates drainage into the collectors. SC, Schlemm canal.

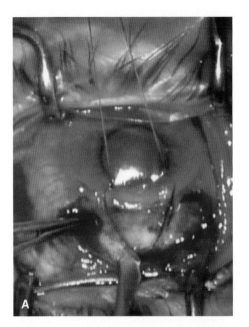
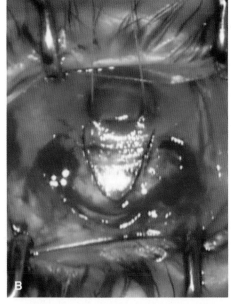

FIGURE 26-2. **Scleral dissection.** A guarded blade is used to create a 300-μm partial-thickness groove (**A** and **B**), followed by sharp dissection to create a sclerocorneal flap (**C**).

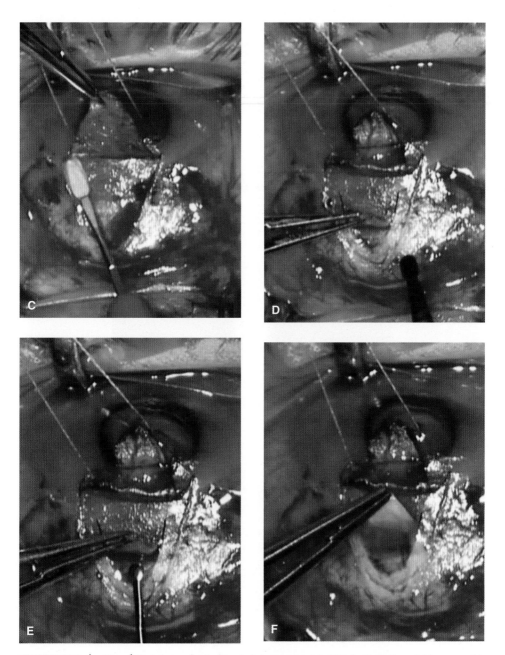

FIGURE 26-2. (*continued*) **D.** A deeper flap is dissected at approximately 99% depth. **E.** Once Schlemm canal is unroofed, a modified Drysdale spatula is used to bluntly dissect the inner corneoscleral flap from Descemet membrane with careful attention not to rupture and enter the anterior chamber. **F.** The appearance of both dissected flaps; there is some blood reflux from each end of the exposed Schlemm canal.

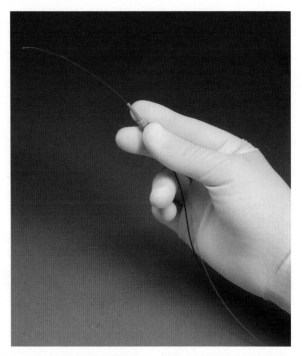

FIGURE 26-3. iTrack 250A canaloplasty microcatheter. The 200-μm-diameter catheter with a 250-μm tip is attached to a battery-powered light source with a second attachment to facilitate injecting viscoelastic to dilate the canal upon removal. (Courtesy of iScience Interventional.)

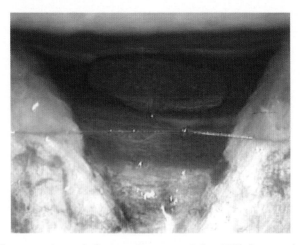

FIGURE 26-4. Prolene suture in canal adjacent to Descemet window. With the removal of the microcannula, the two ends of the attached prolene suture are tied tight. Note the large clear Descemet window after excising the deep scleral flap.

TRABECULAR MESHWORK ABLATING PROCEDURES: TRABECTOME, KAHOOK DUAL BLADE, AND GONIOSCOPY-ASSISTED TRANSLUMINAL TRABECULOTOMY

These procedures represent ab interno procedures designed to reduce IOP by enhancing drainage into the canal by removing the TM. They can be combined with cataract surgery or be done as stand-alone procedures. Trabectome (NeoMedix Inc., Tustin, CA) was the first widely adopted TM ablating procedure, becoming commercially available in 2006 (Fig. 26-5). It allows the surgeon to remove about 100 to 120 degrees of the nasal TM with the use of plasma-mediated ablation. GATT (Ellex Medical Lasers Ltd, Adelaide, Australia) and KDB (New World Medical, Rancho Cucamonga, CA) represent newer approaches to the same procedure. GATT accomplishes an ab interno 360-degree incision of the TM using the iTrack catheter or prolene suture passed through an ab interno incision of the TM. The KDB acts in a manner similar to that of Trabectome using a dual blade rather than plasma-mediated ablation to remove a similar portion of the TM.

Mechanism of Action

- It is generally agreed that the primary site of resistance in open-angle glaucoma resides in the juxtacanalicular area. These procedures ablate or incise the juxtacanalicular area to eliminate the area of resistance, creating a direct flow into the canal and collectors.

- The absence of resistance has other implications. In settings of elevated episcleral pressure (as might occur when a patient's head is positioned lower than the heart), there is concern about blood reflux from the collector channels back into the canal and anterior chamber and potentially inducing a hyphema.

Technique: Trabectome

- The surgery uses a Swan-Jacob gonioprism for direct visualization. To maximize the angle structures, the patient's head is positioned opposite to the eye receiving treatment.

- After creating a clear corneal paracentesis site, a viscoelastic is used to maintain anterior chamber depth.

- The electrosurgical pulse is applied through the handpiece to remove 3 to 6 clock hours of TM.

- The Trabectome handpiece simultaneously irrigates, ablates, and aspirates the treated area (Fig. 26-6).

Technique: Gonioscopy-assisted transluminal trabeculotomy

- Similar to the Trabectome, the surgery uses a gonioprism for direct visualization of the TM.

- After creating a paracentesis site that will later be used to pass the suture or iTrack microcatheter, a viscoelastic is used to maintain anterior chamber depth after which a main corneal incision is made in the temporal clear cornea.

- The microcatheter or prolene is placed through the paracentesis. An incision is then made in the nasal TM. The microcatheter or 5-0 prolene suture is then inserted into the meshwork through this incision and passed 360 degrees around the canal until the tip exits out the other side of the incision.

- The two ends are grasped and the meshwork is incised for 360 degrees (Fig. 26-7).

Technique: Kahook Dual Blade

- Similar to other ab interno procedures, a surgical gonioprism is used for direct visualization of the TM.

- After creating a clear corneal paracentesis site, viscoelastic is used to maintain anterior chamber depth after which a main corneal incision is made in the temporal clear cornea.

• The KDB is then introduced through the main incision and the TM is engaged with the tip of the blade. An incision is created removing 100 to 120 degrees of meshwork. Often, this generates a strip of TM that can be removed with microforceps (**Figs. 26-8** and 9).

Outcomes

• A case series of Trabectome suggested an IOP reduction of 40% for up to 2 years. Success rates (defined as a decrease in IOP by 20% and decrease in medications to achieve target IOP) were 78% and 64% at 6 and 12 months, respectively. However, sample size attrition was a significant issue.

• A subsequent Trabectome study showed a much lower success rate of between 30% at 1 year, with success being defined as a decrease in IOP <21 mm Hg and >20% from baseline as well as the lack of hypotony or need for additional glaucoma surgery.

• A retrospective review of 85 patients who underwent GATT showed a pressure reduction of 11.1 mm Hg and a decrease in glaucoma medications of 1.1 at 12 months in the POAG group (*n* = 57). The procedure seems to be even more effective in the secondary glaucoma group, achieving an IOP reduction of 19.2 mm Hg and a decrease in glaucoma medications by 1.9 (*n* = 28). Transient hyphemia was seen in 30% of patients at 1 week.

• Other studies have shown the utility of both GATT and KDB in congenital glaucoma and juvenile open-angle glaucoma.

• The presence of blood reflux at the conclusion of the procedure is confirmation of reduced outflow resistance. This is a transient complication that usually resolves within 1 to 2 weeks.

• Other possible complications such as infection, wound leak, and choroidal effusion are seldom seen.

• The value of these procedures is their relative technical ease performing the surgery. Also, these ab interno procedures allow sparing of the conjunctiva; thus, future filtering or drainage device surgery will not be compromised.

BIBLIOGRAPHY

Francis BA, Minckler DS, Dustin L, et al. Combined cataract extraction and trabeculectomy by internal approach for coexisting cataract and open-angle glaucoma. *J Cataract Refract Surg.* 2008;34:1096–1103.

Francis BA, See RF, Rao NA, et al. Ab interno trabeculectomy: development of a novel device (Trabectome) and surgery for open-angle glaucoma. *J Glaucoma.* 2006;15:68–73.

Grover DS, Godfrey DG, Smith O, et al. Gonioscopy-assisted transluminal trabeculotomy, ab interno trabeculotomy: technique report and preliminary results. *Ophthalmology.* 2014;121:855–861.

Grover DS, Smith O, Fellman RL, et al. Gonioscopy assisted transluminal trabeculotomy: an ab interno circumferential trabeculotomy for the treatment of primary congenital glaucoma and juvenile open angle glaucoma. *Br J Ophthalmol.* 2015;99:1092–1096.

Jea SY, Francis BA, Vakili G, et al. Ab interno trabeculectomy (Trabectome) versus trabeculectomy for open angle glaucoma. *Ophthalmology.* 2012;119:36–42.

Jea SY, Mosaed S, Vold SD, et al. Effect of failed Trabectome on subsequent trabeculectomy. *J Glaucoma.* 2012;21(2):71–75.

Khouri AS, Wong SH. Ab interno trabeculectomy with a dual blade: surgical technique for childhood glaucoma. *J Glaucoma.* 2017;26(8):749–751.

Minckler DS, Baerveldt G, Alfaro MR, et al. Clinical results with the Trabectome for treatment of open-angle glaucoma. *Ophthalmology.* 2005;112:962–967.

Minckler DS, Baerveldt G, Ramirez MA, et al. Clinical results with the Trabectome, a novel surgical device for the treatment of open-angle glaucoma. *Trans Am Ophthalmol Soc.* 2006;104:40–50.

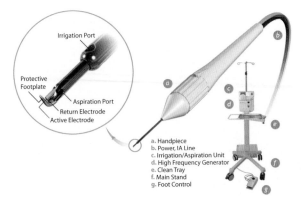

Irrigation Port

Protective
Footplate

Aspiration Port

Return Electrode

Active Electrode

a. Handpiece
b. Power, IA Line
c. Irrigation/Aspiration Unit
d. High Frequency Generator
e. Clean Tray
f. Main Stand
g. Foot Control

FIGURE 26-5. Trabectome handpiece and setup. The irrigation sleeve ends 5 mm above the tip. The footplate is 800 μm heel to tip, with a maximum width of 230 μm and maximum thickness of 110 μm. The gap between the electrocautery pole and the footplate is 150 μm. (Courtesy of NeoMedix Corporation, Tustin, CA.)

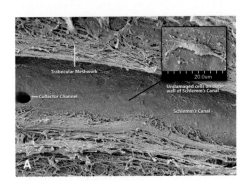

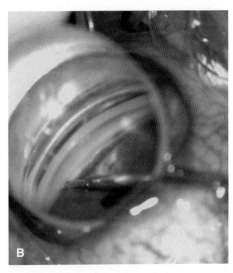

FIGURE 26-6. Trabectome. A. Canal view following Trabectome procedure exposing the trabecular meshwork and collectors. (Courtesy of NeoMedix Corporation, Tustin, CA.) **B.** Intraoperative view of Trabectome procedure. The tip is within Schlemm canal and moving to the left. Behind the probe, the opalescent colored outer wall of Schlemm canal can be seen extending from the right of the probe to the edge of the mirror.

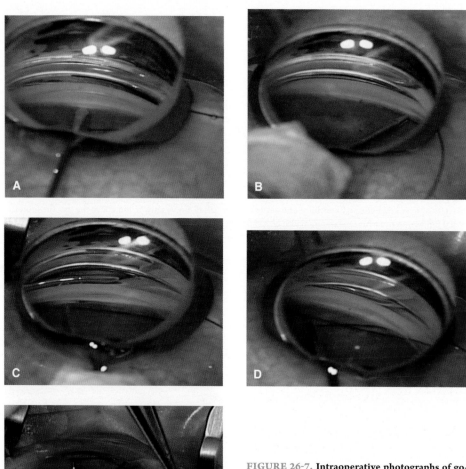

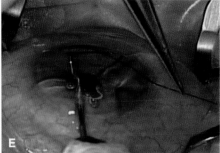

FIGURE 26-7. **Intraoperative photographs of gonioscopy-assisted transluminal trabeculotomy.** The incision is made in the trabecular meshwork under gonioscopic view (**A**). The prepared prolene suture is placed into the canal and advanced 360 (**B** and **C**). The ends are grasped (**D**) and removed (**E**), creating a 360 degree trabeculotomy. (Courtesy of Davinder S. Grover, Glaucoma Associates of Texas, Dallas, TX.)

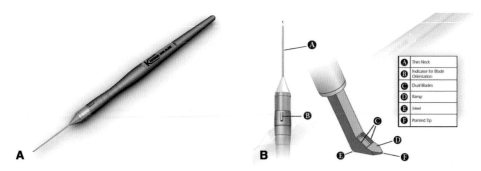

FIGURE 26-8. Kahook Dual Blade. A. Wide view of blade with handle. **B.** Blade details, showing the dual blade and the ramp, heel, and tip. (Courtesy of New World Medical, Rancho Cucamonga, CA.)

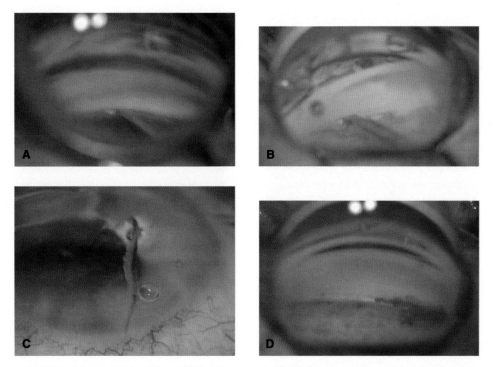

FIGURE 26-9. Intraoperative photos of Kahook Dual Blade. The blade is advanced toward the trabecular meshwork (**A**) and the trabecular meshwork is engaged. Once properly seated in the canal, the blade is advanced through the canal, creating a strip of excised meshwork (**B**). The removed strip reveals both pigmented and nonpigmented trabecular meshwork (**C**). Blood reflux is visualized following removal of the nasal trabecular meshwork (**D**).

iSTENT

The iStent trabecular micro-bypass system (Glaukos, Laguna Hills, CA) is also a minimally invasive ab interno device placed through the canal. It is a heparin-coated, nonferromagnetic, surgical-grade titanium stent approximately 0.3 mm in height (Fig. 26-10) that is considered the smallest implant placed in humans.

Mechanism of Action

• While small, the stent is of sufficient size to maintain a stable position in the TM, yet also allowing for multiple implants (Fig. 26-11). When successfully placed through the TM, the iStent reestablishes outflow and reduces IOP.

• Studies have suggested that placing more than one stent provides greater IOP lowering.

Technique

• The iStent is inserted through a small temporal clear corneal incision, generally, in the nasal quadrant.

• With one lumen extending into the anterior chamber and the other into the canal, the resistance imposed by the TM is reduced (Fig. 26-12).

Outcomes

• The iStent appears to be safe and effective.

• It is often placed at the time of cataract surgery. Implanting the iStent in conjunction with cataract surgery resulted in a mean IOP reduction of 5.1 mm Hg. The stent also reduced the mean number of medications (1.1 fewer medications).

• At 1 year, 66% of eyes treated with combined cataract surgery and the iStent achieved 20% IOP reduction without medication.

• Adverse events reported include stent lumen obstruction, iris touch by device, and malpositioning of the stent. Hyphema was reported to be transient.

• No changes were noted in the endothelium; no hypotony, flat chambers, or choroidal effusion.

BIBLIOGRAPHY

Bahler CK, Smedley GT, Zhou J, et al. Trabecular bypass stents decrease intraocular pressure in cultured human anterior segments. *Am J Ophthalmol.* 2004;138:988–994.

Samuelson TW, Katz LJ, Wells JM, et al. Randomized evaluation of the trabecular micro-bypass stent with phacoemulsification in patients with glaucoma and cataract. *Ophthalmology.* 2011;118:459–467.

Spiegel D, Wetzel W, Neuhann T, et al. Coexistent primary open-angle glaucoma and cataract: interim analysis of a trabecular micro-bypass stent and concurrent cataract surgery. *Eur J Ophthalmol.* 2009;19:393–399.

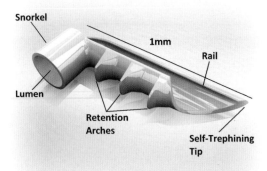

FIGURE 26-10. **iStent.** Surgical-grade titanium with two openings and ridged tube to provide greater retention in the canal. (Courtesy of Glaukos, Laguna Hills, CA.)

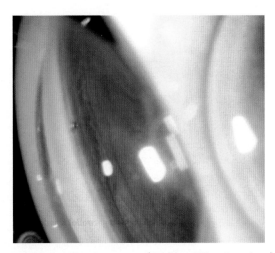

FIGURE 26-11. **iStent.** Postoperative iStent appearance. (Courtesy of Tom Samuelson.)

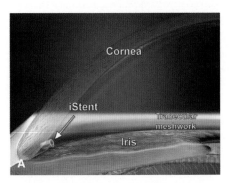
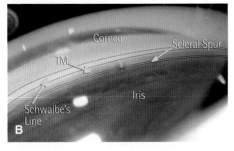

FIGURE 26-12. **iStent positioning. A.** Optimal position of the stent. **B.** iStent placed through the trabecular meshwork positioned in the canal. Note the proximity of the iStent in relation to the landmarks of the angle. (Courtesy of Glaukos, Laguna Hills, CA.)

Cyclodestructive Procedures for Glaucoma

Marisse M. Solano, Shan C. Lin, Geoffrey P. Schwartz, and Louis W. Schwartz ■

INTRODUCTION

Intraocular pressure is the major risk factor for glaucoma that ophthalmologists are able to control. Medically, either eye drops or pills are used to decrease aqueous production or increase aqueous outflow to effectively lower intraocular pressure. Most surgical and laser procedures, including trabeculectomy, tube shunts, goniotomy, iridectomies, laser trabeculoplasty, and laser iridotomy, decrease the intraocular pressure by increasing outflow. Cyclodestructive procedures are designed to destroy the ciliary processes, thereby decreasing aqueous production. Because of the unpredictability of these procedures in lowering intraocular pressure and the complications associated with their use, such cyclodestructive procedures are often considered a surgery of last resort. However, recent studies and practices have employed these procedures as a first-line surgery and even before medication treatment.

INDICATIONS

● Cyclodestruction of the ciliary body has traditionally been reserved for use in patients who have failed previous treatment with medicines or surgeries.

● Exceptions to this rule include patients who are not willing to undergo filtration surgery, those who cannot undergo surgery owing to medical conditions, and patients in underdeveloped countries. In underdeveloped countries, where medical care is expensive and not always available, diode contact transscleral cyclophotocoagulation (CPC), which is portable and relatively easy to use, may be effective and safe as the first line of treatment for glaucoma, although the energy delivered is typically lower than that used in nonseeing eyes.

● Nonpenetrating forms of CPC may have benefit in controlling pain in blind, painful eyes, and may allow the patient to avoid removal of the eye as long as visualization or ultrasound reveals no intraocular tumor.

■ Types of glaucoma that have been treated with varying degrees of success include end-stage open-angle glaucoma; neovascular glaucoma; glaucoma post penetrating keratoplasty; advanced angle closure, both primary and secondary; traumatic glaucoma; malignant glaucoma; silicone oil glaucoma; congenital glaucoma; pseudophakic and aphakic open-angle glaucoma; and secondary open-angle glaucoma.

■ Alternative treatments that are usually considered in this group of patients include filtering surgery with antimetabolite or tube shunts.

● Transscleral CPC, micropulse CPC, and endoscopic cyclophotocoagulation (ECP) have been used in cases of relatively good potential vision.[1,2] In the case of ECP, this is often in the setting of combined cases with cataract surgery.[2] Inflammation and cystoid macular edema (CME) are not infrequent complications and should be anticipated and prevented with appropriate steroid therapy.

CONTRAINDICATIONS

● There are relatively few strict contraindications to the various forms of CPC.

● A phakic patient with good vision has historically been the primary contraindication; however, recent studies have used transscleral CPC and ECP in such cases.[1,2]

● Marked uveitis is a relative contraindication because patients have increased inflammation and risk for CME following the treatment; care should be taken to try to quiet the eye as much as possible before the procedure. However, uveitic glaucoma is one of the secondary glaucomas that have been treated successfully with ECP and transscleral CPC.

● For all of the nonpenetrating forms of CPC, the procedure is usually performed in the office, and patient cooperation is required; inability to cooperate may be a contraindication in such cases.

● For ECP, very poor visual potential (no light perception or hand motions) is a contraindication because there are potential risks for endophthalmitis and choroidal hemorrhage with this intraocular surgery.

● Newer technologies such as micropulse transscleral cyclophotocoagulation (MP TCP) and ECP allow for the use of cyclodestructive procedures in eyes with better visual prognosis.

REFERENCES

1. Egbert PR, Fiadoyor S, Budenz DL, et al. Diode laser transscleral cyclophotocoagulation as a primary surgical treatment for primary open-angle glaucoma. *Arch Ophthalmol.* 2001;119(3):345–350.
2. Chen J, Cohn RA, Lin SC, et al. Endoscopic photocoagulation of the ciliary body for treatment of refractory glaucomas. *Am J Ophthalmol.* 1997;124(6):787–796.

TECHNIQUES

Several techniques are used for cyclodestruction. They include noncontact transscleral CPC, contact transscleral CPC, MP TCP, cyclocryotherapy, transpupillary CPC, and ECP. All of the procedures may be repeated and the nonpenetrating forms may often require multiple treatments.

NONCONTACT TRANSSCLERAL CYCLOPHOTOCOAGULATION

- A neodymium (Nd):YAG laser is used to perform noncontact CPC. In the past, a semiconductor diode laser, Microlase (Keeler, Inc., Broomall, PA), was also utilized.[1]

- Retrobulbar anesthesia is given.

- A lid speculum is placed if a contact lens is not used.

- A contact lens developed by Bruce Shields may or may not be used. The contact lens has the advantages of having markers at 1-mm intervals to better judge the distance from the limbus, blocking some of the laser light from entering the pupil, and blanching an inflamed conjunctiva to decrease superficial charring of the conjunctiva[2] (Fig. 27-1).

- Eight to 10 burns are placed 1 to 3 mm (optimal: 1.5 mm) from the limbus for 180 to 360 degrees, taking care to avoid the 3 and 9 o'clock meridians in order to avoid coagulating the long posterior ciliary arteries and causing anterior segment necrosis. Energy levels of 4 to 8 J are used. The laser beam is focused on the conjunctiva; however, the laser is defocused such that its effect is actually 3.6 mm beyond the conjunctival surface, with most of the energy being absorbed by the ciliary body (Fig. 27-2). In general, the greater the energy levels used, the greater is the inflammation.[3–5]

REFERENCES

1. Hennis HL, Stewart WC. Semi-conductor diode laser transscleral cyclophotocoagulation in patients with glaucoma. *Am J Ophthalmol.* 1992;113:81–85.
2. Simmons RB, Blasini M, Shields MD, et al. Comparison of transscleral neodymium:YAG cyclophotocoagulation with and without a contact lens in human autopsy eyes. *Am J Ophthalmol.* 1990;109:174–179.
3. Frankhauser F, Van der Zypen E, Kwasniewska S, et al. Transscleral cyclophotocoagulation using a neodymium YAG laser. *Ophthalmic Surg Lasers.* 1986;1:125–141.
4. Schwartz LW, Moster MR. Neodymium:YAG laser transscleral cyclodiathermy. *Ophthalmic Laser Ther.* 1986;1:135–141.
5. Crymes BM, Gross RL. Laser placement in noncontact Nd:YAG cyclophotocoagulation. *Am J Ophthalmol.* 1990;110:670–673.

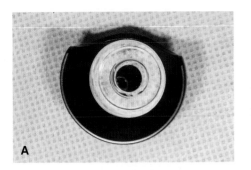
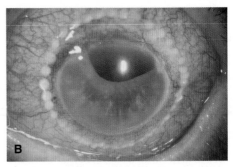

FIGURE 27-1. Noncontact transscleral cyclophotocoagulation. A. Shields lens. Shields lens for noncontact transscleral cyclophotocoagulation. **B.** Placement of laser burns 1.5 mm from the limbus. Note blanching of inflamed conjunctiva.

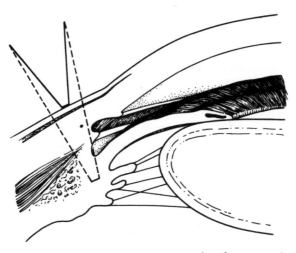

FIGURE 27-2. Noncontact transscleral cyclophotocoagulation (CPC). Diagram of noncontact transscleral CPC showing that the laser energy is actually focused within the ciliary body.

CONTACT TRANSSCLERAL CYCLOPHOTOCOAGULATION

- This technique is currently the most popular nonpenetrating cyclodestructive procedure. It uses a contact diode laser probe that is relatively small and portable (G-Probe; IRIDEX Corporation, Mountain View, CA). Krypton and Nd:YAG lasers have also been used to perform contact transscleral CPC.[1-3]

- In this technique, retrobulbar anesthesia is given and a lid speculum is placed.

- The patient is placed in the supine position.

- The "heel edge" (as opposed to the tip portion) of the probe is placed at the limbus. Because of the design of the G-probe, the energy is actually delivered 1.2 mm from the limbus; approximately 30 applications of 1.5 to 2.0 W of energy are applied for 1.5 to 2 seconds over 360 degrees, avoiding the 3 and 9 o'clock positions (Fig. 27-3).

- The energy level is titrated to be slightly below (250 mW lower) the audible pop, because audible pops are associated with greater inflammation and hyphema.[4]

REFERENCES

1. Schuman JS, Puliafito CA, Allingham RR, et al. Contact transscleral continuous wave neodymium:YAG laser cyclophotocoagulation. *Ophthalmology*. 1990;97:571–580.
2. Schuman JS, Bellows AR, Shingleton BJ, et al. Contact transscleral Nd:YAG laser cyclophotocoagulation: midterm results. *Ophthalmology*. 1992;99:1089–1095.
3. Immonen IJ, Puska P, Raitta C. Transscleral contact krypton laser cyclophotocoagulation for treatment of glaucoma. *Ophthalmology*. 1994;101(5):876–882.
4. Allingham RR, DeKater AW, Bellows AR, et al. Probe placement and power levels in contact transscleral neodymium:YAG cyclophotocoagulation. *Arch Ophthalmol*. 1990;109:738–742.

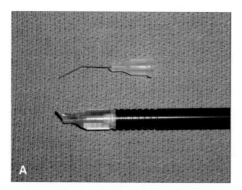
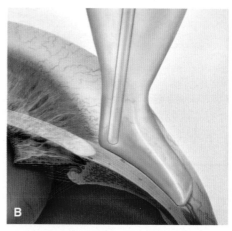

FIGURE 27-3. Contact transscleral cyclophotocoagulation. A. G-probe for diode laser treatment. **B.** Diagram showing the placement of the G-probe relative to the limbus, so that laser application is at the ciliary body.

MICROPULSE TRANSSCLERAL CYCLOPHOTOCOAGULATION

- MP TPC was approved by the U.S. Food and Drug Administration in 2015 (IRIDEX Laser Systems, IRIDEX Corporation, Mountain View, CA).

- A circular probe delivers the energy by applying laser approximately 2 mm behind the limbus, with a continuous movement back and forth from the limbus at the horizontal meridian.

- Transscleral diode laser is delivered in repetitive microsecond pulses interspersed with intermittent rest periods.[1–3]

- It can be performed under retrobulbar or general anesthesia.[1–3]

- Energy used is 2,000 mW for 80 seconds on each hemisphere of the eye (for a total of 160 seconds[1–3]; some clinicians have "double treated" for a total of 320 seconds.

- The 3 and 9 o'clock positions should be left untreated (Fig. 27-4).

REFERENCES

1. Tan AM, Chockalingam M, Aquino MC, et al. Micropulse transscleral diode laser cyclophotocoagulation in the treatment of refractory glaucoma. *Clin Exp Ophthalmol.* 2010;38:266–272.
2. Aquino MC, Barton K, Tan AM, et al. Micropulse versus continuous wave transscleral diode cyclophotocoagulation in refractory glaucoma: a randomized exploratory study. *Clin Exp Ophthalmol.* 2015;43(1):40–46.
3. Kuchar S, Moster M, Reamer C, et al. Treatment outcomes of micropulse transscleral cyclophotocoagulation in advanced glaucoma. *Lasers Med Sci.* 2016;31:393–396.

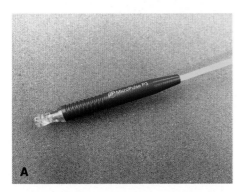
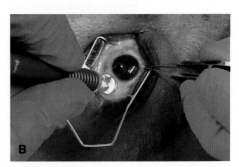

FIGURE 27-4. Micropulse transscleral cyclophotocoagulation. A. MP3 probe used to deliver micropulse laser. **B.** Probe is placed perpendicularly to the eye surface 2 mm behind the limbus, laser is delivered by a sweeping motion avoiding the 3 and 9 o'clock positions.

CYCLOCRYOTHERAPY

- A nitrous oxide cryosurgical unit is used to cool the 2.5-mm probe to $-80°C$, which is placed approximately 1 mm posterior to the limbus for 60 seconds.

- Two to three quadrants are treated with four spots per quadrant, avoiding the 3 and 9 o'clock positions (Fig. 27-5).[1]

REFERENCE

1. Bietti G. Surgical intervention on the ciliary body: new trends for the relief of glaucoma. *JAMA.* 1950;142:889–897.

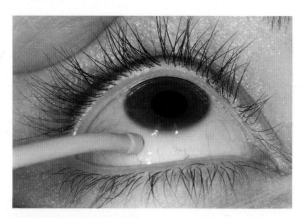

FIGURE 27-5. **Cyclocryotherapy (CCT).** Photograph demonstrating CCT. The probe is placed approximately 1 mm posterior to the limbus.

TRANSPUPILLARY CYCLOPHOTOCOAGULATION

- A continuous-wave argon laser is delivered via a biomicroscope. The concept behind this technique is to apply the laser energy directly to the ciliary processes instead of having to go through other structures, such as the conjunctiva and sclera.

- To visualize the ciliary processes, a Goldmann-type gonioprism and scleral depression are necessary. Wide dilation of the pupil, iridectomy, or both are usually required for visualization.

- Laser settings of 50- to 100-μm spot size, 700 to 1,000 mW, for 0.1 second, with the energy level being adjusted to create a whitening of the tissue, are used to treat all visible ciliary processes (Fig. 27-6).

- The major disadvantage of this technique is visualization problems.[1] It is rarely used for this reason.

REFERENCE

1. Shields S, Stewart WC, Shields MD. Transpupillary argon laser cyclophotocoagulation in the treatment of glaucoma. *Ophthalmic Surg Lasers*. 1988;19:171–175.

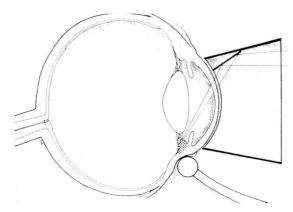

FIGURE 27-6. Transpupillary cyclophotocoagulation (CPC). Diagram showing transpupillary CPC. The laser energy is being focused by a mirrored lens onto the ciliary body, which has been moved into view by scleral depression.

ENDOSCOPIC CYCLOPHOTOCOAGULATION

- This technique is performed in the operating room under local retrobulbar, sub-Tenon's, or topical anesthesia.

- There are two different approaches: limbal and pars plana.

- In the limbal approach, the pupil is maximally dilated, an incision approximately 2.5 mm in width is made with a keratome, and viscoelastic is introduced between the iris and the crystalline lens or the pseudophakic posterior chamber lens to access the ciliary processes. A maximum of 180 degrees can be treated through an incision with a straight probe or up to 270 degrees with a curved probe. A second incision can be made directly opposite the original one to treat the remaining untreated processes. Viscoelastic is irrigated out after the procedure and the wound closed with 10-0 nylon suture. A cataract extraction may be combined with this procedure at the same time, usually with the ECP following the extraction.

- When performing the ECP through the pars plana incision, the patient must be aphakic or pseudophakic. A typical pars plana incision is made 3.5 to 4.0 mm from the limbus, an anterior vitrectomy is performed, and the laser endoscope is inserted. Two incisions can be created if more than 180 to 270 degrees of processes are to be treated. The sclerotomies are closed with 7-0 Vicryl suture. The laser endoscope has camera imaging, He–Ne aiming beam, light source, and laser delivery transmitted through an 18-, 19-, or 20-gauge endoprobe. The probe is connected to a video camera, light source, and video monitor. There is a 110-degree view in standard probes; however, a new line of high-resolution endoprobes have a 170-degree field. An advantage of the 18-gauge probe is its sturdiness and greater potential for multiple uses. A semiconductor diode laser at 810 nm wavelength can deliver energy continuously or as timed pulses. Applications are typically from 0.5 to 5 seconds, 300 to 900 mW, to achieve an end point of whitening and shrinkage of each ciliary process (Fig. 27-7). To avoid a visible explosion (pop) of the ciliary process, laser power, duration, or both can be decreased. The surgeon performs the procedure by viewing the video monitor.[1]

REFERENCE

1. Chen J, Cohn RA, Lin SC, et al. Endoscopic photocoagulation of the ciliary body for treatment of refractory glaucomas. *Am J Ophthalmol.* 1997;124(6): 787–796.

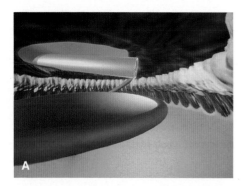 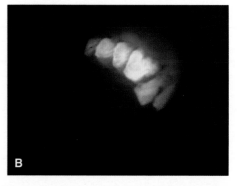

FIGURE 27-7. Endoscopic cyclophotocoagulation. A. Diagram showing an endolaser probe delivering energy to the ciliary body. (Courtesy of Martin Uram, MD.) **B.** View through the endoscopic camera of the whitened, shrunken ciliary processes on the left following delivery of the laser energy. The processes on the right have not received treatment but one process has the red He–Ne beam focused on its tip.

POSTPROCEDURE CARE

- In all of these treatments, topical steroids are used postoperatively at varying frequencies depending on the inflammation level and risk for CME or uveitis.

- Sub-Tenon's steroids are often given to blunt the inflammation and prevent CME.

- Cycloplegic and nonsteroidal anti-inflammatory drops may also be recommended. Analgesics and ice packs are sometimes prescribed for pain.

COMPLICATIONS

- **Table 27-1** lists the complications of cyclodestructive procedures.

- The most feared of these complications are chronic hypotony leading to phthisis, which occurs in 5% to 10% of patients treated by transscleral CPC, and sympathetic ophthalmia, which is extremely rare and may be secondary to other prior intraocular surgeries.

- Significant pain occurs in about 50% of patients treated by the transscleral route and may last for several hours to several weeks, the usual duration being 2 to 3 days, following the procedure. One cannot predict from the type of glaucoma which patients will have this significant pain. It can be treated with analgesics and ice.

- With ECP, the most common vision-threatening complication is CME, occurring in 10% of cases from a large series.[1]

TABLE 27-1. Potential Complications of Cyclodestructive Procedures*

Uveitis–iritis (hypopyon)
Cystoid macular edema (with ECP)
Vitritis
Chronic flare
Pain
Hyphema
Vitreous hemorrhage
Corneal edema
Thinning of the sclera (with transscleral CPC)
Retinal detachment
Sympathetic ophthalmia (controversial)
Malignant glaucoma
Anterior segment necrosis or ischemia
Decreased vision
Blindness
Chronic hypotony
Phthisis
Traumatic cataract (with ECP)
Endophthalmitis (with ECP)
Choroidal hemorrhage (with ECP)

*Those that are specific to the transscleral or endoscopic approach are noted.
CPC, cyclophotocoagulation; ECP, endoscopic cyclophotocoagulation.

REFERENCE

1. Chen J, Cohn RA, Lin SC, et al. Endoscopic photocoagulation of the ciliary body for treatment of refractory glaucomas. *Am J Ophthalmol.* 1997;124(6):787–796.

Late Complications of Glaucoma Surgery

Nathan Radcliffe, Gabriel Chong, Francisco Fantes, and Paul F. Palmberg ∎

INTRODUCTION

In most cases, glaucoma-filtering surgery is safe and effective at lowering intraocular pressure. However, this treatment is not always perfect. Some of the undesired outcomes of filtering surgery are caused by technical failures or by an undesirable wound healing response (**Table 28-1**). Reproducible, methodical, and safe surgical techniques combined with attempted modulation of the biologic response may minimize some of these undesired outcomes. Despite our best efforts, however, delayed problems can occur (**Table 28-2**).

The goal of this chapter is to review some of the more common delayed complications of

glaucoma-filtering surgery and discuss possible treatment strategies. Some of the treatment strategies are more strongly established and have passed the test of time. Other procedures and alternatives are newer and may have helped one or more of the authors to solve some individual problems. The newer or somewhat infrequent procedures may not yet have passed the tests of rigorous research and time because of the rarity of the situations in which they have been applied.

TABLE 28-1. Factors That Can Influence Wound Healing

Impeccable and precise surgical techniques
Use of antimetabolites
Etiology of glaucoma, such as uveitic or neovascular cause
Use of postoperative anti-inflammatory medications
Other biologic factors, such as genetics, age, and race

TABLE 28-2. Undesirable Outcomes as a Result of a Vigorous or Inadequate Healing Response

Vigorous Healing Response
Loss of filter due to scarring
Inadequate filtration
Bleb encapsulation
Inadequate Healing Response
Hypotony
Choroidal effusion
Macular folds
Flat chambers
Bleb leaks
Bleb-related infections
Giant blebs

HYPOTONY

- Hypotony can result in reduced vision from corneal striae, maculopathy, choroidal effusion, and delayed suprachoroidal hemorrhages.

- It is often the result of insufficient scleral flap resistance that many times will require resuturing the flap in trabeculectomies performed with antimetabolites. Alternative therapies have also been described[1-4]; however, these therapies are probably less likely to be successful in cases in which antimetabolites have been used, or a rapid result is needed, such as patients with a flat chamber, maculopathy, or the so-called kissing choroidals. When there is overfiltration with a necrotic-looking scleral flap, sutures may not provide enough resistance to flow. In these cases, donor tissue may be needed as a roof to the flap to achieve the desired resistance. It is advisable to have donor tissue available whenever one is attempting to revise a scleral flap or to repair a leaking bleb.

- Chronic hypotony, which persists for at least 3 months, can lead to hypotony maculopathy and loss of vision.[5] Dr. Palmberg employs a method using transcorneal sutures to treat hypotony at the slit lamp. The technique involves passing 10-0 nylon sutures through the cornea, through the scleral flap, and then back through the conjunctiva at the slit lamp with the objective of increasing resistance at the scleral flap to raise intraocular pressure (Fig. 28-1).

Hypotony Maculopathy

- Hypotony maculopathy is a condition in which folds in the choroid or retina, or both, involving the foveal region cause blurred vision in the setting of hypotony. The mechanism is probably scleral contraction.

- The maculopathy does not occur in all cases of hypotony, but is more likely to occur in eyes of patients who are young and myopic, and those with marked reductions in intraocular pressure.

- It is best to treat this condition quickly, because it can become permanent, although there are reports of success after years of involvement[6] (Fig. 28-2A and B).

- The best therapy is prevention, such as the cornea safety valve incision as devised by Palmberg.[7]

- Palmberg also described a technique for bleb revisions to fix maculopathies, whereby two sets of sutures are added. The first set of two sutures adjusts the outflow from the flap to an intraocular pressure of 8 to 12 mm Hg. The second set is adjusted to an intraocular pressure of 20 to 25 mm Hg.[7] It is important to keep in mind the possibility that donor tissue may be needed when revising a flap (see Fig. 28-2C and D).

Shallow and Flat Anterior Chamber

- Depending on the etiology, flat chambers can be associated with high or low intraocular pressures (Table 28-3; Fig. 28-3). With a postoperative flat or shallow chamber, the clinical history, examination, and intraocular

TABLE 28-3. Causes of Altered Intraocular Pressure and a Flat Anterior Chamber

High Intraocular Pressure and Flat Chamber
Aqueous misdirection syndrome (i.e., malignant glaucoma)
Suprachoroidal hemorrhage
Pupillary block
Low Intraocular Pressure and Flat Chamber
Overfiltration caused by insufficient flap resistance
Uveal–scleral outflow tract due to choroidal detachment
Cyclodialysis cleft
A true flat chamber with lens–cornea or intraocular lens–cornea touch (should be fixed immediately)

pressure guide the examiner in making the diagnosis.

- The indications for draining a choroidal effusion include the following:

    - Flat chamber resulting in lens–corneal contact or significant iridocorneal contact that is likely to lead to permanent synechiae

    - So-called kissing choroidals (retina–retina contact between the choroidal swellings) to avoid fibrin adherence between the overlying retina

    - Persistence (after treating with cycloplegics or topical steroids)

- It is appropriate to observe these eyes for several weeks so long as neither of the first two conditions is present.

Strategies for Reformation of the Anterior Chamber

- Tamponade via pressure or Simmons' shell or symblepharon ring: The strategy is likely to be more successful in surgeries without antimetabolites, and is to be used in situations of overfiltration.

- Viscoelastic injection into the anterior chamber: This strategy is more likely to have success in filters without antimetabolites.

- Resuturing the flap: This may end up being the definitive solution when antimetabolites were used.

Draining Choroidal Effusions

- A paracentesis is placed temporally (Figs. 28-4 and 28-5A).

- Conjunctival incisions are made at 4:30 and 7:30 meridians from 2 to 7 mm from the limbus, or a limbal peritomy from the 4 to 8 o'clock positions.

- A half-thickness radial incision of 2 mm is made, beginning 3 mm from the limbus as measured by calipers.

- The edge of the flap is grasped by a toothed forceps for countertraction.

- With a sharp blade, the incision is slowly and carefully deepened until the suprachoroidal space is opened (Fig. 28-5B).

- The incision is enlarged with a Kelly punch (Fig. 28-5C).

- If the incision is over a pocket of fluid, it will begin the outflow, which can be helped by infusing balanced salt solution through the paracentesis, lifting the edges of the flap, and rolling a cotton-tipped swab along the scleral surface.

- If the incision is not over a pocket of fluid and fluid is not mobilized to the incision, a cyclodialysis spatula can be used to separate the choroids gently from the scleral wall to obtain communication to an adjacent pocket of fluid. This dissection should be done extremely carefully, and not more than a few millimeters from the incision.

- Indirect ophthalmoscopy could be used at this time to look at the flattened retina. The anterior chamber should be deep, as well, and iridocorneal adhesions should be released with a cyclodialysis spatula if necessary.

- The conjunctival incisions should be closed, leaving the punched incisions open (Fig. 28-5D).

Delayed Suprachoroidal Hemorrhages

- A suprachoroidal hemorrhage is a condition in which bleeding occurs in the suprachoroidal space separating the uvea from the sclera. These hemorrhages can occur intraoperatively as well as in the postoperative period.

    - If bleeding occurs intraoperatively, the posterior pressure can cause extrusion of the contents of the eye (e.g., expulsive hemorrhage). The delayed suprachoroidal hemorrhages can be the result of de novo bleeding into the suprachoroidal space or of bleeding into a preexisting choroidal effusion.

- The risk factors include marked decompressions of the intraocular pressure, multiple previous eye surgeries, myopia, previous vitrectomy, and systemic hypertension.

- A suprachoroidal hemorrhage often presents as sudden, severe pain associated with a brown-colored choroidal elevation in one side of the vitreous cavity. It is advisable to manage the patient with vitreoretinal surgery if possible.

- Serial B-scan ultrasounds are helpful to show the location of the hemorrhage and monitor the clot for lysis; this usually occurs 5 to 10 days after the onset of the hemorrhage.

- Many surgeons prefer waiting until the clot liquefies (lyses) before draining the hemorrhage. The technique is the same as described earlier for drainage of a choroidal effusion.

- Smaller suprachoroidal hemorrhages may reabsorb spontaneously in about 1 month with good visual results. While the clot is liquefying, the intraocular pressure should be controlled medically to the best degree possible.

- An extremely elevated intraocular pressure could force an earlier intervention.

REFERENCES

1. Akova YA, Dursun D, Aydin P, et al. Management of hypotony maculopathy and a large filtering bleb after trabeculectomy with mitomycin C: success with argon laser therapy. *Ophthalmic Surg Lasers.* 2000;31(6):491–494.
2. Marzeta M, Toczolowski J. Administration of autologous blood to a patient via intrableb injection as a method for treating hypotony after trabeculectomy. *Klin Oczna.* 2000;102(3):199–200.
3. Okada K, Tsukamoto H, Masumoto M, et al. Autologous blood injection for marked overfiltration early after trabeculectomy with mitomycin C. *Acta Ophthalmol Scand.* 2001;79(3):305–308.
4. Yieh FS, Lu DW, Wang HL, et al. The use of autologous fibrinogen concentrate in treating ocular hypotony after glaucoma filtration surgery. *J Ocul Pharmacol Ther.* 2001;17(5):443–448.
5. Azuara-Blanco A, Katz LJ. Dysfunctional filtering blebs. *Surv Ophthalmol.* 1998;43(2):93–126.
6. Delgado MF, Daniels S, Pascal S, et al. Hypotony maculopathy: improvement of visual acuity after 7 years. *Am J Ophthalmol.* 2001;132(6):931–933.
7. Palmberg P. Surgery for complications. In: Albert D, ed. *Ophthalmic Surgery: Principles and Techniques.* Vol. 1. London, UK: Blackwell Science; 1999.

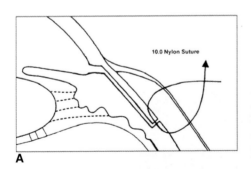

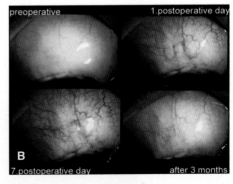

FIGURE 28-1. Transcorneal sutures. A. Diagram of the technique. (From Eha J, Hoffman E, Pfeiffer N. *Graefes Arch Clin Exp Ophthalmol.* 2008;246:869–874.) **B.** Photo montage of the effect of transcorneal sutures over time.

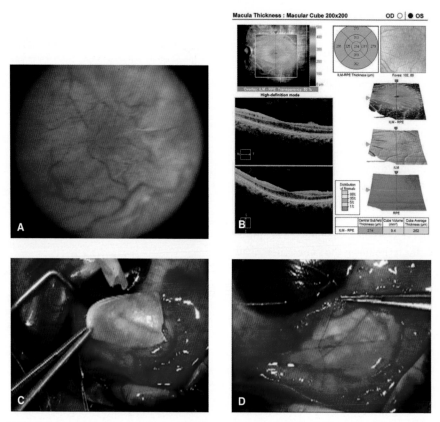

FIGURE 28-2. **Hypotony. A.** Dramatic example of hypotony causing folds in the choroid and retina involving the foveal region. **B.** Example of trace cystic changes and subtle folds in the internal limiting membrane in a patient with hypotony maculopathy as shown in optical coherence tomography. **C.** Intraoperative video still frame showing a cut piece of donor cornea being used to cover a flap. **D.** Intraoperative video still frame showing a compression suture of 10-0 nylon being used over the piece of donor cornea to increase the scleral resistance to aqueous outflow. ILM, internal limiting membrane; RPE, retinal pigment epithelium.

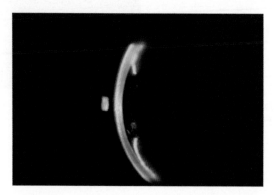

FIGURE 28-3. **Shallow anterior chamber slit-beam photograph showing a shallow anterior chamber.** There is significant iridocorneal touch; however, neither the pupillary border nor intraocular lens is in contact with the cornea.

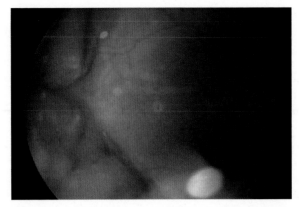

FIGURE 28-4. Peripheral choroidal effusions. Fundus photograph showing peripheral choroidal effusions (left).

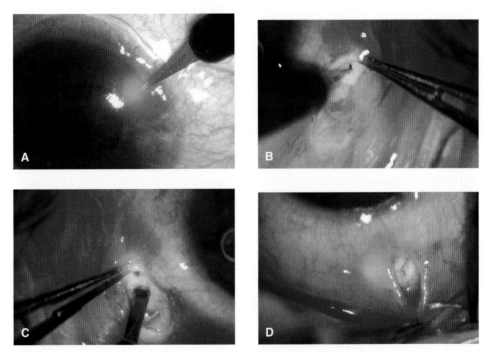

FIGURE 28-5. Repair of choroidal effusion. Intraoperative video still photographs of a repair of choroidal effusion. **A.** Paracentesis side port using a sharp point number 75 blade is made at the corneoscleral limbus. **B.** A sharp blade is used to gently enter the suprachoroidal space at the base of the partial-thickness radial scleral incision. **C.** Once the suprachoroidal space is entered, the incision is widened using a Kelly punch; at the base of the incision, a hole created by the punch can be seen. **D.** The conjunctival incision is closed using 7-0 Vicryl sutures; the sclerotomy is left open.

BLEB LEAKS

● A bleb leak is a tiny hole in the wall of the bleb causing leakage of aqueous. This is a direct communication between the exterior world and the interior of the bleb. The use of intraoperative antimetabolites is a risk factor for the development of a bleb leak.

● The mechanism of a bleb leak is thought to be as follows. Ischemic blebs are stretched and surrounded by heavily scarred tissue, which limits the ability of the aqueous to flow beyond the scarred tissue. The bleb expands locally, producing a tractional hole when the tissue overreaches its maximal stretch.

● The bleb leaks are best detected by applying fluorescein to the surface of the bleb and viewing it under a slit lamp with a cobalt blue filter in place. A positive Seidel test consists of a change in the color of the dye to green-yellow, in response to the outflow of aqueous from the leak. Sometimes a leak can only be detected after applying gentle pressure to the globe.

● Leaks increase the risk of infection and endophthalmitis; therefore, early detection and management could be critical.[1-4] The reported incidence of late postoperative bleb-related infections after a trabeculectomy ranges from 0.4% to 9.6% at 2 to 6 years.[5,6] It is also estimated that blebitis occurs with an incidence of 5.7% per year, whereas the incidence of endophthalmitis ranges from 0.8% to 1.3% per year.[5]

● Careful surgical techniques during surgery are critical in decreasing the risk of bleb leaks. Special attention has to be paid to technique in the trabeculectomy—in suturing the conjunctiva; in the time, area, and washout of the antimetabolites; and to being methodical when applying laser suture lysis.[7]

Treatment

Conservative Management

● Following are some of the techniques described to manage wound healing in eyes with bleb leaks. These techniques have the advantage of sparing the patient from surgery. The disadvantage is that they are not always successful and leaks can recur. Although these treatments are not operative procedures, each has its own set of risks.

■ Use of 28-mm soft contact lenses for 2 weeks[7]

■ Use of butyryl methacrylate glue and a silicon disc[7]

■ Infusion of autologous blood into the bleb[8]

■ Application of compression sutures[7]

■ Pressure eye patching, oral carbonic anhydrase inhibitor, and topical autologous serum[5]

■ Chemical irritants (trichloroacetic acid, sodium nitrate)[9]

■ Cryopexy and diathermy[10]

■ Argon laser, thermal Nd:YAG laser[11,12]

Surgical Treatment

● Options

■ Closing the trabeculectomy with a scleral or corneal patch graft and replacing with a glaucoma drainage device (GDD)—in severe cases, corneal lamellar grafting has been described as a "final" solution to a dysfunctional bleb whereby the scarred conjunctiva and weakened spongy sclera are dissected away and replaced with round lamellar preserved donor corneal tissue.[13]

■ Conjunctival advancement—this has been demonstrated to be highly successful. Patients with late bleb leaks managed with conjunctival advancement were more likely to have successful outcomes and less likely to have serious intraocular infections than those managed more conservatively.[14-18]

■ Free conjunctival graft[19]—free conjunctival autologous graft is a safe and successful procedure for bleb repair and bleb reduction. However, patients should be aware of the possibility of requiring postoperative medical or surgical intervention for intraocular pressure control after the revision.

■ Amniotic membrane (AM)[14]—in cases in which the conjunctival tissue available is considered by the surgeon to be very limited (e.g., as a result of thinning or scarring), or there is already some degree of ptosis present, an AM graft could be an alternative. The technique described next is slightly different from the one described by Budenz et al.[14] In this technique, the graft is folded upon itself, leaving the basement layer outward, and the stromal layer on the inside (Fig. 28-6).

● The technique of suturing AM is as follows:

■ The conjunctiva surrounding the ischemic bleb is freed (Fig. 28-7A and B).

■ The old ischemic bleb is excised (Fig. 28-7C).

■ The donor AM is removed and folded upon itself (see Fig. 28-6).

■ The anterior edges of the graft are sutured at the corners to corneal limbus using 9-0 nylon.

■ The posterior edge of the AM underneath the free undermined anterior conjunctiva (Fig. 28-7D)

■ The graft is tightly sutured to the anterior edge of the patient's free conjunctiva using a running 8-0 Vicryl suture (Fig. 28-7E).

■ A 9-0 nylon compression suture is placed at the anterior edge of the graft, at the level of the limbus (Fig. 28-7F).

■ The site is checked for wound leaks with fluorescein strips.

■ The anterior compression suture can be removed after 1 month (Fig. 28-8).

● A variation of this technique could be applied to free conjunctival grafts as well, adding the steps of cutting the tissue from the selected site, and without folding the free graft.

Results and Prognosis

● The study of AM transplantation by Budenz et al.[14] does not offer an effective alternative to conjunctival advancement for repair of leaking glaucoma-filtering blebs. The cumulative survival rate for AM transplant was 81% at 6 months, 74% at 1 year, and 46% at 2 years. The cumulative survival rate was 100% for conjunctival advancement throughout follow-up.

● Although Budenz et al.'s study showed that AM grafts were less successful than results of the standard conjunctival advancement, their study showed that they could be successful in certain situations, providing an alternative treatment for bleb leaks in special circumstances.

● The long-term results of the study of Budenz et al. were published in 2007 with a median follow-up of 80 months.[20] Almost half of 15 patients who received AM transplantation developed failures, 4 required reoperation for bleb leakage, and 3 required reoperation for uncontrolled intraocular pressure.[20] Four of 15 patients with conjunctival advancement experienced failure, with 1 requiring another operation for a bleb leak and 3 patients requiring glaucoma intervention.[20] Although not statistically significant, the Kaplan-Meier long-term survival curves trended toward earlier failure with the AM transplant group.[20]

● Other groups have had more success with AMs, including a group in Japan (Nagai-Kusuhara et al.) that reported six patients who underwent AM transplantation–assisted bleb revision for leaking blebs; and all six patients had their leaks resolved without complications.[21]

■ However, another group, also in Japan, concluded that the use of AM transplant did not improve the overall surgical outcome for their patients.[22] Their Kaplan-Meier survival curves showed a success rate of

58.3% at 6 months and 21.9% after 1 year for the AM transplant group compared to 74.8% success in their control group from 6 to 12 months.[22]

- In addition, if an AM graft fails, conjunctival advancement is still a possibility. It may even be possible to make modifications in the surgical technique that could alter the outcomes. This last point is only speculative; it will need to be proved by a randomized clinical trial comparable to the Budenz et al. trial and, of course, by the final test of time.

REFERENCES

1. Jampel HD, Quigley HA, Kerrigan-Baumrind LA, et al. Risk factors for late-onset infection following glaucoma filtration surgery. *Arch Ophthalmol.* 2001;119(7):1001–1008.
2. Lehmann OJ, Bunce C, Matheson MM, et al. Risk factors for development of post-trabeculectomy endophthalmitis. *Br J Ophthalmol.* 2000;84(12):1349–1353.
3. Liebmann JM, Ritch R. Bleb related ocular infection: a feature of the HELP syndrome. Hypotony, endophthalmitis, leak, pain. *Br J Ophthalmol.* 2000;84(12): 1338–1339.
4. Soltau JB, Rothman RF, Budenz DL, et al. Risk factors for glaucoma filtering bleb infections. *Arch Ophthalmol.* 2000;118(3):338–342.
5. Sharan S, Trope GE, Chipman M, et al. Late-onset bleb infections: Prevalence and risk factors. *Can J Ophthalmol.* 2009;44(3):279–283.
6. Song A, Scott IU, Flynn HW Jr, et al. Delayed-onset bleb-associated endophthalmitis: clinical features and visual acuity outcomes. *Ophthalmology.* 2002;109(5):985–991.
7. Palmberg P. Surgery for complications. In: Albert D, ed. *Ophthalmic Surgery: Principles and Techniques.* Vol. 1. London: Blackwell Science; 1999.
8. Okada K, Tsukamoto H, Masumoto M, et al. Autologous blood injection for marked overfiltration early after trabeculectomy with mitomycin C. *Acta Ophthalmol Scand.* 2001;79(3):305–308.
9. Gehring JR, Ciccarelli EC. Trichloracetic acid treatment of filtering blebs following cataract extraction. *Am J Ophthalmol.* 1972;74(4):622–624.
10. Douvas NG. Cystoid bleb cryotherapy. *Am J Ophthalmol.* 1972;74(1):69–71.
11. Bettin P, Carassa RG, Fiori M, et al. Treatment of hyperfiltering blebs with Nd:YAG laser-induced subconjunctival bleeding. *J Glaucoma.* 1999;8(6):380–383.
12. Fink AJ, Boys-Smith JW, Brear R. Management of large filtering blebs with the argon laser. *Am J Ophthalmol.* 1986;101(6):695–699.
13. Fukuchi T, Matsuda H, Ueda J, et al. Corneal lamellar grafting to repair late complications of mitomycin C trabeculectomy. *Clin Ophthalmol.* 2010;4:197–202.
14. Budenz DL, Barton K, Tseng SC. Amniotic membrane transplantation for repair of leaking glaucoma filtering blebs. *Am J Ophthalmol.* 2000;130(5):580–588.
15. Budenz DL, Chen PP, Weaver YK. Conjunctival advancement for late-onset filtering bleb leaks: indications and outcomes. *Arch Ophthalmol.* 1999;117(8): 1014–1019.
16. Burnstein AL, WuDunn D, Knotts SL, et al. Conjunctival advancement versus nonincisional treatment for late-onset glaucoma filtering bleb leaks. *Ophthalmology.* 2002;109(1):71–75.
17. O'Connor DJ, Tressler CS, Caprioli J. A surgical method to repair leaking filtering blebs. *Ophthalmic Surg.* 1992;23(5):336–338.
18. Wadhwani RA, Bellows AR, Hutchinson BT. Surgical repair of leaking filtering blebs. *Ophthalmology.* 2000;107(9):1681–1687.
19. Schnyder CC, Shaarawy T, Ravinet E, et al. Free conjunctival autologous graft for bleb repair and bleb reduction after trabeculectomy and nonpenetrating filtering surgery. *J Glaucoma.* 2002;11(1):10–16.
20. Rauscher FM, Barton K, Budenz DL, et al. Long-term outcomes of amniotic membrane transplantation for repair of leaking glaucoma filtering blebs. *Am J Ophthalmol.* 2007;143(6):1052–1054.
21. Nagai-Kusuhara A, Nakamura M, Fujioka M, et al. Long-term results of amniotic membrane transplantation-assisted bleb revision for leaking blebs. *Graefes Arch Clin Exp Ophthalmol.* 2008;246(4):567–571.
22. Kiuchi Y, Yanagi M, Nakamura T. Efficacy of amniotic membrane-assisted bleb revision for elevated intraocular pressure after filtering surgery. *Clin Ophthalmol.* 2010;4:839–843.

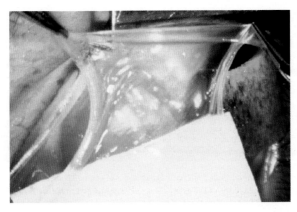

FIGURE 28-6. **A single layer of amniotic membrane being peeled from the supporting membrane.** The stromal layer is against the paper and sticky. The basement membrane layer is shiny and nonsticky.

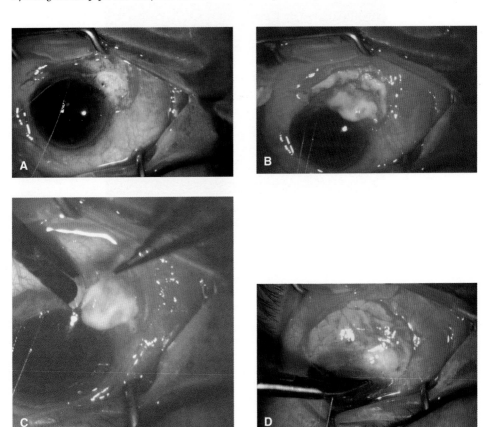

FIGURE 28-7. **Amniotic membrane (AM) graft technique. A.** The conjunctival tissue surrounding the ischemic bleb has been cut along the margins of the bleb; a superiorly placed 7-0 Vicryl corneal traction suture is also seen. **B.** The conjunctival-Tenon's flap has been bluntly undermined to mobilize the tissue. **C.** The ischemic bleb is excised using a number 67 blade. **D.** The posterior layer of the AM sandwich is pushed and now lying underneath the conjunctival-Tenon's flap.

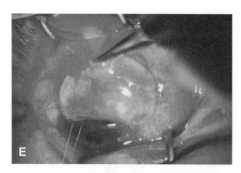
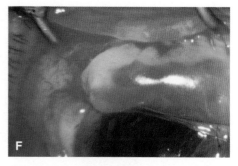

FIGURE 28-7. (*continued*) **E.** The conjunctival-Tenon's flap and AM sandwich are sutured together using a running 8-0 Vicryl suture. **F.** At the corneal edge of the graft, a 9-0 nylon compression suture is used to obstruct flow from underneath the AM graft at the limbus.

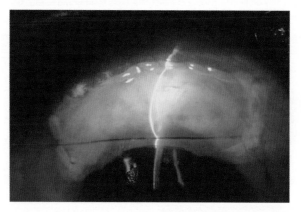

FIGURE 28-8. **Appearance after bleb revision.** Postoperative appearance of the same eye shown in Figure 28-7 following bleb revision using a double-layer amniotic membrane graft.

GIANT BLEBS

Giant blebs can grow over the cornea, creating dellen and producing irregular astigmatism and loss of best-corrected visual acuity. The management of a giant bleb should be in a stepwise manner, moving from the simplest to more complex solutions.

Treatment

- Options
  - Cleavage and pushing technique—a cleavage plane of the hanging bleb is found using a dull spatula; this is then pushed back posterior to the limbus.
  - Same technique with compression stitch—the same technique is followed, placing a compressive stitch as the limbus that will encourage permanent contraction.
  - Amputation of the corneal portion in spongy-looking blebs—this approach is useful for spongy-looking blebs over the cornea. The exuberant portion is cut with Vannas scissors.
  - Amputation of the whole bleb—this is generally unnecessary.
- There are always exceptions. The following clinical study describes an exceptional case. The patient was a 55-year-old African-American man who had only one functioning eye in which multiple surgeries had been performed, including the latest, a successful mitomycin C trabeculectomy for advanced glaucoma. The other eye had been lost to glaucoma.
  - The patient developed corneal edema and underwent cornea transplant when his visual acuity decreased from 20/30 to 20/200 in the functional eye. We performed a corneal transplant, and his visual acuity improved to a baseline of 20/30 after 6 months.
  - The trabeculectomy also remained functional and kept the intraocular pressure

controlled throughout the postoperative course. After 1 year, the patient began to develop a larger bleb that invaded the cornea, significantly reducing his visual acuity (**Fig. 28-9A**).

- The patient was managed as previously described, but the bleb always returned, growing larger. Eventually his visual acuity worsened to 20/400, resulting in an eye that was barely functional. In response to the patient's frustration, and after a long discussion with him about the risks of surgery, we decided to take the unusual step of revising the whole bleb.

- In this case, the patient had another problem—a lack of free, unscarred conjunctiva surrounding the bleb, or in that eye, for that matter. As a result, we decided to excise the bleb and to rebuild it with a double layer of AM donor graft. A small bleb with minimal vascularization formed, and this has maintained the intraocular pressure under good control for over 4 years (**Fig. 28-9B**).

Bleb-related Infections and Use of Corneal Patches

- Bleb leaks and inferior blebs are risk factors for infections. The infections can be localized to the bleb (**Fig. 28-10**), produce necrosis of the surrounding tissue (**Fig. 28-11**), or progress to full-blown endophthalmitis. Inferior location of the bleb should be considered a high risk factor for infections (around 1% in superior blebs versus around 8% in inferior blebs in several studies)[1-3]; so consideration should be made to their closure, especially when there has been a history of infection or leaks.

- In the case of bleb-related endophthalmitis, *Streptococcus* species and *Staphylococcus* species are the most common causative organisms.[4] Although results from the Endophthalmitis Vitrectomy Study (postcataract endophthalmitis was studied) have been applied by clinicians as a paradigm to treat bleb-related endoph-thalmitis, there is growing evidence that those results cannot be directly applied because of differences in the virulence of the pathogens involved between postcataract endophthalmi-tis and bleb-related endophthalmitis, in partic-ular the *Streptococcus* species.

- Regardless of prompt treatment (tap and inject vs. vitrectomy), visual prognosis is poor; final visual acuities are >20/400 in only 22% to 53% of patients.[4] Several stud-ies also report conflicting results regarding treatment modality, with Song et al. reporting worse visual outcomes with vitrectomy treat-ment and Busbee et al. reporting the oppo-site.[4,5] Smiddy et al.[6] reported 34 cases from Bascom Palmer with neither tap injection nor tap injection with vitrectomy proving superior in the management of bleb-related endophthalmitis.

Corneal Patching

- Corneal tissue that is not of transplant qual-ity can be preserved in glycerin and used for patching, as follows:

  ▪ The donor cornea is cut to the needed size.

  ▪ Descemet membrane is peeled off with two large-toothed forceps.

  ▪ The bed is cleaned of necrotic tissue.

  ▪ The cornea patch is sutured with 9-0 nylon sutures and compressive sutures, as needed.

  ▪ The patch is covered by conjunctiva. If little conjunctiva is available, the surgeon may consider covering it with AM, with the stromal layer inside, in direct contact with the patch.

  ▪ To close the filtration permanently, the surgeon can consider placing more than one tight compression stitch, and leaving the stitches in place until they become loose, or for 6 to 8 weeks if they are reason-ably well tolerated.

- In one case, a patient developed necrotizing blebitis (see Fig. 28-10), which required use of a corneal patch graft, covered by an AM graft. At the same time, a GDD was placed superiorly (**Fig. 28-12**).

Bleb Dysesthesia

- On occasion, blebs can be associated with a certain degree of discomfort. The etiology of the pain is attributed to the height and shape of the bleb, which disturbs the spread of the tear film, producing dellen.[7,8] This condition has been associated with the presence of bubbles at the slit-lamp examination, by the capture of air bubbles within the tears as the upper eyelid moves over the irregular bleb (**Fig. 28-13**).

- Eyes with glaucoma-filtering blebs expe-rience more dysesthesia than do eyes with-out filtering blebs. Budenz et al. identified young age, supranasal bleb location, poor lid coverage, and bubble formation as being associated with glaucoma-filtering–bleb discomfort.[7]

- Some blebs that produce dysesthesia have been described as ischemic, thin-walled, and associated with low-normal pressures. Palmberg described a technique in which, by using compressing stitches for 3 weeks over the bleb, there is a change in the offending profile of the bleb, thereby re-ducing discomfort for up to 83% of patients tested with this technique.[9] The technique is as follows:

  ▪ If the bleb is very thin, and the sutures could traumatize the surface, the surgeon may consider aspirating a small amount of aqueous with a 30-gauge needle from the anterior chamber to decompress the bleb (**Fig. 28-14A**).

  ▪ One or more 9-0 nylon mattress sutures are anchored in the cornea.

  ▪ Sutures are passed posteriorly over the portion of the bleb to be compressed, and passed again over the bleb to tie the knot (Fig. 28-14B).

■ The knot is tied tightly and rotated into the cornea, making sure that the area targeted is well compressed.

■ Sutures are left in place from 1 to 4 weeks, and then removed (Fig. 28-14C).

REFERENCES

1. Greenfield DS, Suner IJ, Miller MP, et al. Endophthalmitis after filtering surgery with mitomycin. *Arch Ophthalmol.* 1996;114(8):943–949.
2. Higginbotham EJ, Stevens RK, Musch DC, et al. Bleb-related endophthalmitis after trabeculectomy with mitomycin C. *Ophthalmology.* 1996;103(4):650–656.
3. Wolner B, Liebmann JM, Sassani JW, et al. Late bleb-related endophthalmitis after trabeculectomy with adjunctive 5-fluorouracil. *Ophthalmology.* 1991;98(7):1053–1060.
4. Song A, Scott IU, Flynn HW Jr, et al. Delayed-onset bleb-associated endophthalmitis: Clinical features and visual acuity outcomes. *Ophthalmology.* 2002;109(5):985–991.
5. Busbee BG, Recchia FM, Kaiser R, et al. Bleb-associated endophthalmitis: Clinical characteristics and visual outcomes. *Ophthalmology.* 2004;111(8):1495–1503; discussion 503.
6. Ba'arah BT, Smiddy WE. Bleb-related endophthalmitis: Clinical presentation, isolates, treatment and visual outcome of culture-proven cases. *Middle East Afr J Ophthalmol.* 2009;16(1):20–24.
7. Suner IV, Greenfield DS, Miller MP, Nicolela MT, Palmberg PF. Hypotony maculopathy following filtering surgery with mitomycin C: Incidence and treatment. *Ophthalmology.* 1977;104:207–214.
8. Soong HK, Quigley HA. Dellen associated with filtering blebs. *Arch Ophthalmol.* 1983;101(3):385–387.
9. Palmberg P. Surgery for complications. In: Albert D, ed. *Ophthalmic Surgery: Principles and Techniques.* Vol. 1. London: Blackwell Science; 1999.

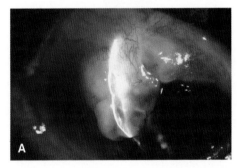 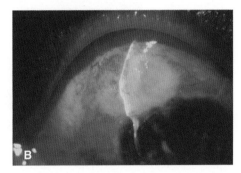

FIGURE 28-9. Giant bleb. A. An ischemic, giant cystic bleb can be seen overhanging onto the cornea. A dell can be seen at the anterior edge of the overhanging bleb. **B.** Postoperative appearance of the eye following bleb revision.

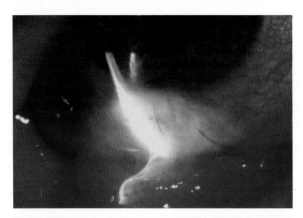

FIGURE 28-10. Bleb-related infection. An inferiorly located bleb with blebitis. The overlying conjunctival tissue is clear, showing hazy bleb fluid beneath.

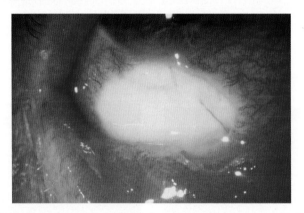

FIGURE 28-11. Bleb-related infection. An inferiorly located bleb, which is ischemic, and a necrotic bleb with opaque conjunctival tissue overlying the bleb.

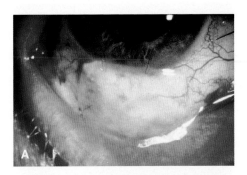

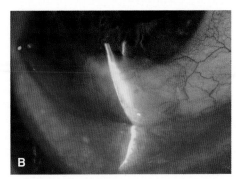

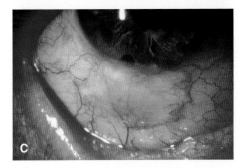

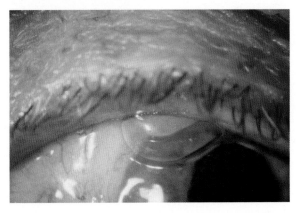

FIGURE 28-12. **Corneal patch. A.** Postoperative appearance at 6 weeks; the clear corneal tissue gives the illusion that a bleb is present. **B.** Slit-beam photograph shows that there is no fluid beneath the conjunctiva. **C.** Postoperative appearance at 1 year.

FIGURE 28-13. **Bleb dysesthesia.** An air bubble can be seen extending from the bleb and the upper lid.

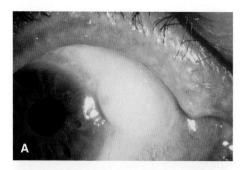

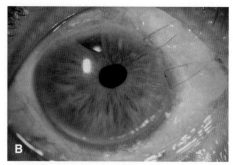

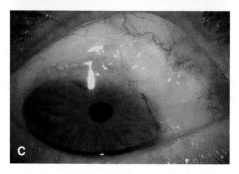

FIGURE 28-14. Dysesthetic bleb. A. Preoperative appearance of a large dysesthetic bleb. **B.** Two 9-0 nylon mattress sutures (or compression sutures) can be seen delimiting the size and height of the bleb. **C.** Postoperative appearance of the eye following removal of the compression sutures; the bleb is smaller.

THE FAILING BLEB: ENCAPSULATION

There are many reasons why trabeculectomies fail. The filter may stop functioning for external causes, such as encapsulation (Fig. 28-15) or scarring. It may fail because of internal causes, as when the ostium becomes occluded as a result of different etiologies, such as membrane formation, iris clot, or vitreous.

Treatment and Results

- Medical management consists simply of antiglaucoma medications, topical steroids, and digital compression. Mandal, in a retrospective study of 503 patients, noted that 18 patients developed encapsulation and 15 of those patients responded well to conservative treatment alone. Three who did not respond underwent excisional bleb revision with mitomycin.[1] Ophir's findings emphasize inflammation as the etiology of encapsulation.[2]

- Meyer et al. showed that bleb needling was effective in reducing intraocular pressure in one-third of the cases for more than 6 months. They also showed that reneedlings are as successful as the first one.[3]

- Dr. Palmberg has devised a transcorneal flap revision technique. A 30-gauge needle is bent in a Z configuration (Fig. 28-16A) and used to enter the anterior chamber through clear cornea (Fig. 28-16B). The needle is then directed to the underside of the scleral flap from the anterior chamber aspect and swept from side to side to break any adhesions and improve flow (Fig. 28-16C and D). The advantage to the corneal approach is avoiding any trauma to the conjunctiva and thus avoiding leaks.

- Excisional bleb revision may possibly be augmented with antimetabolites. This could be a last alternative in cases where medical management and needling prove unsuccessful.

REFERENCES

1. Mandal AK. Results of medical management and mitomycin C-augmented excisional bleb revision for encapsulated filtering blebs. *Ophthalmic Surg Lasers.* 1999;30(4):276–284.
2. Ophir A. Encapsulated filtering bleb. A selective review–new deductions. *Eye (Lond).* 1992;6(Pt 4):348–352.
3. Meyer JH, Guhlmann M, Funk J. How successful is the filtering bleb "needling"? *Klin Monbl Augenheilkd.* 1997;210(4):192–196.

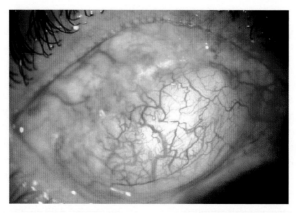

FIGURE 28-15. Encapsulated bleb. An encapsulated bleb; the tense appearance and thickened appearance of the wall of the "cyst" can be seen. Also note the increased vascularization of the overlying conjunctiva.

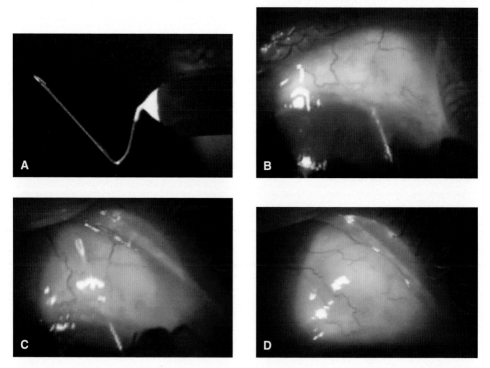

FIGURE 28-16. Transcorneal flap revision. A. A 30-gauge needle is bent into a "Z" configuration. **B.** The needle is then guided through clear cornea into the anterior chamber. **C.** The needle tip is seen protruding out underneath the scleral flap, visible under clear conjunctiva. **D.** There is a nice elevation of the bleb after the needle has been used to sever any fibrous adhesions, freeing the flap.

CIRCUMFERENTIAL BLEB

The use of antimetabolites leads to the potential development of thin-walled, avascular blebs. Aqueous can spread more readily in thin-walled blebs, leading to large, exuberant circumferential blebs that can be irritating to patients (**Fig. 28-17A**). Patients with circumferential blebs may complain of foreign body sensation, photophobia, and tearing.[1]

Treatment

- Rahman and Thaller described a technique termed bleb-limiting conjunctivoplasty for the treatment of circumferential blebs.[2]

  ■ Briefly, a number 75 blade is used to incise the conjunctiva and Tenon's capsule down to sclera in a circumferential bleb, bisecting the bleb.

  ■ The two cut edges of Tenon's capsule are then sutured back down onto bare sclera.

  ■ Once the circumferential bleb has been split into two blebs, the lower bleb that is no longer connected to the aqueous

filtering from the flap is reabsorbed, leaving behind a much smaller filtering bleb.

- Bovie handheld cautery has also been described as a technique to treat circumferential blebs in the office setting.[3]

- Cautery is applied to the bleb at the slit lamp after local anesthesia (**Fig. 28-17B**).

- Excess fluid from the bleb is drained through the cautery puncture wounds, which then self-seal from the heat (**Fig. 28-17C**).[3] The heat seals the edge of the bleb at the location specified by the clinician. The rest of the bleb that is now sealed off from the aqueous is reabsorbed and a smaller filtering bleb is the final result.

REFERENCES

1. Anis S, Ritch R, Shihadeh W, et al. Surgical reduction of symptomatic, circumferential, filtering blebs. *Arch Ophthalmol.* 2006;124(6):890–894.
2. Rahman R, Thaller VT. Bleb-limiting conjunctivoplasty for symptomatic circumferential trabeculectomy blebs. *J Glaucoma.* 2003;12(3):272–274.
3. Schwartz AL, Albano M. Application of handheld cautery for reduction of symptomatic circumferential trabeculectomy blebs. *J Glaucoma.* 2010;19(7):497–498.

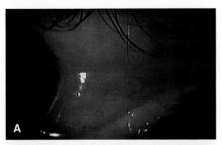
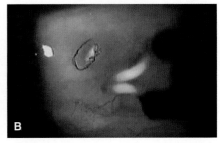
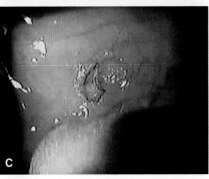

FIGURE 28-17. Circumferential bleb. A. Slit-lamp image of a circumferential bleb. **B.** Cautery is applied to the bleb to allow drainage of fluid. **C.** A cotton tip applicator is used to express fluid from the bleb. The heat from the cautery results in a self-sealing wound.

TUBE SHUNT EROSIONS

GDDs have proved to be useful for lowering intraocular pressure and treating glaucoma. Some of these devices are valveless and need a ligature to avoid hypotony until a capsule has formed around the plate to provide resistance (Fig. 28-18). These devices, however, are not without their own unique complications. One such complication, although uncommon (30% in the past but now <5%), is erosion of the tube (Fig. 28-19) and/or drainage plate through any reinforcing graft tissue and the conjunctiva.[1] An exposed tube or plate can be a nidus for infection and ultimately lead to endophthalmitis.[2–4] During the initial surgery, sclera, dura, fascia, pericardium, or split-thickness cornea (Fig. 28-20B) is used as a patch graft to prevent tube erosion.[5] The use of a long (perhaps 6 mm) needle-generated scleral tunnel without a patch graft has been reported to avoid erosions in a pediatric population.

Treatment

• Initial management of any tube erosion should include rapid surgical intervention consisting of replacing the patch graft, usually with the same material initially used to prevent possible infection.

• Any signs of infection should include management by prompt culture and treating the infection with topical antibiotics.[1]

• Causes of tube erosion are varied but not well defined and likely consist of several factors, including poor tissue turgor and mechanical factors such as mechanical rubbing from the lid.[1]

• Dr. Budenz recommends routing the tube directly at 12 o'clock when entering the anterior chamber to place the entire tube and patch graft completely underneath the upper lid to minimize mechanical trauma.[1] In cases of recurrent erosion, several groups have studied uses of materials such as double-layered AM,[6] double-thickness–processed pericardium patch graft,[7] and buccal mucous membrane grafts.[8] Five of six cases using buccal mucous membrane did not re-erode, all the patients with a double-layered AM graft were treated successfully, and none of the patients with double-thickness pericardium had tube exposure.

■ The basic premise behind all these ideas is to minimize mechanical factors and use a patch graft material to cover the tube and prevent the tube from eroding through the conjunctiva and exposing the patient to possible infection.

REFERENCES

1. Heuer DK, Budenz D, Coleman A. Aqueous shunt tube erosion. *J Glaucoma.* 2001;10(6):493–496.
2. Al-Torbak AA, Al-Shahwan S, Al-Jadaan I, et al. Endophthalmitis associated with the Ahmed glaucoma valve implant. *Br J Ophthalmol.* 2005;89(4):454–458.
3. Bayraktar Z, Kapran Z, Bayraktar S, et al. Delayed-onset Streptococcus pyogenes endophthalmitis following Ahmed glaucoma valve implantation. *Jpn J Ophthalmol.* 2005;49(4):315–317.
4. Gedde SJ, Scott IU, Tabandeh H, et al. Late endophthalmitis associated with glaucoma drainage implants. *Ophthalmology.* 2001;108(7):1323–1327.
5. Sarkisian SR Jr. Tube shunt complications and their prevention. *Curr Opin Ophthalmol.* 2009;20(2):126–130.
6. Ainsworth G, Rotchford A, Dua HS, et al. A novel use of amniotic membrane in the management of tube exposure following glaucoma tube shunt surgery. *Br J Ophthalmol.* 2006;90(4):417–419.
7. Lankaranian D, Reis R, Henderer JD, et al. Comparison of single thickness and double thickness processed pericardium patch graft in glaucoma drainage device surgery: A single surgeon comparison of outcome. *J Glaucoma.* 2008;17(1):48–51.
8. Rootman DB, Trope GE, Rootman DS. Glaucoma aqueous drainage device erosion repair with buccal mucous membrane grafts. *J Glaucoma.* 2009;18(8):618–622.
9. Albis-Donado O, Gil-Carrasco F, Romero-Quijada R, Thomas R. Evaluation of Ahmed glaucoma valve implantation through a needle-generated scleral tunnel in Mexican children with glaucoma. *Indian J Ophthalmol.* 2010;58(5):365–373.

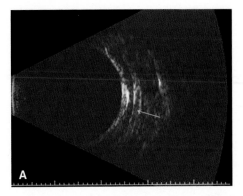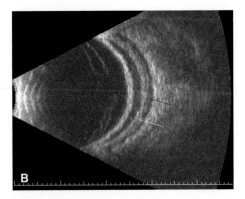

FIGURE 28-18. Ultrasound imaging of glaucoma drainage device (GDD). A. A Baerveldt GDD before capsule formation. The plate is indicated by the *yellow arrow.* **B.** A Baerveldt GDD after tube opening with fluid (*red arrow*) overlying the plate (*yellow arrow*).

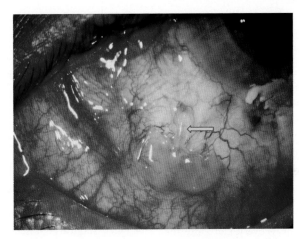

FIGURE 28-19. Tube exposure. An exposed glaucoma drainage device tube as indicated by the *yellow arrow.*

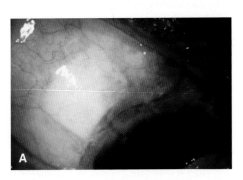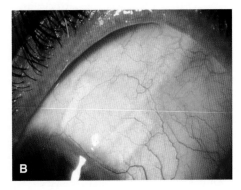

FIGURE 28-20. Patch graft. A. Scleral patch graft. **B.** Clear corneal patch graft.

Supraciliary Microstent Surgery

Steven D. Vold ▪

INTRODUCTION

Microincisional glaucoma surgery is quickly becoming a popular surgical option in the management of glaucoma. Ike Ahmed coined the acronym MIGS to describe what he termed micro-invasive (or minimally invasive) glaucoma surgery. Per his definition, MIGS has the following characteristics: (1) ab interno surgical approach; (2) minimal tissue trauma; (3) superior safety and low complication profile; (4) at least modest intraocular pressure (IOP) lowering efficacy; and (5) rapid patient recovery. Currently, the only FDA-approved supraciliary microstent surgery available to surgeons is the CyPass microstent (Alcon Laboratories, Fort Worth, TX) (Figs. 29-1 to 29-3). In the near future, the iStent supra (Glaukos Corporation, Laguna Hills, CA) will potentially be another supraciliary device available to ophthalmic surgeons.

CYPASS MICROSTENT

Indications

● Currently only FDA approved for treatment of mild to moderate primary open-angle glaucoma in the setting of cataract surgery

● Under evaluation as stand-alone procedure

Contraindications

● Secondary glaucomas

● Angle closure glaucomas

Instrumentation and Supplies

● Lidocaine 1% or tetracaine 0.5%

● Intraocular acetylcholine or carbachol

● Direct surgical gonioscope (modified Swan-Jacob, Hill or Alcon Vold goniolens)

● Ophthalmic viscosurgical device (OVD)

● CyPass loading and insertion devices

Surgical Procedure

1. Procedure is generally performed after phacoemulsification.

2. Examine the anterior chamber angle carefully before bringing the patient to surgery. Understanding the patient's angle anatomy is critical to CyPass surgical success.

3. Handle the loaded CyPass insertion device with care. Personally remove the

apparatus from the packaging and make a significant effort to avoid hitting the CyPass on the corneal wound.

4. Tilt the microscope toward you and the patient's head away from you by approximately 30 to 45 degrees to allow for good angle visualization using a modified Swan-Jacob or Hill lens. The Transcend Vold goniolens is designed to reduce the need for microscope and patient head tilt to achieve proper angle visualization.

5. Before implantation of the CyPass, remove the cataract via phacoemulsification and consider injecting an intraocular acetacholine or carbachol to induce miosis. Hyperinflate the anterior chamber with a cohesive OVD to facilitate safe placement of the CyPass.

6. Enter the anterior chamber through the temporal clear cornea cataract incision holding the CyPass parallel to the iris to avoid having the CyPass catch on the corneal wound lip and to prevent CyPass touch of the iris and intraocular lens.

7. When the CyPass is fully within the anterior chamber, rotate the CyPass microstent into a position radial to the iris and trabecular meshwork. From an approximately 60-degree-angle approach, gently press the guidewire tip of the CyPass insertion device against the scleral spur and begin to guide the CyPass posteriorly into the supraciliary space (Fig. 29-4).

8. Using a smooth, slow forward motion, guide the CyPass as radially as possible into the supraciliary space until approximately 75% of its 6.35-mm length is well positioned within the supraciliary space. No resistance should be encountered during microstent insertion. If resistance is encountered or a cyclodialysis appears to be developing, withdraw the device

and reimplant the CyPass in a different nasal quadrant.

9. Deploy the CyPass retracting the guidewire from the CyPass insertion device. Use the tip of the insertion device to position the proximal end of the CyPass between the pigmented trabecular meshwork and Schwalbe line (Fig. 29-5). Devices too anteriorly positioned should be gently tapped to ensure the CyPass is posterior to the Schwalbe line. Overinserted CyPass microstents can be retracted into proper position using intraocular micrograsping forceps.

10. Avoid placing the CyPass near larger iris angle vessels in the nasal quadrants if possible. Accurate radial CyPass placement prevents formation of larger cyclodialysis cleft.

11. Evacuate the cohesive OVD and any anterior chamber blood from the eye using automated irrigation and aspiration to prevent postoperative pressure spikes. Keep the automated irrigation and aspiration tip at least 2 to 3 mm from the CyPass to avoid possibly creating or enlarging any cyclodialysis cleft.

12. Pressurize the eye between 20 and 25 mm Hg with balanced salt solution to prevent reflux of blood into the anterior chamber.

13. Test corneal wound with Weck-cel sponge to ensure the wound is water-tight. If not, place a single 10-0 nylon suture in the wound.

14. Be aware of three key things when implanting the CyPass: (1) your angle anatomy; (2) the wound (lifting up on the wound, depressing down on the wound) can cause to lose your visualization; (3) relaxing your hand, to relieve lateral forces before depressing the trigger to release the CyPass under control.

Postoperative Care

1. Examine eye and check IOP within 24 hours of procedure.

2. Discontinue glaucoma medications in immediate postoperative period unless early postoperative IOP elevation due to retained OVD.

3. Use topical antibiotic for approximately 1 to 2 weeks postoperatively.

4. Prescribe one of the following steroids in treated eye:

   ▪ Loteprednol 0.5% four times a day for approximately 4 weeks

   ▪ Prednisolone acetate 1% four times a day for 2 weeks followed by taper over 2 to 4 weeks

   ▪ Difluprednate 0.05% two times a day for 4 weeks

5. Perform additional follow-up examinations within 2 weeks of the procedure and then 4 to 6 weeks after the procedure (**Figs. 29-6** and **29-7**).

Complications

- Malpositioning of the microstent
- Iris incarceration within microstent
- Endophthalmitis
- Hyphema
- Peripheral anterior synechiae
- Chronic uveitis
- Iridodialysis or cyclodialysis
- Descemet detachment
- Elevated IOP

BIBLIOGRAPHY

Francis BA, Singh K, Lin SC, Hodapp E, Jampel HD, Samples JR. Novel glaucoma procedures: a report by the American Academy of Ophthalmology. *Ophthalmology.* 2011;118(7):1466–1480.

Saheb H, Ahmed II. Micro-invasive glaucoma surgery: current perspectives and future directions. *Curr Opin Ophthalmol.* 2012;23(2) 96–104.

Shareef S, Alward W, Crandall A, Vold S, Ahmed I. Intra-operative gonioscopy: a key to successful angle surgery. *Expert Rev Ophthalmol.* 2014;9:515–527.

Vold SD, Ahmed II, Craven ER; CyPass Study Group. Two-Year COMPASS trial results: supraciliary microstenting with phacoemulsification in patients with open-angle glaucoma and cataracts. *Ophthalmology.* 2016;123(10):2103–2112.

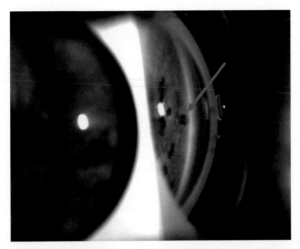

FIGURE 29-1. Gonioscopic view of well-positioned CyPass in the angle. The *blue arrow* points to the proximal end of the stent that is visible in the nasal anterior chamber.

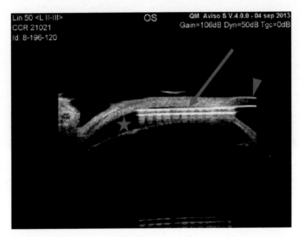

FIGURE 29-2. Ultrasound biomicroscopy image of CyPass in the angle. The *blue arrow* shows the CyPass in the suprachoroidal space. The *blue star* shows a subscleral lake of fluid. The *arrow head* indicates the cornea.

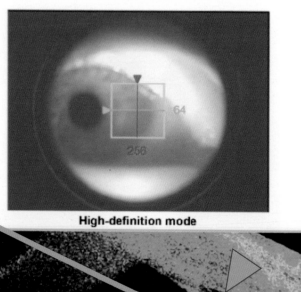

High-definition mode

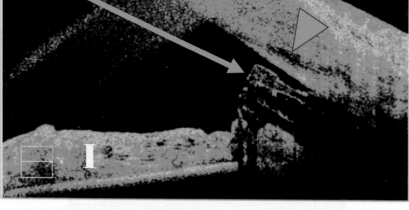

FIGURE 29-3. **Ocular coherence tomography (OCT) of CyPass in the angle.** Anterior segment OCT of a well-positioned CyPass with the proximal end (*blue arrow*) adjacent to the trabecular meshwork. The *blue arrowhead* indicates Schlemm canal. I, iris.

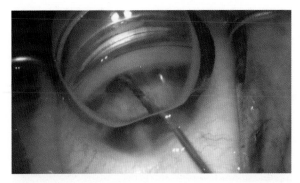

FIGURE 29-4. **Intraoperative view of CyPass placement.** Direct gonioscopic view using a Jacob gonioprism showing the initial insertion of the guide wire into the ciliary body face just below the scleral spur.

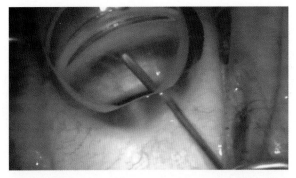

FIGURE 29-5. **Intraoperative view of CyPass placement:** after advancing the device into the suprachoroidal space, the device is released from the inserter by retraction of the guide wire. The CyPass is manually advanced by gentle tapping so that the proximal end is adjacent to the trabecular meshwork.

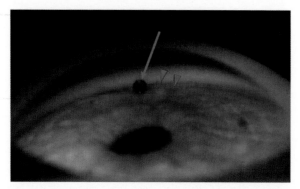

FIGURE 29-6. Gonioscopic photo postoperatively of well-positioned CyPass: The *blue arrow* shows the proximal end of the CyPass adjacent to the pigmented band of the trabecular meshwork (*blue arrowhead*). The tip of the *red arrowhead* indicates scleral spur.

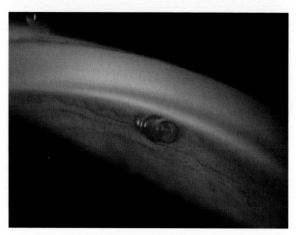

FIGURE 29-7. Higher magnification view of well-positioned CyPass in the angle. The proximal two rings are visible.

Index

Note: Locators followed by 'f' and 't' refer to figures and tables respectively.

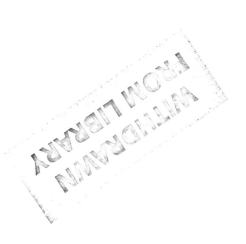

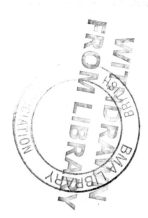